Sustainable Environment Monitoring Systems for Medical Care

Calin Ciufudean
https://orcid.org/0000-0002-2145-8219
Stefan cel Mare University of Suceava, Romania

IGI Global
Scientific Publishing
Publishing Tomorrow's Research Today

Published in the United States of America by
IGI Global Scientific Publishing
701 East Chocolate Avenue
Hershey, PA, 17033, USA
Tel: 717-533-8845 | Fax: 717-533-7115
Website: https://www.igi-global.com E-mail: cust@igi-global.com

Library of Congress Cataloging-in-Publication Data

Names: Ciufudean, Calin, 1962- editor
Title: Sustainable environment monitoring systems for medical care / edited by: Calin Ciufudean.
Description: Hershey PA : IGI Global Scientific Publishing, [2026] | Includes bibliographical references. | Summary: "The book aims to explore advanced applications that illustrate these concepts and makes a significant contribution to the development of the next generation of intelligent hybrid biostructures"-- Provided by publisher.
Identifiers: LCCN 2025032424 (print) | LCCN 2025032425 (ebook) | ISBN 9798337356365 hardcover | ISBN 9798337356372 paperback | ISBN 9798337356389 ebook
Subjects: LCSH: Medical care--Data processing | Medical informatics
Classification: LCC R858 .S87 2026 (print) | LCC R858 (ebook)
LC record available at https://lccn.loc.gov/2025032424
LC ebook record available at https://lccn.loc.gov/2025032425

British Cataloguing in Publication Data
A Cataloguing in Publication record for this book is available from the British Library.

Table of Contents

Preface xi

Chapter 1
Environmental Impact of Healthcare Facilities: Energy, Waste, Water, Emissions 1
M. Vinayaka, Visvesvaraya Technological University, Belagavi, India
B. Lokeshappa, University BDT College of Engineering, India
Shanmukha N. T., Government Engineering College, Krishnarajpet, India

Chapter 2
IoT-Based Environmental Monitoring to Reduce Healthcare Facilities' Environmental Impact: Mitigating the Effects of Healthcare Infrastructure on Ecosystems and Public Health 17
Kholis Kholis Ernawati, Universitas YARSI, Indonesia

Chapter 3
An Agentic Approach to Sustainable Environmental Monitoring Systems in Healthcare 49
Cristina Elena Turcu, Ştefan cel Mare University of Suceava, Romania
Corneliu Octavian Turcu, tefan cel Mare University of Suceava, Romania

Chapter 4
AI-Driven Environmental Monitoring Systems in Smart Hospitals: Enhancing Patient Outcomes and Sustainable Care 89
Muhammad Usman Tariq, Abu Dhabi University, UAE & University College Cork, Ireland

Chapter 5
Empowering Sustainable Medical Care Through Data Analytics, Visualization, and Intelligent Decision Support 117
Gaganpreet Kaur, CGC University, Mohali, India
Amandeep Kaur, CGC University, Mohali, India
Ramandeep Sandhu, Lovely Professional University, India

Chapter 6
Designing Real-Time Interactive Dashboards for City-Wide Health and Environmental Monitoring: A Data Visualization Approach to Sustainable Medical Care 139
C. V. Suresh Babu, Hindustan Institute of Technology and Science, India
V. Karunya Lydia, Hindustan Institute of Technology and Science, India
M. Jeevananthan, Hindustan Institute of Technology and Science, India
S. Sidharth, Hindustan Institute of Technology and Science, India

Chapter 7
IoT Governance in Healthcare: Privacy, Security, and Regulatory 165
Renu Mishra, Department of CSE, SSCSE, Sharda University, India
Adarsh Tiwari, Sharda University, India
Sneha Sinha, Sharda University, India
Anmol Kr. Sah, Sharda University, India
Mamta Narwaria, Sharda University, India

Chapter 8
Earlier Glaucoma Detection Using Optimised Blood Vessel Segmentation With CNN 189
A. Sindhu, JCT College of Engineering and Technology, India

Chapter 9
Staff Safety and Well-Being 211
S. C. Vetrivel, Kongu Engineering College, India
N. Rajavel, Selvamm Arts and Science College, India
V. P. Arun, JKKN College of Engineering and Technology, India

Chapter 10
Psychological Impacts of Natural Disasters: Recent Understandings and Future Directions 241
Guddo, Lovely Professional University, Punjab, India
Belinda Nyarkoh, Lovely Professional University, Punjab, India
Shikha Pandey, University of Lucknow, India

Compilation of References 271

About the Contributors 317

Index 323

Detailed Table of Contents

Preface xi

Chapter 1
Environmental Impact of Healthcare Facilities: Energy, Waste, Water, Emissions 1
M. Vinayaka, Visvesvaraya Technological University, Belagavi, India
B. Lokeshappa, University BDT College of Engineering, India
Shanmukha N. T., Government Engineering College, Krishnarajpet, India

The healthcare industry, which should be the most nature-friendly, is ironically one of the biggest causes of environmental degradation. Worldwide, healthcare is responsible for about 4.4% of the total greenhouse gas emissions, which puts it among the major contributors of climate change. This chapter, through a systems-based analytical framework combining Life Cycle Assessment (LCA), Material Flow Analysis (MFA), and Multi-Criteria Decision Analysis (MCDA), reveals the Healthcare Environmental Paradox the conflict of health promotion resulting in environmental harm. It also talks about the healthcare sector's primary causes of the environmental crisis that include energy consumption, waste generation, water utilization, and emissions from healthcare operations. Pointing out the current shifts in the healthcare sustainability landscape, the chapter wraps up by enumerating the climate change mitigation measures and the upcoming research topics related to the circular economy, green chemistry, digital health, and climate-resilient healthcare infrastructure.

Chapter 2
IoT-Based Environmental Monitoring to Reduce Healthcare Facilities' Environmental Impact: Mitigating the Effects of Healthcare Infrastructure on Ecosystems and Public Health 17
Kholis Kholis Ernawati, Universitas YARSI, Indonesia

Healthcare facilities are vital to public health, but they also significantly impact the environment through energy and water consumption, medical waste, and pollutant emissions. This article explores the role of Internet of Things (IoT)-based environmental monitoring systems in minimizing hospitals' ecological footprint. IoT systems use real-time data from smart sensors to track air and water quality, energy usage, and waste volume. The analysis is framed by Cyber-Physical Systems (CPS), the One Health approach, and the Technology-Organization-Environment

(TOE) model. A narrative literature review (2019–2024) highlights IoT's potential to improve pollution control, resource efficiency, and environmental compliance in healthcare settings. Despite clear benefits, implementation faces barriers such as high costs, cybersecurity risks, limited digital skills, and regulatory gaps. The article concludes that IoT offers a strategic path toward sustainable healthcare, aligned with Sustainable Development Goals (SDGs) 3, 6, 11, and 13.

Chapter 3
An Agentic Approach to Sustainable Environmental Monitoring Systems in Healthcare 49
Cristina Elena Turcu, Ştefan cel Mare University of Suceava, Romania
Corneliu Octavian Turcu, tefan cel Mare University of Suceava, Romania

This chapter explores the transformative role of agentic AI in sustainable environmental monitoring for healthcare. The need for this shift arises from the sector's considerable environmental footprint and the challenge of ensuring contaminant-free spaces vital for patient safety and preventing Healthcare-Associated Infections (HAIs). The chapter introduces the theoretical foundations, architecture, and capabilities of AI agents, highlighting their contribution to "smart healthcare". A conceptual multi-agent system is then proposed to integrate intelligent agents into sustainable monitoring. The model covers functional requirements such as real-time monitoring and predictive analysis, as well as non-functional ones like scalability, security, and adherence to sustainability principles. The discussion concludes by addressing key technical, ethical, and regulatory challenges that must be overcome to fully harness agentic AI's potential in building proactive, personalized, and environmentally sustainable healthcare ecosystems.

Chapter 4
AI-Driven Environmental Monitoring Systems in Smart Hospitals: Enhancing Patient Outcomes and Sustainable Care 89
Muhammad Usman Tariq, Abu Dhabi University, UAE & University College Cork, Ireland

The convergence of artificial intelligence (AI), the Internet of Medical Things (IoMT), and advanced environmental surveillance in intelligent hospitals represents a transformative leap in healthcare. Continuing analysis of data on air quality, temperature, humidity, particle levels, and energy consumption optimizes KI-controlled environmental monitoring systems to support sustainable care. These intelligent systems actively identify deviations from optimal environmental conditions, reducing the risk of infection, improving patient comfort and recovery rates, and minimizing energy consumption and waste. Hospitals can utilize real-time views, adaptive controls, and predictions to deliver safer, greener, more cost-effective, and more effective services. This chapter examines key technologies, integration issues, regulatory considerations, and practical implementations worldwide that support these systems. Future discussions on in-depth research and analysis outline the path to an intelligent hospital ecosystem that prioritizes both patient outcomes and environmental responsibility.

Chapter 5
Empowering Sustainable Medical Care Through Data Analytics, Visualization, and Intelligent Decision Support 117
Gaganpreet Kaur, CGC University, Mohali, India
Amandeep Kaur, CGC University, Mohali, India
Ramandeep Sandhu, Lovely Professional University, India

The growing emphasis on sustainable medical environments has intensified the need for intelligent systems that can monitor, interpret, and respond to environmental data in real-time. This chapter explores the transformative role of data analytics, visualization, and decision support systems (DSS) in building sustainable environment monitoring frameworks for medical care. In modern healthcare settings, vast volumes of environmental data ranging from air quality indices and humidity levels to noise pollution and biohazard alerts are generated continuously. Harnessing this data through advanced analytics and machine learning algorithms enables early detection of risks, efficient resource allocation, and predictive maintenance of medical facilities. This proactive approach not only enhances operational efficiency but also supports eco-conscious medical practices. Visualization tools such as interactive dashboards, heatmaps, and real-time graphs convert complex datasets into actionable insights, allowing healthcare administrators and clinical teams to monitor trends, spot anomalies, and make faster, evidence-based decisions. When integrated with DSS, these technologies provide intelligent recommendations that support infection control, energy management, and patient safety in a seamless, automated manner. This chapter offers an in-depth discussion on innovative models and real-world case studies where sustainable environment monitoring systems powered by data analytics and visualization have significantly improved clinical and environmental outcomes. It also addresses challenges related to data integration, scalability, and user training, offering strategic insights for future-ready smart hospitals. By linking sustainability with technology and healthcare, the chapter highlights how data-driven strategies can empower greener, smarter, and safer medical environments.

Chapter 6
Designing Real-Time Interactive Dashboards for City-Wide Health and Environmental Monitoring: A Data Visualization Approach to Sustainable Medical Care 139
C. V. Suresh Babu, Hindustan Institute of Technology and Science, India
V. Karunya Lydia, Hindustan Institute of Technology and Science, India
M. Jeevananthan, Hindustan Institute of Technology and Science, India
S. Sidharth, Hindustan Institute of Technology and Science, India

The research presents a Smart Health and Environment Dashboard which merges patient health monitoring with environmental measurements to foster sustainable healthcare practices. The platform solves the issues of previous systems while speeding up decision processes by uniting sensor-based data collection with AI-driven analysis and interactive visualization. The study implemented design science methodology through prototyping and user simulations and complete evaluation against neuroergonomics and user experience standards. The research revealed substantial improvements in overall system usability together with enhanced system responsiveness and precise monitoring which delivers for public health management. The team successfully conducted investigations into telehealth systems and mobile applications together with predictive AI functionality and expansion to other metropolitan regions. The findings demonstrate that real-time data infrastructures play an essential role in transforming contemporary urban healthcare systems toward sustainable and effective healthcare delivery.

Chapter 7
IoT Governance in Healthcare: Privacy, Security, and Regulatory 165
Renu Mishra, Department of CSE, SSCSE, Sharda University, India
Adarsh Tiwari, Sharda University, India
Sneha Sinha, Sharda University, India
Anmol Kr. Sah, Sharda University, India
Mamta Narwaria, Sharda University, India

The Internet of Things (IoT) has changed how patients are cared for by making it possible to monitor patients from a distance, connect smart diagnoses, and even do real-time nursing analytics. It also creates new problems with privacy, security, and following the rules. This paper states the current IoT governance models in healthcare and evaluates the integration of privacy-preserving technologies, cybersecurity frameworks, and legal compliance relationship. A thorough literature review of twenty empirical studies identifies best practices and gaps in the governance of secure IoT health systems and proposes a comprehensive, evidence-based governance model for the implementation of IoT technologies that integrates both technical and policy-related approaches to the governance of IoT health systems.

Chapter 8
Earlier Glaucoma Detection Using Optimised Blood Vessel Segmentation With CNN 189
A. Sindhu, JCT College of Engineering and Technology, India

Glaucoma, being one of the major causes of irreversible blindness, is largely asymptomatic in its early stages, and therefore, early detection is the hour of need. Traditional diagnostic techniques are time-consuming and are prone to variability. In response to this problem, we introduce a deep learning-based approach that efficiently segments the glaucoma-sensitive optic disc (OD) and optic cup (OC) using an ensemble of convolutional neural networks (CNNs). To ensure increased accuracy of predictions, the system uses majority voting and state-of-the-art Attention U-Net models with pre-trained ResNet34, Inceptionv3, and DenseNet121 backbones. Following training of the ensemble over a heterogeneous dataset of REFUGE, Drishti-GS, and RIM-ONE images, the ensemble outperforms in glaucoma classification and fundus image segmentation. The novelty lies in the complementary use of ensemble learning and backbone-specific Attention U-Nets, which improve segmentation accuracy and reduce model overfitting. Traditional preprocessing methods, Gaussian noise removal, and a CNN-based classification pipeline further enhance the accuracy of predictions. The system finally offers an efficient and automated way to enable early glaucoma screening and diagnosis.

Chapter 9
Staff Safety and Well-Being 211
S. C. Vetrivel, Kongu Engineering College, India
N. Rajavel, Selvamm Arts and Science College, India
V. P. Arun, JKKN College of Engineering and Technology, India

In healthcare environments, the safety and well-being of staff are fundamental to ensuring high-quality medical care and sustainable operations. With the increasing complexity of healthcare delivery systems, professionals are exposed to a wide range of risks, including infectious diseases, chemical exposure, workplace violence, ergonomic hazards, and psychological stress. This chapter explores the development of sustainable environment monitoring systems tailored to safeguard healthcare staff while promoting their physical and mental well-being. It emphasizes the integration of advanced technologies—such as IoT-based sensors, wearable devices, artificial intelligence, and real-time data analytics—to detect and mitigate occupational hazards within medical care facilities. The chapter also examines the importance of designing proactive monitoring frameworks that not only identify potential risks but also enable timely interventions to prevent incidents.

Chapter 10
Psychological Impacts of Natural Disasters: Recent Understandings and Future Directions 241
Guddo, Lovely Professional University, Punjab, India
Belinda Nyarkoh, Lovely Professional University, Punjab, India
Shikha Pandey, University of Lucknow, India

This chapter examines the complex psychological impact of natural disasters on individuals and communities across different contexts and populations. Drawing on interdisciplinary research from clinical psychology, public health, disaster management, and social sciences, the chapter provides an integrative analysis of the psychological sequelae of natural disasters, ranging from immediate stress responses to long-term mental health outcomes. Particular attention is given to vulnerable populations, factors influencing psychological resilience, current intervention frameworks, and cultural variations in psychological responses. The chapter identifies critical gaps in current understanding, highlighting the need for more culturally responsive, trauma-informed approaches to disaster mental health. Finally, it proposes evidence-based recommendations for strengthening psychological resilience at individual, community, and systems levels, emphasising the importance of integrating mental health considerations into broader disaster preparedness, response, and recovery frameworks.

Compilation of References 271

About the Contributors 317

Index 323

Preface

Healthcare systems are increasingly challenged to deliver high-quality medical care while responding to escalating environmental, technological, and societal pressures. The healthcare sector's substantial consumption of energy and resources, combined with its responsibility to protect vulnerable populations, places sustainability at the core of modern medical practice. *Sustainable Environment Monitoring Systems for Medical Care* addresses this imperative by examining how intelligent monitoring, data-driven decision making, and emerging digital technologies can reduce environmental impact while enhancing patient safety, staff well-being, and overall healthcare outcomes.

ORGANIZATION OF BOOK

The book brings together interdisciplinary perspectives spanning environmental science, healthcare engineering, artificial intelligence, data analytics, and public health. Early chapters establish a foundational understanding of the environmental footprint of healthcare facilities, highlighting energy use, waste generation, water consumption, and emissions, and framing these challenges within sustainability and systems-based analytical approaches. Subsequent chapters explore the role of IoT, cyber-physical systems, and smart sensing infrastructures in enabling real-time environmental monitoring and resource optimization within healthcare settings.

A central theme of the volume is the integration of advanced intelligence—ranging from machine learning and agentic AI to predictive analytics and decision support systems—into sustainable healthcare environments. These contributions demonstrate how intelligent monitoring systems can proactively manage risks, improve infection control, support vulnerable patient populations, and optimize operational efficiency. The book also emphasizes visualization and dashboard-based interfaces that translate complex environmental and health data into actionable insights for clinicians, administrators, and policymakers.

Beyond technological innovation, the volume addresses critical cross-cutting issues including governance, privacy, security, regulatory compliance, staff safety, and psychological well-being. By incorporating perspectives on occupational health, disaster impacts, and ethical deployment of digital systems, the book underscores that sustainability in healthcare is not solely an environmental or technical concern, but a human-centered one.

Collectively, the chapters offer both conceptual frameworks and practical directions for researchers, practitioners, and decision makers seeking to design resilient, intelligent, and environmentally responsible healthcare systems. This book aims to contribute to the ongoing transition toward sustainable medical care, where environmental stewardship, technological innovation, and human well-being are mutually reinforcing goals.

Chapter 1
Environmental Impact of Healthcare Facilities: Energy, Waste, Water, Emissions

M. Vinayaka
https://orcid.org/0009-0001-9988-2490
Visvesvaraya Technological University, Belagavi, India

B. Lokeshappa
University BDT College of Engineering, India

Shanmukha N. T.
Government Engineering College, Krishnarajpet, India

ABSTRACT

The healthcare industry, which should be the most nature-friendly, is ironically one of the biggest causes of environmental degradation. Worldwide, healthcare is responsible for about 4.4% of the total greenhouse gas emissions, which puts it among the major contributors of climate change. This chapter, through a systems-based analytical framework combining Life Cycle Assessment (LCA), Material Flow Analysis (MFA), and Multi-Criteria Decision Analysis (MCDA), reveals the Healthcare Environmental Paradox the conflict of health promotion resulting in environmental harm. It also talks about the healthcare sector's primary causes of the environmental crisis that include energy consumption, waste generation, water utilization, and emissions from healthcare operations. Pointing out the current shifts in the healthcare sustainability landscape, the chapter wraps up by enumerating the climate change mitigation measures and the upcoming research topics related to the circular economy, green chemistry, digital health, and climate-resilient healthcare infrastructure.

DOI: 10.4018/979-8-3373-5636-5.ch001

1. INTRODUCTION

Healers are the ones that make up the healthcare industry. But it may exacerbate illness-causing circumstances due to how it functions. One of the biggest problems with modern healthcare is this seeming contradiction. Worldwide, the healthcare industry is the fifth biggest contributor to climate change, accounting for around 4.4% of all net greenhouse gas (GHG) emissions (Karliner et al. 2019). Not only does this have an effect on the environment, but healthcare facilities also use a lot of resources (both electricity and water) and release harmful pollutants into the air and water.

A big issue in public health is the effect of healthcare on the environment. Malnutrition, malaria, diarrhea, and heat stress will cause an additional 250,000 deaths year between 2030 and 2050, according to a World Health Organization study (2018). Making an ethical argument for change may lead many health implications to be worsened by the same industry that prioritized them.

Focusing on complex systems and their interactions, this chapter delves into the environmental effect of healthcare in detail. Researches, healthcare executives, and legislators may use it to better align healthcare operations with health promotion activities by identifying possible change levers.

2. METHODOLOGY AND ANALYTICAL FRAMEWORK

The effects on the healthcare setting are investigated in this research from a systems thinking vantage point. This framework is based on methodology.

Life Cycle Assessment (LCA): From production to final disposal, we calculate the ecological footprint of healthcare goods and services.

Material Flow Analysis (MFA): Tracking the flow of supplies and resources throughout healthcare facilities to identify potential problem areas that need attention.

Greenhouse Gas Protocol: Consistent with the method for identifying and measuring emissions throughout Scopes 1–3.

Multi-Criteria Decision Analysis (MCDA): Evaluation of treatment alternatives taking into account environmental factors, cost, efficacy, and feasibility of implementation.

3. ENERGY CONSUMPTION IN HEALTHCARE FACILITIES

3.1 Drivers of Healthcare Energy Demand

Healthcare facilities are among the business sector's most energy-intensive structures. Even though they only accounted for 2.2% of all commercial floor area, hospitals accounted for 4.3% of all commercial building energy usage in the United States (U.S. EIA, 2022). There are a lot of reasons why we use so much energy.

24/7 Operational Requirements: Nighttime and weekend operations are typically reduced by most business facilities. A hospital center, on the other hand, is never below than 100% capacity. Emergency departments, critical care units, and diagnostic labs must have operational lighting, HVAC systems, and other necessities.

Advanced Medical Technologies: More and more medical equipment means greater and more energy use. According to Harris (2020), the energy consumption of a single magnetic resonance imaging equipment ranges from 12 to 25 kW. In standby mode, this system consumes a significant amount of energy to power the cryogenic cooling systems. Radiation treatment linear accelerators and computed tomography (CT) scanners need a lot of power. Automated laboratory analyzers function in a similar fashion.

Stringent Environmental Controls: To avoid the spread of illness, specialized heating, ventilation, and air conditioning (HVAC) systems with high air exchange rates, precise humidity and temperature regulation, and superior filtration are necessary. Air changes occur twenty to twenty-five times each hour in operating rooms. Regular commercial spaces often only need 2-4 modifications (ASHRAE, 2019). The energy consumption of the heater, air conditioner, and fan is significantly increased as a result of this.

Sterilization and Processing Requirements: Continuous operation is maintained by central sterile supply departments. Autoclaves, which are large steam sterilizers, and low-temperature sterilization devices are available to them. Powering and maintaining them consumes a significant amount of energy.

3.2 Energy Intensity by Department

The amount of power used by different hospital departments varies significantly. We can put measures in place to improve efficiency.

Intensive Care Units (ICUs): The continual illumination, complicated monitoring equipment, and high ventilation rates in intensive care units result in an annual energy consumption of 350 to 400 kWh/m^2, as reported by Garcia-Sanz-Calcedo et al. (2018).

Operating Theaters: Energy consumption in hospitals is highest in operation rooms. They use 500-700 kWh/m^2 of energy every year. Reason being: many high-energy systems are in operation simultaneously, including the HVAC system, operating room lighting, anaesthetic machines, patient monitors, and procedure-specific equipment.

Diagnostic Imaging Departments: Depending on factors such as equipment age, usage rates, and operating methods, the energy consumption of nuclear medicine, MRI, and CT rooms may range from 200 to 300 kWh/m^2/year.

General Patient Rooms: For typical HVAC, lights, and minor medical equipment, the typical annual usage is 100–150 kWh/m^2.

3.3 Comparative International Analysis

Because of differences in climate, medical procedures, and construction rules, the energy intensity of healthcare varies greatly among nations.

United States: In the United States, hospitals use around 259 kWh of electricity and 1,040 MJ of gas each year.

European Union: Because of improvements in room design and a stronger mandate for energy-neutral new construction, hospitals in the European Union use 30% less energy than their international equivalents. (Bouzid et al., 2020).

Developing Countries: A lack of infrastructure and an inconsistent energy supply are two issues that plague healthcare facilities in a number of developing nations. Diesel generators are more harmful to the environment than using energy from the grid as a backup power source.

3.4 Case Study: Energy Audit of a 500-Bed Tertiary Care Hospital

Several trends emerged from MGH's comprehensive energy audit.

Annual Energy Consumption:

- Electricity: 125,000 MWh
- Natural Gas: 850,000 therms
- Steam: 450 million pounds

Carbon Footprint: There are 14,700 vehicles contributing 68,000 metric tons of CO2e annually.

Major Energy End-Uses:

- HVAC Systems: 45%
- Medical Equipment: 25%
- Lighting: 15%
- Domestic Hot Water: 10%
- Other Equipment: 5%

Implementation of a $12 million energy efficiency program yielded:

- Annual energy cost savings: $3.2 million
- Payback period: 3.7 years
- Carbon reduction: 12,500 metric tons CO_2e annually

4. HEALTHCARE WASTE GENERATION AND MANAGEMENT

4.1 Waste Characterization and Classification

Medical facilities produce healthcare hazardous waste when they test, treat, or immunize patients or conduct research with biological substances. What is considered health care waste by the World Health Organization

General (Municipal) Waste (75-90%): Paper, cardboard, food scraps, and non-hazardous packaging are all examples of business or domestic trash. This stream isn't dangerous, but it does have a lot of recyclables that end up in landfills due to contamination.

Hazardous Medical Waste (10-25%):

- **Infectious Waste:** Waste contaminated with blood, bodily fluids, or potentially pathogenic microorganisms. Includes used dressings, swabs, materials from isolation rooms, and discarded cultures.
- **Pathological Waste:** Human tissues, organs, body parts, and fluids from surgery and autopsy.
- **Sharps Waste:** Needles, syringes, scalpels, and other items that could cause percutaneous injury.
- **Chemical Waste:** Solvents, disinfectants, heavy metals from equipment, and laboratory reagents.
- **Pharmaceutical Waste:** Expired, unused, or contaminated medications, including cytotoxic drugs.

- **Genotoxic Waste:** Highly hazardous waste containing cytotoxic drugs used in cancer chemotherapy.
- **Radioactive Waste:** Unsealed sources from diagnostic and therapeutic procedures in nuclear medicine.

4.2 Regional Disparities in Waste Management

There is a wide range of healthcare waste management systems worldwide.:

High-Income Countries: Frequently has advanced systems for monitoring, specialized treatment centers, and regulatory frameworks. The problem of inefficient and incorrect segregation persists. About fifteen to twenty percent of the garbage ends up in (Windfeld & Brooks, 2015).

Low- and Middle-Income Countries: The proper disposal of waste is impossible due to a lack of infrastructure, regulations, and resources. An estimated fifteen percent of all harmful waste is generated inside the health care system, according to the World Health Organization. Notably, out of the 24 developing nations that were examined, only 58% of the institutions had adequate waste management systems. (WHO, 2018).

4.3 Pharmaceutical Waste: A Growing Concern

A new problem has arisen: pharmaceuticals that pollute water systems. Both patients and others dispose of drugs in different ways. Eighty percent of American streams were found to be polluted with pharmaceutical chemicals, according to a comprehensive analysis (Bradley et al., 2020). Included in this category are specific worries.

Antibiotics: Contributing to the spread of microorganisms in the environment that are resistant to antibiotics..

Hormonal Medications: Disruption of aquatic reproduction may occur at doses as low as parts per trillion.

Cytotoxic Drugs: The persistence of powerful carcinogens in wastewater treatment plants.

4.4 Case Study: Waste Stream Analysis in a Multi-Hospital System

An investigation on the composition of garbage from an Ontario healthcare system including ten hospitals.:

Total Waste Generation: A daily average of 8.5 kg, or 12,500 tons per year

Waste Composition:

- General Waste: 78%
- Recyclable Materials (paper, cardboard, plastics): 15%
- Regulated Medical Waste: 6%
- Hazardous Chemical Waste: 1%

Recycling Contamination Rate: A recent study found that 28 percent of the products put into recycling bins were contaminated or not recyclable. Recycling facilities rejected these items due to the high contamination level, drawing attention to a serious problem with current waste management and recycling procedures.

Intervention Impact: The regulated medical waste decreased by 32% and the recycling rates increased by 41% over the course of 18 months after a thorough waste segregation program was implemented. An annual savings of $285,000 was achieved by this program's implementation of staff education, standardized bin placement, and audit input.

5. WATER RESOURCE UTILIZATION IN HEALTHCARE

5.1 Clinical Water Applications

Because of its central role in direct patient care, water requires a wide range of quality criteria.:

Hemodialysis: The most water-intensive therapeutic therapy is dialysis, which uses 300-600 liters of ultra-purified water. According to Connor et al. (2020), a patient who goes through dialysis three times a week would need more water than 45,000 liters a year only for the procedure. Dialysis water purification processes include ultrafiltration, reverse osmosis, and deionization; each liter of dialysis water requires two to three liters of source water.

Sterilization and Medical Processing: Autoclaving, or steam sterilization, uses 1-2 liters of water every cycle to heat the chamber and operate the vacuum. On the other hand, instrument washer-disinfectors have a wide range of water consumption rates, from 40 to 100 liters every cycle, depending on their size and technical characteristics.

Laboratory Operations: A hospital's overall water use may be 5-10% due to automated analyzers, glassware cleaners, and pure water systems, all of which contribute significantly to water consumption in clinical labs.

5.2 Operational Water Demands

Non-clinical water uses represent substantial consumption:

HVAC Systems: Because of evaporation, drift, and blowdown, cooling towers at large healthcare institutions may use millions of gallons of water annually. To be more precise, 5,000 to 10,000 gallons of water may evaporate daily from a cooling tower serving a 500-bed hospital.

Food Services: Food preparation, cleaning, and dishwashing are the three main uses of water in commercial kitchens that serve patients, employees, and visitors.

Laundry Operations: It takes between one and two gallons of water to process one pound of linens, and hospital laundries handle millions of pounds of linens annually.

Sanitation and Hygiene: Consideration of handwashing compliance, surface cleaning, and toilet flushing is critical for establishing the baseline water demand for a business or community. These habits have a major impact on water use and are vital for sustaining sanitation and hygiene standards.

5.3 Water Quality Requirements

Numerous water quality classes are necessary for healthcare institutions.

Potable Water: In order to guarantee safe public consumption and effective sanitation measures, it is vital to meet drinking water requirements.

Critical Care Water: Dialysis treatments, laboratory tests, and sterile processing all need very pure water.

Ultrapure Water: A resistance higher than 18 MΩ·cm is necessary for use in pharmaceutical production and laboratory settings.

5.4 Case Study: Water Conservation in Water-Stressed Regions

Groote Schuur Hospital in Cape Town, South Africa, implemented stringent water conservation measures in response to severe water shortages caused by the 2017–2018 drought.:

Baseline Consumption: About 925,000 gallons per day, or 28,000 cubic meters each month.

Intervention Strategies:

- Installation of water-efficient fixtures (aerators, low-flow toilets)
- Cooling tower optimization and alternative cooling technologies
- Greywater recycling for toilet flushing and irrigation

- Education campaigns targeting staff and visitors
- Leak detection and repair programs

Results: Proven to be feasible without sacrificing patient care by cutting water use by 45% (15,400 cubic meters monthly) in healthcare without affecting clinical operations.

6. EMISSIONS AND ATMOSPHERIC IMPACT

6.1 Greenhouse Gas Accounting Framework

Scopes are the three main ways in which emissions are categorized under the Greenhouse Gas Protocol.

Scope 1 (Direct Emissions): Emissions from sources owned or controlled by the facility, including:

- On-site combustion of natural gas, fuel oil, or propane
- Fugitive emissions from refrigerants and anesthetic gases
- Fleet vehicles (ambulances, transport vans)

Scope 2 (Indirect Emissions from Purchased Energy): The production of steam, heating, and cooling, as well as the power and electricity bought, all contribute significantly to pollution.

Scope 3 (Other Indirect Emissions): A company's indirect emissions are those that come from sources that the company does not directly own or control.

- Supply chain emissions (production of pharmaceuticals, medical devices, food)
- Employee commuting and patient travel
- Waste disposal
- Capital equipment

The emissions profile of the healthcare industry shows that Scope 3 is much more responsible for the majority of emissions (70-80%) compared to other sectors (Karliner et al., 2019).

6.2 Direct Emissions Sources

Anesthetic Gases: The potential for desflurane, sevoflurane, and isoflurane, three inhaled anesthetics, to contribute to global warming is substantial—2,540 times that of CO2 over a century, to be exact. Desflurane anesthesia for one hour is equivalent to the pollution produced by a typical passenger car traveling 250 miles per hour. (Ryan & Nielsen, 2010).

Metered-Dose Inhalers (MDIs): Based on the formulation and use, the carbon footprint per device may range from 18 to 36 kg CO_2, since many MDIs use hydrofluoroalkane (HFA) propellants, which have a high GWP..

Fugitive Refrigerant Emissions: Refrigeration plays a crucial role in healthcare facilities for storing medical supplies and providing comfort cooling. But hydrofluorocarbon (HFC) refrigerants are a major climatic danger due to their leakage; their GWPs are thousands of times higher than CO2.

6.3 Indirect Emissions from Supply Chains

Emissions are most heavily concentrated in the healthcare supply chain.:

Pharmaceuticals: About a quarter of all greenhouse gas emissions come from healthcare manufacturing processes, which use a lot of energy and resources due to complicated chemical synthesis with many stages and usually poor yields.

Medical Devices: The production, packing, and shipping of single-use disposable products, including PPE, are significant sources of pollution. With a 300–400% increase in worldwide PPE usage, the COVID-19 pandemic had a dramatic effect on the environment. (Klemeš et al., 2020).

Food Services: Emissions from farming, processing, transporting, and disposing of food scraps are a byproduct of the cafeteria and patient feeding operations.

6.4 Case Study: Anesthetic Gas Impact Assessment

Anaesthetic gas emissions were the subject of a thorough investigation at the UCSF Medical Center.

Annual Anesthetic Gas Usage:

- Sevoflurane: 1,250 liters
- Desflurane: 480 liters
- Isoflurane: 120 liters
- Nitrous Oxide: 45,000 liters

Carbon Footprint: It's the equivalent of 700 passenger cars' worth of CO_2 emissions per year, at 3,250 metric tons.

Intervention Strategy: Implementation of a multi-faceted program including:

- Default anesthetic machine settings to lower fresh gas flows
- Educational campaign on environmental impact of anesthetic choices
- Protocol encouraging use of sevoflurane over desflurane for routine cases
- Increased utilization of regional anesthesia and total intravenous anesthesia (TIVA)

Achieved 65% reduction in desflurane use and 40% reduction in anesthetic gas emissions within 12 months, with annual cost savings of $75,000 from reduced agent purchases.

7. INTERCONNECTED SYSTEMS ANALYSIS

Because of the interdependencies and trade-offs associated with resource flows, the environmental consequences of healthcare facilities are interrelated.

Energy-Water Nexus: Cooling systems and fuel processing rely heavily on water, while water treatment and distribution rely heavily on electricity. Cooling towers in HVAC systems use both water and electricity, therefore this synergy is apparent in healthcare facilities.

Waste-Emissions Nexus: The handling of waste has a substantial impact on emissions. Unlike landfilling, which releases methane into the atmosphere, incinerating plastic trash sends pollutants into the air. Although recycling often reduces emissions, the energy required for processing and shipping may be somewhat costly.

Supply Chain Interconnections: Waste, water use for cleaning, energy usage for sterilization, and emissions from production and transportation are all factors to consider when deciding between single-use and reusable items.

Clinical Practice-Resource Use Relationships: Choosing to use surgical equipment more than once reduces waste but increases the need for water and energy to sterilize, two examples of how clinical practices affect resource use.

In order to find synergistic treatments that provide numerous benefits and stop problems from moving across different environmental domains, it is necessary to understand how systems are linked.

8. REGULATORY FRAMEWORKS AND POLICY LANDSCAPE

Various regulatory frameworks impact the environmental performance of healthcare.

International Agreements: While the Kigali Amendment to the Montreal Protocol aims to phase down high GWP HFC refrigerants, the Minamata Convention on Mercury focuses on medical devices that contain mercury.

National Regulations: Vary significantly by country but typically include:

- Hazardous waste management standards (e.g., RCRA in the United States)
- Air quality standards regulating incinerator emissions
- Water discharge permits limiting pollutant releases
- Building codes influencing energy and water efficiency

Voluntary Programs: Multiple initiatives support healthcare sustainability:

- Practice Greenhealth (U.S.) and Healthcare Without Harm (global) provide frameworks and recognition programs
- LEED for Healthcare and BREEAM Healthcare offer green building certification
- The Joint Commission (U.S.) includes environmental standards in accreditation

Emerging Policy Trends: Increasing focus on climate resilience, mandatory carbon reporting, extended producer responsibility, and green public procurement.

9. MITIGATION STRATEGIES AND BEST PRACTICES

The healthcare industry may significantly reduce its environmental effect with the use of evidence-based initiatives:

Energy Efficiency:

- Retro-commissioning of HVAC systems typically identifies 5-15% energy savings
- LED lighting retrofits with occupancy sensors
- High-efficiency medical equipment with power management features
- On-site renewable energy generation (solar PV, geothermal)

Waste Reduction:

- Standardized waste segregation programs with staff education
- Transition to reusable products where clinically appropriate
- Reprocessing of single-use devices where approved
- Sustainable procurement policies favoring products with reduced packaging

Water Conservation:

- Water-efficient fixtures and equipment
- Cooling tower optimization and alternative cooling technologies
- Rainwater harvesting and greywater recycling for non-potable uses
- Landscape design with native, drought-tolerant species

Emissions Reduction:

- Anesthetic gas management protocols favoring agents with lower GWP
- Refrigerant management programs to prevent leaks and recover at end-of-life
- Electric vehicle infrastructure for fleet and staff vehicles
- Sustainable procurement policies considering carbon footprint

Integrated Design: New facilities are constructed with integrated design that optimizes resource flows and reduces lifetime environmental impact, including orientation, building envelope, systems selection and material choice.

10. ECONOMIC ANALYSIS OF SUSTAINABILITY INTERVENTIONS

Decisions regarding the execution of sustainability efforts are sometimes impacted by financial considerations.:

Cost-Benefit Analysis: There may be substantial monetary gains from environmental measures.

- Energy efficiency projects typically achieve 20-30% internal rate of return
- Waste reduction programs directly reduce disposal costs
- Water conservation lowers utility bills and may reduce sewer charges

Total Cost of Ownership: When buying services or products, it is important to include the operating cost (energy and water and maintenance), purchase cost, and end-of-life disposal cost in the sustainable buying criteria.

Funding Mechanisms: Various options exist for financing sustainability initiatives:

- Capital budget allocations
- Energy performance contracts where savings pay for improvements
- Grants and incentives from utilities or government programs
- Green revolving funds that reinvest savings into new projects

Example: A comprehensive sustainability project was launched by Cleveland Clinic, which achieved many objectives.

- $65 million in cumulative energy savings since 2010
- 35% reduction in regulated medical waste disposal costs
- 22% water use reduction saving $3.5 million annually
- Demonstrated that environmental and financial goals align in healthcare operations

11. FUTURE DIRECTIONS AND RESEARCH AGENDA

Much is unknown to us.

Closed-loop systems are an essential part of the circular economy model for medical materials. They don't just recycle; they re-think systems to get rid of waste and circulate everything.

We will become carbon neutral during delivery and also in supply networks by making a plan. Healthcare facilities may ensure their functioning is not impaired due to climatic disasters through resilience planning integrated into their design. Another indication is the arrival of extreme weather conditions, water shortages, etc.

The term "digital health environmental impact" describes the broader effects of telemedicine and other forms of digital health technology on the environment, taking into account factors like less travel and higher energy consumption from devices and data centers.

Sustainable clinical practice guidelines are evidence-based standards for medical care that take environmental impacts into account in order to guide procedures that provide the best possible results for patients while making responsible use of available resources.

The field of “Green Chemistry” within the pharmaceutical industry focuses on creating safe, effective, and environmentally friendly pharmaceutical substances and methods of synthesis.

12. CONCLUSION: TOWARD SUSTAINABLE HEALTHCARE DELIVERY

Healthcare facilities' impact on the environment is a pressing concern that needs fixing right now. In this chapter, we take a look at the energy, water, waste, and emissions impacts of healthcare and identify some ways it might be improved. There are several fronts that must be addressed in order to transition to sustainable healthcare.:

- **Individual Level:** Healthcare professionals making environmentally conscious decisions in daily practice
- **Organizational Level:** Healthcare facilities implementing comprehensive sustainability programs
- **System Level:** Policymakers creating regulatory frameworks that incentivize sustainable practices
- **Global Level:** International collaboration to share best practices and develop standards

Healthcare operations and environmental stewardship must be brought into harmony for both practical and ethical reasons. As intended, a virtuous cycle aiding health protection may be achieved if the healthcare industry lessens its impact on the environment. Only by acknowledging these environmental consequences, valuing the connections to other domains, and discussing evidence-based transformative techniques can health care sustainability be achieved.

REFERENCES

ASHRAE. (2019). HVAC Design Manual for Hospitals and Clinics (2nd ed.). American Society of Heating, Refrigerating and Air-Conditioning Engineers.

Bouzid, A., Gendy, M. E., & Leduc, L. (2020). Energy performance benchmarking for healthcare buildings in France. *Energy and Building*, *224*, 110241.

Bradley, P. M., Journey, C. A., & Romanok, K. M.. (2020). Expanded target-chemical analysis reveals extensive mixed-organic-contaminant exposure in U.S. streams. *Environmental Science & Technology*, *54*(18), 11587–11598. PMID: 28401767

Connor, A., Lillywhite, R., & Cooke, M. W. (2020). The carbon footprint of a renal service in the United Kingdom. *QJM: An International Journal of Medicine*, *104*(9), 749–755. PMID: 20719900

EPA. (2023). *Greenhouse Gas Equivalencies Calculator*. United States Environmental Protection Agency.

Garcia-Sanz-Calcedo, J., Al-Kassir, A., & Yusaf, T. (2018). Economic and environmental impact of energy saving in healthcare buildings. *Applied Energy*, *228*, 1354–1363.

Harris, J. (2020). The Energy Burden of Medical Imaging: A Review. *Health Environments Research & Design Journal*, *13*(4), 25–40.

Karliner, J., Slotterback, S., Boyd, R., Ashby, B., & Steele, K. (2019). *Health care's climate footprint: How the health sector contributes to the global climate crisis and opportunities for action*. Health Care Without Harm.

Klemeš, J. J., Fan, Y. V., Tan, R. R., & Jiang, P. (2020). Minimising the present and future plastic waste, energy and environmental footprints related to COVID-19. *Renewable & Sustainable Energy Reviews*, *127*, 109883. PMID: 34234614

Ryan, S. M., & Nielsen, C. J. (2010). Global warming potential of inhaled anesthetics: Application to clinical use. *Anesthesia and Analgesia*, *111*(1), 92–98. PMID: 20519425

U.S. EIA. (2022). *Commercial Buildings Energy Consumption Survey (CBECS)*. U.S. Energy Information Administration.

WHO. (2018). *Health-care waste. Fact Sheet*. World Health Organization.

Windfeld, E. S., & Brooks, M. S. (2015). Medical waste management - A review. *Journal of Environmental Management*, *163*, 98–108. PMID: 26301686

Chapter 2
IoT-Based Environmental Monitoring to Reduce Healthcare Facilities' Environmental Impact:
Mitigating the Effects of Healthcare Infrastructure on Ecosystems and Public Health

Kholis Kholis Ernawati
https://orcid.org/0000-0002-3582-5294
Universitas YARSI, Indonesia

ABSTRACT

Healthcare facilities are vital to public health, but they also significantly impact the environment through energy and water consumption, medical waste, and pollutant emissions. This article explores the role of Internet of Things (IoT)-based environmental monitoring systems in minimizing hospitals' ecological footprint. IoT systems use real-time data from smart sensors to track air and water quality, energy usage, and waste volume. The analysis is framed by Cyber-Physical Systems (CPS), the One Health approach, and the Technology-Organization-Environment (TOE) model. A narrative literature review (2019–2024) highlights IoT's potential to improve pollution control, resource efficiency, and environmental compliance in healthcare settings. Despite clear benefits, implementation faces barriers such as high costs, cybersecurity risks, limited digital skills, and regulatory gaps. The article concludes that IoT offers a strategic path toward sustainable healthcare, aligned with Sustainable Development Goals (SDGs) 3, 6, 11, and 13.

DOI: 10.4018/979-8-3373-5636-5.ch002

INTRODUCTION

Healthcare facilities—such as hospitals, clinics, and rehabilitation centers—strategically improve community wellbeing through promotive, preventive, curative, and rehabilitative functions. However, the operational activities of these institutions generate significant ecological impacts. The high energy demands required to operate heating, ventilation, air conditioning (HVAC) systems, lighting, and advanced medical equipment lead to substantial resource consumption and carbon emissions. Research shows that hospitals can achieve significant energy savings through conservation strategies, with an initial target of a 5% reduction in energy consumption in the first year and 2.5% in each subsequent year (González et al., 2018).

Sustainable architecture and design play a crucial role in reducing the ecological footprint of healthcare facilities. Guidelines such as the Green Guide for Health Care provide practical approaches for operational efficiency, energy and water conservation, and improved resource management (McGain & Naylor, 2014). Additionally, Moldovan et al. (2023) emphasize that integrating sustainability principles into healthcare service accreditation and quality systems is vital to balancing medical care with environmental preservation.

Beyond energy consumption, medical waste management poses a significant challenge. Hospitals produce approximately 0.5 to 2.5 kg of medical waste per patient daily, depending on infrastructure and healthcare management practices (Mominkhan et al., 2023). This waste includes sharps, chemicals, and other hazardous materials from laboratories, patient wards, and isolation units (Ibrahim et al., 2023; Wafula et al., 2019). Improper waste management can lead to soil and water contamination and increase the risk of infectious disease transmission (Han et al., 2024; Mishbahuddin et al., 2021).

The absence of an adequate waste management framework in many developing countries further exacerbates the situation. A study in Ethiopia revealed that most healthcare facilities lack structured waste management systems, resulting in substandard practices that pose health risks to communities (Wassie et al., 2022). Moreover, the global healthcare sector contributes nearly 5% of total carbon dioxide emissions, creating a paradox: institutions aimed at improving health simultaneously contribute to the factors that worsen disease (Mominkhan et al., 2023).

The rising trend in biomedical waste due to population growth, urbanization, and the use of disposable medical devices reinforces the urgency of re-evaluating waste management protocols. Efforts such as reducing single-use materials and transitioning to bioplastics and reusable medical tools have been proven to significantly lower greenhouse gas emissions (Ernawati, et al., 2025; Obubu et al., 2023). Visser et al. (2024) demonstrated that patients respond positively to healthcare institutions that prioritize environmental sustainability, without compromising service satisfaction.

This highlights a shared responsibility between healthcare providers and communities in driving the transition toward a sustainable health system.

Internet of Things (IoT) technology is one emerging solution to address medical waste. Integrating smart sensors and cloud-based monitoring systems enables hospitals to track air and water quality, energy use, and waste volume in real time. These systems support early detection of environmental risks and data-driven decision-making to enhance efficiency and mitigate impact (Ernawati et al., 2024; Ernawati, et al., 2025; Gordon et al., 2023).

The healthcare sector stands at a critical juncture where waste management and carbon emission mitigation challenges must be addressed innovatively and strategically. Transforming healthcare facilities toward environmentally friendly practices is highly relevant within the framework of the Sustainable Development Goals (SDGs), particularly Goal 3 (Good Health and Wellbeing), Goal 6 (Clean Water and Sanitation), and Goal 13 (Climate Action).

THEORETICAL FRAMEWORK

Implementing Internet of Things (IoT) technologies in environmental monitoring systems within healthcare facilities can be conceptualized through Cyber-Physical Systems (CPS). CPS integrates physical components—sensors, actuators, and edge computing devices—with cloud-based digital systems and artificial intelligence to enable real-time synchronization between the physical and virtual worlds (Haque et al., 2014). In hospitals, CPS facilitates the automated and predictive monitoring of environmental parameters, including temperature, humidity, carbon dioxide (CO_2) levels, energy consumption, and waste volume. This integration supports faster, more accurate, and data-driven decision-making processes aimed at mitigating the ecological footprint of healthcare operations.

The One Health approach offers a multidisciplinary framework that emphasizes the interconnectedness of human, animal, and environmental health. Improper medical waste management poses significant threats to healthcare personnel and patients. It contributes to broader ecosystem degradation, such as soil and water pollution and the exacerbation of antimicrobial resistance in the environment (Destoumieux-Garzón et al., 2018). IoT systems capable of comprehensively detecting and managing waste and environmental conditions have the potential to strengthen the institutional implementation of One Health principles within healthcare services.

From a technological adoption standpoint, the Technology-Organization-Environment (TOE) framework provides a more contextualized understanding than classical models such as the Diffusion of Innovation theory. The TOE framework posits that the adoption of new technologies like IoT is influenced by three key dimensions: technological characteristics (e.g., complexity and compatibility), organizational readiness (including human resources and infrastructure), and external environmental pressures from institutional and regulatory environments (Monye et al., 2024). In practice, factors such as budget constraints, unprepared hospital management systems, and weak national regulatory frameworks often hinder the implementation of IoT systems in healthcare facilities, particularly in developing countries.

By integrating the CPS, One Health, and TOE frameworks, this theoretical foundation offers a comprehensive and contemporary basis for understanding how IoT technologies can be effectively leveraged to monitor, prevent, and respond to the environmental impacts of healthcare facility operations systemically and sustainably.

PURPOSE AND FOCUS OF THE ARTICLE

This chapter aims to conceptually and practically explore how Internet of Things (IoT)-based environmental monitoring systems can be effectively implemented in healthcare facilities, particularly in resource-constrained settings in developing countries. Drawing on the theoretical foundations of Cyber-Physical Systems (CPS), One Health, and the Technology-Organization-Environment (TOE) framework, this article analyzes the contribution of digital monitoring systems in minimizing hospitals' ecological footprint while enhancing public health outcomes.

Specifically, the objectives of this article are to:

1. Explain the implementation framework of IoT-based environmental monitoring systems in hospital operations, emphasizing the integration of sensory components, cloud-based systems, and managerial decision-making processes.
2. Analyze the effectiveness of IoT technologies in reducing environmental pollution, energy consumption, and medical waste-related health risks.
3. Formulate strategic recommendations for the sustainable adoption of digital environmental monitoring systems, considering organizational readiness, regulatory frameworks, and policy support in developing countries.

The scope of discussion includes:

1. An analysis of the key environmental impacts of hospital operations, including air and water pollution, solid and liquid waste generation, and inefficient energy consumption.
2. Identification of relevant IoT devices and infrastructure for environmental monitoring in healthcare settings.

3. A review of case studies and conceptual models of integrated monitoring systems that demonstrate either successful implementation or key challenges.
4. An evaluation of the multidimensional benefits of IoT adoption, particularly in terms of environmental sustainability, economic efficiency, and improved public health.
5. A discussion of implementation barriers, including budget constraints, data security concerns, human resource capacity, and the lack of adaptive regulations for environmentally oriented digital transformation.

METHODOLOGY

This sub-chapter adopts a narrative literature review approach to explore the application of Internet of Things (IoT) technologies in environmental monitoring systems within healthcare facilities. The literature search was conducted across major databases—including Scopus, PubMed, and IEEE Xplore—and Google Scholar, focusing on publications from 2019 to 2024. Sources reviewed include peer-reviewed journal articles, policy reports, technical documents from Ministries of Health, and white papers from institutions implementing "green hospital" initiatives, specifically those addressing energy monitoring, air quality, water usage, and waste management.

The literature was selected based on its relevance: only empirical studies discussing the implementation of IoT for environmental monitoring in hospitals or healthcare settings and comprehensive contextual literature reviews were included. Technical articles not directly related to healthcare facilities were excluded. The data were then categorized into four main thematic areas aligned with the article's analytical framework: (1) comparisons between conventional methods and IoT-based automation; (2) IoT system design and architecture; (3) sensor deployment and dashboard implementation; and (4) technical, organizational, and policy-related challenges.

In the synthesis section, the selected studies are narratively integrated: manual monitoring mechanisms are contrasted with real-time IoT-based systems, real-world applications in healthcare facilities are presented, and patterns of strengths and limitations are discussed to support the formulation of practical recommendations for implementation.

RESULTS AND DISCUSSION

1. Environmental Impacts of Healthcare Facility Operations

Healthcare facilities, including hospitals and clinics, are increasingly recognized as significant indirect contributors to environmental degradation due to their resource-intensive operational activities. The environmental impacts include improper medical waste disposal, air pollution, high energy consumption, and pressure on water resources.

a. Medical and Domestic Waste

Medical waste management is critical to healthcare service delivery due to its direct implications for public health and environmental integrity. Hospitals typically generate between 0.5 and 2.5 kg of waste per patient daily, encompassing various categories such as biological materials, chemicals, and sharps. The volume and composition of this waste are influenced by the level of technological intervention and the waste management practices adopted by healthcare institutions (Hosseinzadeh et al., 2023). Hospitals are mandated to comply with strict waste management protocols to mitigate the risks associated with improper disposal, which can result in groundwater contamination, microbiological pollution, and the spread of infectious diseases such as hepatitis and HIV (Ernawati, et al., 2024; Peng et al., 2020).

The composition of hospital waste is strongly associated with the type of institution (public or private) and bed capacity. For example, a study conducted in Tehran revealed that general waste comprised the majority (ranging from 56.3% to 91.6%) of total waste generated by private hospitals, while infectious waste, though representing a smaller proportion (4.1% to 43.2%), still posed substantial risks (Hosseinzadeh et al., 2023).

Hospital staff training and awareness regarding proper waste management procedures are vital to minimizing health risks. A study by Hepsiba and Vijayalakshmi highlighted a significant knowledge gap among sanitation personnel: only 18.75% of staff demonstrated adequate knowledge prior to receiving structured educational interventions, underscoring the urgent need for targeted training in healthcare facilities (Hepsiba & G, 2023). Observational studies across various countries have revealed similar concerning trends: despite the availability of color-coded bins, improper usage often persists, undermining effective waste segregation processes (Ernawati, et al., 2025; Khalid et al., 2021)

The global COVID-19 pandemic has further exacerbated the burden of medical waste, particularly from the widespread use of disposable personal protective equipment (PPE). This surge has intensified the need for more stringent waste management practices to prevent a secondary public health crisis from mismanaged infectious waste (Peng et al., 2020; Wei et al., 2021). The increase in infectious waste volumes has placed considerable pressure on existing waste management infrastructure, demanding a critical reassessment of current practices and the adoption of more comprehensive strategies to safeguard public health and environmental sustainability.

Implementing effective medical waste management practices is essential for mitigating the risks associated with hospital-generated waste. There is an urgent need to strengthen healthcare workforce training programs, ensure strict adherence to established protocols, and pursue systemic reforms in waste handling and disposal strategies to protect public health and environmental quality.

b. Energy Consumption

Hospital operations depend highly on heating, ventilation, air conditioning (HVAC) systems, advanced medical equipment, and intensive lighting systems. These components typically require substantial energy input, presenting significant challenges in managing energy consumption. High energy use in hospitals negatively impacts both operational costs and environmental sustainability. Therefore, the implementation of effective energy efficiency strategies is essential. One study demonstrated that hospitals could reduce their energy consumption by up to 5% in the first year and by 2.5% annually in subsequent years through targeted energy efficiency interventions (Zlateva et al., 2024).

Several energy efficiency strategies can be adopted to optimize HVAC usage in hospital settings. Research highlights the importance of employing technologies to reduce energy consumption, carbon dioxide (CO_2) emissions, and associated operational costs in healthcare facilities (Zlateva et al., 2024). Additionally, the definition and periodic revision of protocols and standards for energy efficiency are necessary to achieve optimal outcomes. Another study found that alternative glazing and shading solutions could result in substantial energy savings—up to 16.3%—indicating that building design and material choices significantly influence energy performance (Kunduracı & İvgin, 2022).

Beyond architectural considerations, the integration of innovative technologies in the management of medical equipment also contributes to energy efficiency. Maintenance management systems that utilize optimization approaches can enhance the effective use of medical devices, reduce equipment downtime, and improve cost efficiency and safety (Ernawati, et al., 2025; Hamdi et al., 2012). Moreover, as explored in recent studies, climate-adaptive energy efficiency models reveal that energy demands vary significantly based on user behavior and climatic conditions, thus increasing the relevance of data-driven techniques for generating actionable insights (Yang et al., 2025).

Developing a comprehensive strategic plan encompassing all dimensions of energy efficiency within hospital settings is critically important. The deployment of intelligent control systems and robust management strategies is expected to yield direct energy savings and create more sustainable and cost-effective hospital environments over the long term.

c. Air Pollution

Air pollution in hospitals—particularly from diesel-powered backup generators and medical waste incinerators—significantly contributes to the increased risk of respiratory illnesses in surrounding communities. Emissions of delicate particulate matter, such as PM2.5, and other hazardous compounds pose serious health threats, especially to vulnerable populations, including children and the elderly. Studies have demonstrated a strong correlation between air pollution and increased hospitalization rates due to respiratory diseases (Zhou et al., 2019).

Diesel generators, commonly used as power backups in hospitals, emit harmful pollutants such as nitrogen oxides and PM2.5 particles, which have been linked to respiratory system damage and cancer (Wu, 2023). These emissions can trigger alveolar inflammation, restrict airflow, and increase the likelihood of asthma attacks and other complications, particularly in individuals with preexisting respiratory conditions. Research indicates that pediatric hospital admissions are associated with exposure to air pollution in residential and school environments, emphasizing the long-term impact of such pollution on vulnerable groups (Zhou et al., 2019).

Medical waste incinerators also contribute significantly to hospital-related air pollution. The combustion of medical waste releases harmful substances into the atmosphere, potentially causing respiratory irritation and increasing disease incidence among healthcare workers, patients, and nearby residents (Albahar et al., 2022). These findings underscore the importance of effective medical waste management and the need for more stringent environmental health policies to protect surrounding communities.

In line with these findings, reducing emissions from primary air pollution sources—such as diesel generators and waste incinerators—is critical to minimizing community health risks. Stricter regulations on using and maintaining polluting equipment and promoting cleaner energy alternatives are expected to reduce hazardous emissions and improve ambient air quality around healthcare facilities (Galushchak et al., 2023).

d. Water Usage

Sterilization of medical instruments, diagnostic laboratories, emergency departments, and sanitation systems demands substantial volumes of clean water. Daily operations in hospitals consume large quantities of water at various stages of sterilization, including cleaning, disinfection, and sterilizing procedures. This becomes a critical concern in water-scarce regions, where the sustainability of clean water supply is under constant threat (Panta et al., 2020).

Sterilization methods such as steam sterilization require additional procedures to ensure efficacy. Research has shown that optimal sterilization conditions require active air removal, such as pre-vacuuming. However, many hospitals—particularly in countries like Nepal—do not adhere to these standards, potentially resulting in contamination and disease transmission due to inadequately sterilized instruments (Panta et al., 2020). These findings highlight the importance of innovation in sterilization techniques and the need for water-efficient technologies.

The material properties of medical instruments also influence sterilization outcomes. Some materials are highly resistant to sterilization processes, while others may undergo significant mechanical changes that compromise safety in clinical settings (Zbyrad et al., 2025). Given this complexity, developing effective and water-efficient sterilization technologies remains a pressing challenge for researchers and healthcare professionals.

Water resource management in this context demands more sustainable strategies. Commitment to reducing water consumption through innovations in cleaning and sterilization processes is increasingly vital, particularly in regions most vulnerable to water scarcity. Improving compliance with best practices in sterilization and adopting technologies that optimize water usage can help mitigate long-term impacts on clean water availability (Panta et al., 2020).

2. Cumulative Environmental Impacts

The paradox of healthcare facilities—intended to heal—contributing to environmental degradation that may trigger new diseases or worsen patient conditions-highlights the urgency of implementing stronger sustainability practices in this sector. Numerous studies show that poor environmental conditions in healthcare institutions directly affect the wellbeing of medical staff and clinical outcomes for patients, creating a vicious cycle of declining service quality that ultimately harms public health.

Sanitation and environmental infrastructure are critical in supporting healthcare workers' wellbeing. A qualitative study in Niger revealed that substandard environmental conditions led to chronic stress and burnout among medical personnel (Anderson et al., 2023). Such dissatisfaction impacts workforce morale and patient care quality, elevating the risks of nosocomial infections and diminishing public trust in health services (Ernawati, et al., 2025; Tantum et al., 2024). These findings directly correlate with poor environmental management and low public health outcomes.

The literature also calls for enhanced training of healthcare personnel on the links between climate change and health. Environmental-aware health professionals are better equipped to address climate-related challenges (Santos et al., 2019). Environmental health practitioners are pivotal in facilitating community-based adaptation strategies to climate impacts, strengthening public health system resilience.

This approach is further reinforced by appeals for medical professionals—including specialists such as radiologists—to recognize their responsibility in climate change mitigation without compromising the quality of care (Brown et al., 2025). Environmental education for medical personnel is crucial to cultivating a generation of health professionals capable of consistently applying environmentally responsible practices.

Ethical considerations also come to the fore, as professional associations and regulatory bodies are increasingly expected to protect public health from climate crisis threats actively. Rising frustration among medical workers reflects the urgent need for institutional accountability and concrete action (Yassaie & Brooks, 2025). Neglecting environmental sustainability risks undermining the very foundations of public health.

Integrating technology-based monitoring systems and a renewed focus on environmental sustainability within healthcare facilities can mitigate adverse health impacts while enhancing the health system's capacity to respond to the global climate crisis. A synergistic approach between healthcare service delivery and environmental stewardship underscores the need for systemic transformation that aligns environmental consciousness with patient care excellence.

Table 1. Environmental Impacts of Healthcare Facilities

Impact Aspect	Source of Issue	Environmental Impact	Health Impact	References
Medical Waste	Mixed infectious and domestic waste	Soil and water contamination	Risk of HIV, Hepatitis transmission	Hosseinzadeh et al., 2023; Peng et al., 2020
Energy Consumption	HVAC systems, medical devices, and lighting	CO_2 emissions, energy inefficiency	High operational burden, staff fatigue	Zlateva et al., 2024; Hariadi et al., 2016
Air Pollution	Incinerators, diesel generators	PM2.5, NOx, local air pollution	Asthma, lung cancer, respiratory disorders	Wu, 2023; Al-Bahar et al., 2022

continued on following page

Table 1. Continued

Impact Aspect	Source of Issue	Environmental Impact	Health Impact	References
Water Usage	Sterilization and routine cleaning processes	Water depletion, wastewater discharge	Infection risk from improperly sterilized medical instruments	Panta et al., 2020; Zbyrad et al., 2025
Cumulative Impact	Combination of all poor environmental factors	Decline in environmental quality of care settings	Staff burnout, nosocomial infection risk	Anderson et al., 2023; Tantum et al., 2024; Ernawati et al., 2025
Climate Unpreparedness	Inadequate curriculum and training	Lack of readiness for climate crisis	Medical personnel unprepared for climate-related health impacts	Santos et al., 2019; Brown et al., 2025
Ethical & Social Aspects	Lack of engagement by associations and regulators	Systemic disregard for environmental sustainability	Medical staff frustration, erosion of public trust	Yassaie & Brooks, 2025

Table 1 summarizes key environmental impact aspects of healthcare facility operations, including medical waste, energy consumption, air pollution, water usage, and cumulative effects on workplace and community environments. These factors are directly linked to environmental degradation, public health risks, and the quality of healthcare services. The empirical references cited emphasize the urgent need for a systematic and comprehensive environmental management approach within the healthcare sector.

3. IoT-Based Environmental Monitoring Systems

Integrating Internet of Things (IoT) technologies into environmental monitoring systems represents a transformative approach to collecting, analyzing, and utilizing air and water quality data, energy consumption, and waste management. IoT-based environmental monitoring systems are characterized by their capacity to deploy diverse sensors that continuously measure specific environmental parameters and transmit data to a centralized platform for analysis and visualization. Core components include air quality sensors, water and wastewater sensors, energy sensors, solid waste sensors, and cloud-based dashboards that are fully integrated to enable effective environmental surveillance.

Air quality is a critical parameter for public health and environmental sustainability. IoT-enabled air sensors can detect major pollutants—such as CO_2, PM2.5, and other hazardous gases—in real-time, thereby supporting rapid-response strategies (Blinova et al., 2024). Their compact design and cost-effectiveness facilitate wide-scale deployment in urban areas. Wireless technologies enable swift data transmission and public access via online platforms, enhancing community awareness and participation in environmental health initiatives (Ernawati, et al., 2025; Sunarno et al., 2020).

Water quality monitoring is another essential component of these systems. IoT sensors for water can measure parameters such as pH, Chemical Oxygen Demand (COD), and Biological Oxygen Demand (BOD), allowing for early detection of contamination and the prevention of further environmental damage (Barbaro et al., 2024). These tools also support automated detection of leakage and pollution, ultimately enhancing drinking water safety and environmental protection.

In energy management, IoT sensors provide valuable data regarding energy consumption and equipment efficiency, enabling the identification of anomalies in electrical load patterns. This monitoring promotes energy conservation and supports broader sustainability goals by optimizing operational performance across residential, commercial, and industrial sectors. Likewise, solid waste management is significantly enhanced through IoT technology, allowing for volume measurement, waste type classification (e.g., infectious, chemical, domestic), and automated documentation to ensure regulatory compliance. Implementing smart waste sensors facilitates route optimization, operational efficiency, and a reduction in environmental impact (Gulraiz et al., 2024).

The cloud-based dashboard serves as the central control unit of the monitoring system, functioning as a platform for data visualization, trend forecasting, and decision-making support. By aggregating data from various sensors, the dashboard provides regulators and urban managers with a comprehensive view of current environmental conditions and emerging trends. This data-driven approach promotes proactive management strategies and cross-sector stakeholder collaboration (Barbaro et al., 2024; Tundjungsari et al., 2020).

IoT systems are rapidly evolving as the demand for integrated environmental monitoring solutions grows. The challenges of urbanization, climate change, and pollution necessitate continuous innovation in sensor technology, data analytics, and cloud computing. These developments open opportunities for interdisciplinary collaboration among engineers, environmental scientists, and policymakers to address increasingly complex environmental challenges.

Beyond conventional environmental monitoring, IoT applications extend to sectors such as smart agriculture, where IoT systems track environmental variables that affect crop yields—demonstrating IoT's broad applicability and transformative potential across industries (Fajar et al., 2023). The implications for public health, sustainability, and climate resilience are substantial, underscoring the importance of integrating IoT into broader environmental strategies.

IoT-based environmental monitoring systems represent a significant advancement in effectively managing environmental parameters. Their key components—air, water, energy, waste sensors, and a cloud dashboard—generate real-time data that empowers stakeholders to make evidence-based decisions. In the face of global environmental crises, the integration and optimization of such systems are an inevitable strategic imperative.

Table 2. IoT-Based Environmental Monitoring Parameters in Healthcare Facilities

Parameter	IoT Sensor	Function	Output	References
Air Quality	CO_2, PM2.5 sensors	Air pollution monitoring	Real-time alerts	Blinova et al., 2024; Ernawati et al., 2025; Sunarno et al., 2020
Water Quality	pH, COD, BOD sensors	Wastewater contamination detection	Automated responses	Barbaro et al., 2024
Energy Consumption	Electrical load sensors	Anomaly detection & energy efficiency	Energy usage data	Gulraiz et al., 2024
Solid Waste	Volume and type sensors	Waste collection optimization & classification	Waste classification data	Gulraiz et al., 2024

As summarized in Table 2, IoT-based environmental monitoring systems rely on sensors capable of measuring key environmental indicators in real time. Air and water quality sensors are crucial in detecting pollution threats to public health. In contrast, energy and solid waste sensors support operational efficiency and environmentally responsible resource management within hospitals. Integrating all parameters into a cloud-based dashboard provides robust data support for strategic environmental management in healthcare facilities.

4. Case Studies

Implementing the Internet of Things (IoT) in the healthcare sector, particularly at the Jakarta Regional General Hospital (RSUD), has significantly impacted operational efficiency. Research indicates that IoT-based devices improve the quality of healthcare services, with nurses' perceptions of technology adoption reflecting positive changes in the healthcare system (Nurmalia & Khoirinnissa, 2021). Reports indicate a 12% reduction in electricity consumption in the first six months after implementation, aligning with trends emphasizing the role of IoT in energy management. This achievement is attributed mainly to IoT-based temperature and humidity sensors managing the heating, ventilation, and air conditioning (HVAC) system, enhancing operational performance (Hasić et al., 2022).

The integration of advanced sensors and IoT technologies not only reduces energy consumption but also improves data collection systems. By monitoring water usage and waste volumes, hospitals can enhance operational efficiency, avoid environmental penalties from regulatory bodies, and demonstrate commitment to sustainable healthcare management (Hasić et al., 2022; Nižetić et al., 2020). With an implementation cost of approximately IDR 300 million for primary hospitals, the system offers a promising return on investment, potentially saving up to IDR 100 million annually (Hasić et al., 2022).

Innovative waste management solutions are a critical component of the IoT ecosystem. Research shows that IoT applications in waste management enable real-time monitoring of biomedical waste, thereby improving waste collection logistics and safety protocols for handling hazardous materials (Ishaq et al., 2023). These implementations have demonstrated positive environmental impacts, such as waste volume reduction and lower operational risks, contributing to more sustainable hospital environments.

IoT systems optimize resource management by automating data analysis related to hospital operations. For instance, energy management can be improved using intelligent algorithms that predict usage patterns and automatically adjust output (Udendhran et al., 2023). This capability is critical in high-cost healthcare settings, where operational efficiency is paramount. Integrating IoT with machine learning opens new avenues for research and underscores the need for cutting-edge technologies to maintain hospital competitiveness and efficiency (Nižetić et al., 2020; Udendhran et al., 2023).

Despite the initial cost barriers, technology landscape analyses indicate a rising trend in hospitals' adoption of IoT innovations. Recent studies emphasize the importance of IoT maturity models that support gradual transitions, capability development, and readiness for change (Hasić et al., 2022). This highlights the need for technological investment and cultivating an innovation-supportive organizational culture.

The momentum toward IoT-driven operational excellence is growing, as healthcare facilities face increasing pressure to meet efficiency standards. The convergence of IoT and big data technologies enables hospitals to extract meaningful insights from operational data, thereby improving understanding of institutional dynamics and patient needs (Hasić et al., 2022; Nižetić et al., 2020). Although upfront costs may be significant, long-term benefits—such as enhanced service quality, environmental compliance, and operational cost savings—provide a compelling rationale for strategic IoT adoption.

Exploring IoT applications must align with sustainability goals. Amid escalating environmental challenges, the healthcare sector's adoption of IoT is a vital step toward a more sustainable future. Implementing these systems enables hospitals to reduce their carbon footprint and enhance the efficient use of resources (Ishaq et al., 2023; Udendhran et al., 2023). These advancements fulfill regulatory demands and reflect the growing social responsibility expected by patients, service providers, and governing authorities.

5. Analysis of Benefits and Efficiency

Implementing Internet of Things (IoT)-based environmental monitoring systems in healthcare facilities generates significant benefits across three key environmental, social, and economic dimensions. This approach addresses operational challenges and aligns with the global commitment to the Sustainable Development Goals (SDGs).

a. Environmental Benefits

Integrating IoT technologies into healthcare systems substantially contributes to environmental sustainability, particularly by reducing carbon footprints produced by heating, ventilation, and air conditioning (HVAC) systems and improving electricity and water use efficiency. Real-time monitoring via IoT sensors allows hospitals to optimize energy usage, minimizing waste. Studies have demonstrated that IoT implementation enables healthcare facilities to manage equipment workloads more efficiently, reducing energy demands and lowering greenhouse gas emissions (Shaw & Dey, 2023; Verdejo Espinosa et al., 2021). Specifically, Espinosa et al. (2021) confirmed that IoT devices enhance energy efficiency and promote overall operational optimization in healthcare systems.

IoT-based automated monitoring systems can also track wastewater and air quality—two critical factors in preventing environmental pollution near healthcare facilities. This proactive approach is vital to avoid the release of hazardous pollutants such as heavy metals and delicate particulate matter (PM2.5), typically emitted during medical waste incineration. Espinosa et al. (2021) further emphasized the importance of such monitoring systems in maintaining local ecosystem integrity and public health, while supporting compliance with environmental standards.

Beyond short-term operational efficiency, IoT solutions offer strategic advantages in the context of sustainable development. According to Abaee et al. (2024), the convergence of public health initiatives and energy efficiency through IoT applications significantly contributes to achieving the SDGs, underscoring the importance of integrating innovative technologies into healthcare systems. Healthcare facilities can expand their capacity to meet sustainability targets by leveraging IoT connected to cloud computing platforms.

b. Social Benefits

The social benefits of IoT-based environmental monitoring systems are substantial, particularly in enhancing the quality of life in urban communities. The system's real-time ability to monitor air and water quality is critical in early detection and prevention of environmentally related health issues. Research shows that exposure to poor environmental conditions can result in respiratory illnesses, skin infections, and gastrointestinal diseases such as diarrhea (Mahajan, 2022). Furthermore, implementing accessible, citizen-centered monitoring frameworks can strengthen community engagement and promote active participation in environmental advocacy and policy decision-making.

Air quality improvements affect health outcomes and influence patient care results and satisfaction with healthcare services. Studies have revealed correlations between clean environments and increased healthcare worker satisfaction. Improved air quality is linked to reduced nosocomial infections, ultimately decreasing workloads and fostering more conducive working conditions for medical personnel (Sathyamoorthy et al., 2024). This correlation underscores that environmental health is integral to human health, especially in densely populated areas where healthcare facilities are the backbone of public health infrastructure.

IoT technologies have revolutionized how environmental data is collected and utilized. High-resolution data equipped with geospatial information from innovative tools—such as portable air pollution sensors—enables research that informs effective mitigation strategies for pollution-related health risks (Park et al., 2021). This capability supports evidence-based policymaking and increases public awareness and education around environmental health risks.

The ease of use and accessibility of IoT devices also empower public participation, including among non-experts, in environmental monitoring activities. This democratization of data collection and analysis processes enhances inclusivity and collective awareness (Okafor et al., 2024). As this technology evolves, its potential to improve environmental quality and public health outcomes will continue to grow, promoting a more sustainable urban living paradigm.

c. Economic Benefits

Integrating IoT technologies across operational domains—particularly healthcare and environmental management—has shown considerable economic benefits. Several studies indicate that this efficiency can lead to a 10–15% annual reduction in operational costs, primarily due to decreased energy and water consumption, and enhanced waste management systems that reduce the risk of penalties for regulatory violations (Huang et al., 2024). With IoT systems, organizations can proactively identify and resolve issues such as water leaks or excessive electricity usage, resulting in significant long-term cost savings (Suherman et al., 2023).

A practical example of this can be seen at Jakarta Regional General Hospital, where implementing IoT-based monitoring systems reduced energy consumption by 12% within just six months. Despite an initial investment of approximately IDR 300 million, the system demonstrated annual savings potential of up to IDR 100 million, making it economically viable over the medium term (Bandaru et al., 2024). This case underscores the potential for IoT investments to yield substantial returns through improved energy management.

Moreover, IoT applications enhance the efficiency of logistical operations, particularly in managing medical waste. Using volume-sensing devices and automated tracking systems enables more efficient waste collection processes, reducing collection frequency and operational costs typically incurred by inefficient manual methods. The optimization provided by IoT in this area also contributes to environmental impact reduction and improved compliance with waste management regulations, ultimately helping institutions avoid costly penalties (Huang et al., 2024).

6. Implementation Challenges

The deployment of Internet of Things (IoT)-based environmental monitoring systems in healthcare facilities presents numerous advantages, yet also involves a complex array of implementation challenges. The following sections outline the primary obstacles identified, contextual explanations, and proposed mitigation strategies.

a. Upfront and Maintenance Costs

Implementing IoT-based environmental monitoring systems in healthcare settings faces considerable financial challenges that hospital administrators must address to ensure successful adoption. One of the most pressing barriers is the high initial capital expenditure required to deploy IoT infrastructure. These expenses include sensor installations, cloud system development, and reliable network construction—costs that can be especially prohibitive for facilities operating under limited budgets, particularly in low- and middle-income countries. Frimpong et al (2023) observe that many hospitals prioritize immediate operational needs over technological innovation, often resulting in inadequate budget allocations for digital initiatives.

In addition to initial installation costs, ongoing maintenance—such as sensor calibration, infrastructure updates, and device replacement—further strains healthcare budgets. While return on investment (ROI) estimates may vary, studies suggest that creative financing strategies—such as public-private partnerships or government incentives—are essential to support the adoption of this technology (Abdulmalek et al., 2022; Senbekov et al., 2020). Innovative funding mechanisms are critical, as traditional public sector financing often falls short of meeting the extensive needs of health infrastructure digitalization (Senbekov et al., 2020).

Furthermore, IoT integration demands significant cultural and operational shifts among healthcare workers. Successful implementation requires technological investment and comprehensive staff training to adapt to new workflows and platforms. A lack of familiarity with advanced digital systems may lead to resistance among personnel, ultimately impeding integration and effective utilization.

b. Data Security

The increasing use of IoT in healthcare services generates vast amounts of data, including sensitive patient information. This raises serious concerns about data privacy and cybersecurity. By nature, IoT's interconnectivity and data-sharing capabilities render systems vulnerable to various threats, including data breaches, unauthorized manipulation, and targeted cyberattacks (Bentameur & Iguenane, 2023; Pal et al., 2018). Given these vulnerabilities, healthcare organizations must implement robust security measures.

Suherman et al. (2023) underscore the importance of deploying advanced cybersecurity technologies to safeguard sensitive medical data. Blockchain, in particular, holds promise in ensuring immutable transaction records, thereby enhancing data integrity and trust within the healthcare ecosystem. Two-factor authentication (2FA) also serves as an effective barrier against unauthorized access, offering additional protection. Continuous training for IT personnel in this sector is critical; well-trained staff are better equipped to recognize and mitigate security risks, reinforcing healthcare systems against evolving digital vulnerabilities (Bozic, 2023).

Encryption plays a central role in securing health data. Implementing hybrid encryption technologies can effectively block unauthorized access and manipulation of medical records. With the increasing use of electronic health records (EHRs), maintaining the balance between secure data storage and efficient access for healthcare delivery is essential (Zengyu et al., 2021).

Access control policies must also evolve alongside the growing dependence on IoT in healthcare. Pal et al. (2018) advocate for fine-grained access control frameworks to enhance security in innovative healthcare systems. These frameworks ensure that only authorized personnel can access sensitive data, without compromising operational efficiency. Moreover, adopting advanced technologies such as artificial intelligence (AI) in integrated risk management can aid in detecting threats and automating incident responses, contributing to a proactive cybersecurity strategy (Knight et al., 2024).

Integrating cybersecurity technologies, effective encryption strategies, and stringent access control policies is essential to securing IoT-generated healthcare data. Ongoing education and training for IT staff further reinforce these protections, establishing a comprehensive defense against the ever-evolving landscape of cyber threats.

c. Human Resource Capacity

The increasing use of the Internet of Things (IoT) in healthcare services generates vast amounts of data, including highly sensitive patient information. The integration of this technology raises serious concerns regarding privacy and data security. IoT's inherent characteristics—such as interconnectivity among devices and seamless data sharing—make such information particularly vulnerable to a range of cyber threats, including data breaches, unauthorized manipulation, and targeted cyberattacks (Bentameur & Iguenane, 2023; Pal et al., 2018). In light of these vulnerabilities, healthcare organizations must implement robust security measures.

Suherman et al. (2023) highlight the importance of deploying advanced cybersecurity technologies to protect sensitive medical data. One notable solution is using blockchain systems, which offer immutable transaction records, enhancing data integrity and building trust within the healthcare ecosystem. In addition, two-factor authentication (2FA) is an effective barrier to unauthorized access, helping safeguard sensitive information from cyber threats. Ongoing training for IT personnel in the healthcare sector is also critical; well-trained staff are more capable of recognizing and mitigating security risks, thus strengthening the system's defenses against digital vulnerabilities (Bentameur & Iguenane, 2023).

Encryption plays a vital role in securing healthcare data. Implementing hybrid encryption technologies can prevent unauthorized access and manipulation of medical information. Jiang et al. (2019) emphasize that secure encryption techniques enable healthcare providers to process and manage sensitive patient data without compromising confidentiality during transmission across interconnected devices. With the increasing adoption of electronic medical records, maintaining the security of such data while ensuring efficient access and information sharing is essential (Zengyu et al., 2021; Zhang et al., 2023).

Access control policies must evolve alongside growing reliance on IoT in the healthcare sector. Pal et al. (2018) advocate for fine-grained access control frameworks, which can significantly enhance the security of innovative healthcare systems. These frameworks ensure that only authorized personnel can access sensitive data without compromising operational efficiency. Furthermore, adopting advanced technologies such as artificial intelligence (AI) in integrated risk management can help identify threats and automate responses to security incidents, reinforcing a proactive approach to risk mitigation (Bozic, 2023; Knight et al., 2024).

Integrating cybersecurity technologies, effective encryption strategies, and stringent access control policies is essential for safeguarding IoT-generated healthcare data from various potential threats. Continuous education and training for IT staff within the healthcare sector further reinforce these measures, establishing a comprehensive defense against the evolving challenges of cybersecurity.

d. Regulatory Frameworks

The regulatory landscape governing IoT in healthcare, especially in developing countries like Indonesia, presents critical gaps. The absence of comprehensive national standards and sector-specific regulations creates legal ambiguities regarding data accountability, licensing of technology providers, and compliance with safety and privacy norms. This regulatory uncertainty hinders the broader adoption of IoT solutions that could otherwise greatly enhance healthcare services (Mittal, 2019; Tenepalli & T M, 2024).

The convergence of IoT and blockchain technologies can address some of these regulatory challenges. Blockchain can enhance security, accountability, and trust in healthcare applications by providing immutable transaction records and ensuring compliance with regulatory standards (Kamangar et al., 2023; Sharma et al., 2022). In particular, integrating IoT with blockchain allows for secure real-time monitoring and management of patient data while safeguarding sensitive health information (Kamangar et al., 2023). Given that IoT requires secure and accessible infrastructure, regulations must also address specific needs such as identity verification mechanisms and data integrity protocols—both of which are critical in clinical contexts (Kamangar et al., 2023; Sharma et al., 2022).

Understanding how healthcare practitioners and stakeholders perceive and adopt emerging technologies is essential for successful implementation (Hasan et al., 2023). Disparities in technology acceptance and use across regions—especially in low-resource settings—underscore the need for targeted regulatory and educational initiatives to support IoT integration in healthcare (Edu, 2024; Hasan et al., 2023).

Establishing a comprehensive regulatory framework for IoT in Indonesian healthcare is urgently needed. Such a framework would address the current legal uncertainties hindering adoption and foster collaboration among ministries and key stakeholders to support the sustainable integration of transformative technologies into healthcare practice.

CONCLUSION AND RECOMMENDATIONS

Conclusion

The Internet of Things (IoT)-based environmental monitoring system represents a strategic innovation that bridges the need for quality medical services with the responsibility of environmental stewardship. This technology enables real-time monitoring of air and water quality, energy consumption, and waste generation while supporting rapid, data-driven, and accurate decision-making in hospital management.

The integrated implementation of IoT systems has been shown to reduce the ecological footprint of healthcare facilities, enhance operational efficiency, and strengthen the resilience of health systems against environmental threats and climate change. With adequate regulatory support, enhanced human resource capacity, and integration into hospital management systems, IoT-based monitoring holds the potential to become a cornerstone of sustainable digital transformation in the healthcare sector—particularly in developing countries.

Recommendations

To enhance the effectiveness of IoT-based environmental monitoring systems in healthcare facilities, the following strategic recommendations are proposed:

1. National Regulations and Standards

Governments and health authorities should develop and adopt national standards concerning the technical specifications, data security protocols, and operational procedures for hospital IoT-based environmental monitoring systems.

2. Fiscal Incentives and Budgetary Support

Fiscal incentives or accessible financing schemes should be provided to hospitals that demonstrate commitment to implementing environmentally friendly digital monitoring systems.

3. Data System Integration

Data generated from IoT systems must be systematically integrated into hospital annual management reports and utilized as a foundation for strategic planning and evidence-based hospital decision-making.

4. Human Resource Training and Technical Capacity

Regular training and technical assistance should be conducted for environmental officers, technicians, and hospital managers on using, analyzing, and applying data from IoT systems.

REFERENCES

Abdulmalek, S., Nasir, A., Jabbar, W. A., Almuhaya, M. A. M., Bairagi, A. K., & Khan, Md. (2022). IoT-Based Healthcare-Monitoring System towards Improving Quality of Life: A Review. *Health Care, 10*(10). Advance online publication. DOI: 10.3390/healthcare10101993 PMID: 36292441

Albahar, S., Li, J., Al-Zoughool, M., Al-Hemoud, A., Gasana, J., Aldashti, H., & Alahmad, B. (2022). Air Pollution and Respiratory Hospital Admissions in Kuwait: The Epidemiological Applicability of Predicted PM2.5 in Arid Regions. *International Journal of Environmental Research and Public Health, 19*(10), 5998. DOI: 10.3390/ijerph19105998 PMID: 35627536

Anderson, D. M., Mahamane, E., Bauza, V., Mahamadou, K. O. B., Tantum, L., & Salzberg, A. (2023). Effects of environmental conditions on healthcare worker wellbeing and quality of care: A qualitative study in Niger. *PLOS Global Public Health, 3*(12), e0002590. DOI: 10.1371/journal.pgph.0002590 PMID: 38117837

Barbaro, A., Chiavassa, P., Fissore, V. I., Servetti, A., Raviola, E., Ramírez-Espinosa, G., Giusto, E., Montrucchio, B., Astolfi, A., & Fiori, F. (2024). Data Acquisition, Processing, and Aggregation in a Low-Cost IoT System for Indoor Environmental Quality Monitoring. *Applied Sciences (Basel, Switzerland), 14*(10), 4021. DOI: 10.3390/app14104021

Bentameur, K., & Iguenane, B. (2023). Impact of Information Security on Online Operations: The Mediating Role of Risk Management. *International Journal of Computations* [IJCIM]. *Information and Manufacturing, 3*(1), 27–34. DOI: 10.54489/ijcim.v3i1.224

Blinova, T., Singh Chauhan, S., Singla, T., Bansal, S., Mittal, A., & Yellanki, V. S. (2024). Performance Evaluation of IoT Sensors in Urban Air Quality Monitoring: Insights from the IoT Sensor Performance Test. *BIO Web of Conferences, 86*, 01088. https://doi.org/DOI: 10.1051/bioconf/20248601088

Bozic, V. (2023). Integrated Risk Management and Artificial Intelligence in Hospital. *Journal of AI, 7*(1), 63–80. DOI: 10.61969/jai.1329224

Brown, M. J., Forster, B. B., McInnes, M. D. F., Komar, M. A., Amin, P., Atwal, S., Chen, S., Hamwi, M., Ladak, R., Malik, A., McKee, H., Wang, M., Yang, J., Hamel, C., & Hanneman, K. (2025). Canadian Association of Radiologists Statement on Planetary Health Education in Radiology. *Canadian Association of Radiologists Journal, 76*(2), 212–220. DOI: 10.1177/08465371241279359 PMID: 39313910

Cilasun Kunduracı, A., & İvgin, S. (2022). Energy Saving Opportunities through Glazing and Shading Alternatives. *Iconarp International. Nihon Kenchiku Gakkai Keikaku-Kei Rombunshu*. Advance online publication. DOI: 10.15320/ICONARP.2022.211

Destoumieux-Garzón, D., Mavingui, P., Boetsch, G., Boissier, J., Darriet, F., Duboz, P., Fritsch, C., Giraudoux, P., Le Roux, F., Morand, S., Paillard, C., Pontier, D., Sueur, C., & Voituron, Y. (2018). The One Health Concept: 10 Years Old and a Long Road Ahead. *Frontiers in Veterinary Science, 5*. Advance online publication. DOI: 10.3389/fvets.2018.00014 PMID: 29484301

dos Santos, M., Howard, D., Kruger, P., Banos, A., & Kornik, S. (2019). Climate Change and Healthcare Sustainability in the Agincourt Sub-District, Kruger to Canyons Biosphere Region, South Africa. *Sustainability, 11*(2), 496. DOI: 10.3390/su11020496

Edu, A. S. (2024). Configural paths for IoTs and big data analytics acceptance for healthcare improvement: A fuzzy-set qualitative comparative analysis. *Aslib Journal of Information Management, 76*(5), 800–821. DOI: 10.1108/AJIM-10-2022-0465

Ernawati, K., Aslichan, A., Albar, A. S., Al Khaliel, A. T., & Al Fatich, A. S. F. (2025). *Green Leadership Strategy to Encourage Pro-Environmental Behavior*. IGI Global., DOI: 10.4018/979-8-3373-2106-6.ch006

Ernawati, K., Burhan, A., Albar, A. S., Al Khaliel, A. T., & Al Fatich, A. S. F. (2024). *Professional Development of Environmental Health Workers*., DOI: 10.4018/979-8-3693-4334-0.ch010

Ernawati, K., Burhan, A., Syawqi Albar, A., Al-Khaliel, A. T., & Fawwaz Al-Fatich, A. S. (2024). Health Education for Sustainable E-Waste Management. In *International Journal of Engineering, Science and Information Technology* (Vol. 4, Issue 3, pp. 128–131). https://doi.org/DOI: 10.52088/ijesty.v4i3.556

Ernawati, K., Hayurani, H., Karimulloh, K., Haryanti, S. C., & Utami, S. P. (2025). Development of a home health assessment application and website-based family disease registration. *International Journal of Innovative Research and Scientific Studies, 8*(3), 4471–4477. DOI: 10.53894/ijirss.v8i3.7538

Ernawati, K., Mardhiyah, D., Wulansari, R., Rifqatussaadah, R., & Utami, S. (2025). *AI's Role in Environmental Health and Tackling Ecological Impacts Through Multidimensional Views*., DOI: 10.4018/979-8-3373-0680-3.ch005

Fajar, M., Chandra, F. B., & Arfandy, H. (2023). Applying Use Case 2.0 Approach to The Development of IoT-Based Rainfall Monitoring System. [JANAPATI]. *Jurnal Nasional Pendidikan Teknik Informatika, 12*(2), 244–252. DOI: 10.23887/janapati.v12i2.61529

Frimpong, B. A., Barbosa, C., & Raed A Abd, A. (2023). The Impact of the Internet of Things (IoT) on Healthcare Delivery: A Systematic Literature Review. *Journal of Techniques, 5*(3), 84–91. DOI: 10.51173/jt.v5i3.1433

Galushchak, O., Burlaka, S., Kupchuk, I., Bondarenko, V., & Gontaruk, Y. (2023). Environmental indicators of the operation of a diesel generator running on a mixture of biofuels. *Polityka Energetyczna – Energy Policy Journal, 26*(4), 195–208. https://doi.org/DOI: 10.33223/epj/170759

González, A., García-Sanz-Calcedo, J., & Rodríguez Salgado, D. (2018). Evaluation of Energy Consumption in German Hospitals: Benchmarking in the Public Sector. *Energies, 11*(9), 2279. DOI: 10.3390/en11092279

Gordon, L. B., Liu, K. T., Hudak, N. C., & Auerbach, A. (2023). Assessing hospitalists' opinions regarding the role of environmental health within the practice of hospital medicine. *Journal of Hospital Medicine, 18*(7), 588–594. DOI: 10.1002/jhm.13098 PMID: 37039588

Gulraiz, A., Gulraiz, H., Zia, M., Badar, S., & Zaidi, S. S. H. (2024). Utilizing IoT and Cloud Computing for Weather-Health Monitoring Application. *International Journal of Electrical Engineering and Computer Science, 6*, 152–158. DOI: 10.37394/232027.2024.6.18

Hamdi, N., Oweis, R., Abu Zraiq, H., & Abu Sammour, D. (2012). An Intelligent Healthcare Management System: A New Approach in Work-order Prioritization for Medical Equipment Maintenance Requests. *Journal of Medical Systems, 36*(2), 557–567. DOI: 10.1007/s10916-010-9501-4 PMID: 20703695

Han, S., Jeong, Y., Lee, K., & In, J. (2024). Environmental sustainability in health care: An empirical investigation of US hospitals. *Business Strategy and the Environment, 33*(6), 6045–6065. DOI: 10.1002/bse.3790

Haque, S. A., Aziz, S. M., & Rahman, M. (2014). Review of Cyber-Physical System in Healthcare. *International Journal of Distributed Sensor Networks, 10*(4), 217415. DOI: 10.1155/2014/217415

Hasan, N., Bao, Y., Miah, S. J., & Fenton, A. (2023). Factors influencing the young physicians' intention to use Internet of Things (IoT) services in healthcare. *Information Development, 39*(4), 902–919. DOI: 10.1177/02666669211064114

Hasić, F., Beirens, B., & Serral, E. (2022). Maturity Model for IoT Adoption in Hospitals. *Computer Information, 41*(1), 213–232. DOI: 10.31577/cai_2022_1_213

Hepsiba, J., & G, V. (2023). Effectiveness of Teaching Programme on Knowledge Regarding Hospital Waste Management a mong House Keeping Employees. *JOURNAL OF CLINICAL AND BIOMEDICAL SCIENCES, 13*(3), 81–84. https://doi.org/ DOI: 10.58739/jcbs/v13i3.23.24

Hosseinzadeh, A., Reshadi, M. A. M., Nazaripour, M., & Rezaei, M. (2023). Medical Waste Management in Private Hospitals in Tehran. *Journal of Advances in Environmental Health Research, 11*(3), 142–146. DOI: 10.34172/jaehr.1274

Huang, C., Chen, Q., Lin, Z., Su, W., Zhang, Z., & Liu, S. (2024). The Economic Impact and Application Challenges of IoT Technology in Smart Home and Infrastructure. *Journal of Innovation and Development, 6*(1), 35–39. DOI: 10.54097/y54jkp60

Ibrahim, M., Kebede, M., & Mengiste, B. (2023). Healthcare Waste Segregation Practice and Associated Factors among Healthcare Professionals Working in Public and Private Hospitals, Dire Dawa, Eastern Ethiopia. *Journal of Environmental and Public Health, 2023*, 1–7. DOI: 10.1155/2023/8015856 PMID: 36747502

Ishaq, A., Mohammad, S. J., Bello, A.-A. D., Wada, S. A., Adebayo, A., & Jagun, Z. T. (2023). Smart waste bin monitoring using IoT for sustainable biomedical waste management. *Environmental Science and Pollution Research International*. Advance online publication. DOI: 10.1007/s11356-023-30240-1 PMID: 37878175

Kamangar, Z. U., Memon, R. A., Murtaza Memon, G., & Kamangar, U. A. (2023). Integration of Internet of Things and blockchain technology in healthcare domain: A systematic literature review. *International Journal of Communication Systems, 36*(16). Advance online publication. DOI: 10.1002/dac.5582

Khalid, S., Haq, N., Sabiha, Z.-A., Latif, A., Khan, M. A., Iqbal, J., & Yousaf, N. (2021). Current practices of waste management in teaching hospitals and presence of incinerators in densely populated areas. *BMC Public Health, 21*(1), 1340. DOI: 10.1186/s12889-021-11389-1 PMID: 34233645

Knight, E., Yolou, I., Li, J., Kockan, C., Jensen, M., & Gerstein, M. (2024). *Homomorphic Encryption: An Application to Polygenic Risk Scores*. https://doi.org/DOI: 10.1101/2024.05.26.595961

Mahajan, S. (2022). Design and development of an open-source framework for citizen-centric environmental monitoring and data analysis. *Scientific Reports, 12*(1), 14416. DOI: 10.1038/s41598-022-18700-z PMID: 36002580

McGain, F., & Naylor, C. (2014). Environmental sustainability in hospitals – a systematic review and research agenda. *Journal of Health Services Research & Policy*, *19*(4), 245–252. DOI: 10.1177/1355819614534836 PMID: 24813186

Mishbahuddin, A. A., Fadli, Justicia, A. K., & Ernawati, K. (2021). Understanding islamic commandments to maintain people's health and environment: A critical review on literature. In *International Journal of Health Sciences* (Vol. 5, Issue 2, pp. 202–211). Universidad Tecnica de Manabi. https://doi.org/DOI: 10.29332/ijhs.v5n2.1427

Mittal, P. (2019). A Survey on Internet of Things (IoT) Based Healthcare Monitoring System. *International Journal of Advanced Trends in Computer Science and Engineering*, *6*(4), 1646–1653. DOI: 10.30534/ijatcse/2019/90842019

Moldovan, F., Moldovan, L., & Bataga, T. (2023). The Environmental Sustainability Assessment of an Orthopedics Emergency Hospital Supported by a New Innovative Framework. *Sustainability*, *15*(18), 13402. DOI: 10.3390/su151813402

Mominkhan, D., Alamri, F. A., Balharith, M., Alharbi, M., Alshebli, A., Alshareef, S. Y., Khairaldain, A., Almutairi, N., Abusit, A., Almuzaini, Y., Alahmari, A. A., & Alabdulaali, M. K. (2023). The current state and potential evolution of carbon emissions in the healthcare sector: A narrative review article. *Frontiers in Sustainable Energy Policy*, *2*. Advance online publication. DOI: 10.3389/fsuep.2023.1230253

Monye, S. N., Monye, S. I., Afolalu, S. A., Okokpujie, I. P., Adetunla, A. O., Ikumapayi, O. M., Aderemi, K. B., Nwankwo, S. O., & Okpako, E. A. (2024). A Conceptual Framework for the Adoption of IoT in the Energy Sector: Technology-Organization-Environment Framework Approach. *2024 International Conference on Science, Engineering and Business for Driving Sustainable Development Goals (SEB4SDG)*, 1–6. https://doi.org/DOI: 10.1109/SEB4SDG60871.2024.10629924

Naga Rani Bandaru, V., Gayatri Sarman Kaligotla, V. S. H., Dhana Satya Prathap Varma, U., Prasadaraju, K., & Sugumaran, S. (2024). A Enhancing Data Security Solutions for Smart Energy Systems in IoT-Enabled Cloud Computing Environments through Lightweight Cryptographic Techniques. *IOP Conference Series. Earth and Environmental Science*, *1375*(1), 012003. DOI: 10.1088/1755-1315/1375/1/012003

Nižetić, S., & Šolić, P., López-de-Ipiña González-de-Artaza, D., & Patrono, L. (2020). Internet of Things (IoT): Opportunities, issues and challenges towards a smart and sustainable future. *Journal of Cleaner Production*, *274*, 122877. DOI: 10.1016/j.jclepro.2020.122877 PMID: 32834567

Nurmalia, D., & Khoirinnissa, N. (2021). Persepsi Perawat Tentang Integrasi Perangkat Berbasis Teknologi Internet of Things (IoT) Dalam Pelayanan Kesehatan Di Rumah Sakit. *Jurnal Kepemimpinan Dan Manajemen Keperawatan*, *4*(2), 199–206. DOI: 10.32584/jkmk.v4i2.1074

Obubu, M., Chuku, N., Ananaba, A., Sadiq, F. U. S., Sambo, E., Kolade, O., Oyekanmi, T., Olaosebikan, K., & Serrano, O. (2023). Lagos State Hospital Waste Management Practices: A Descriptive Overview with Stakeholders' Role and Key Recommendations. *Journal of Environmental Protection*, *14*(02), 108–125. DOI: 10.4236/jep.2023.142008

Okafor, N., Ingle, R., Saunders, M., & Delaney, D. (2024). *Assessing and Improving the Quality of IoT Sensor Data in Environmental Monitoring Networks: A Focus on Peatlands*. https://doi.org/DOI: 10.36227/techrxiv.170905846.67456956/v1

Pal, S., Hitchens, M., Varadharajan, V., & Rabehaja, T. (2018). Fine-Grained Access Control for Smart Healthcare Systems in the Internet of Things. *EAI Endorsed Transactions on Industrial Networks and Intelligent Systems*, *4*(13), 154370. DOI: 10.4108/eai.20-3-2018.154370

Panta, G., Richardson, A. K., Shaw, I. C., & Coope, P. A. (2020). Compliance of primary and secondary care public hospitals with standard practices for reprocessing and steam sterilization of reusable medical devices in Nepal: Findings from nationwide multicenter clustered audits. *BMC Health Services Research*, *20*(1), 923. DOI: 10.1186/s12913-020-05788-0 PMID: 33028325

Park, Y. M., Sousan, S., Streuber, D., & Zhao, K. (2021). GeoAir—A Novel Portable, GPS-Enabled, Low-Cost Air-Pollution Sensor: Design Strategies to Facilitate Citizen Science Research and Geospatial Assessments of Personal Exposure. *Sensors (Basel)*, *21*(11), 3761. DOI: 10.3390/s21113761 PMID: 34071590

Peng, J., Wu, X., Wang, R., Li, C., Zhang, Q., & Wei, D. (2020). Medical waste management practice during the 2019-2020 novel coronavirus pandemic: Experience in a general hospital. *American Journal of Infection Control*, *48*(8), 918–921. DOI: 10.1016/j.ajic.2020.05.035 PMID: 32504761

Sathyamoorthy, S., Matthew, U. O., Adekunle, T. S., & Okafor, N. U. (2024). Advances and Challenges in IoT Sensors Data Handling and Processing in Environmental Monitoring Networks. *HAFED POLY Journal of Science. Management and Technology*, *5*(2), 40–60. DOI: 10.4314/hpjsmt.v5i2.3

Senbekov, M., Saliev, T., Bukeyeva, Z., Almabayeva, A., Zhanaliyeva, M., Aitenova, N., Toishibekov, Y., & Fakhradiyev, I. (2020). The Recent Progress and Applications of Digital Technologies in Healthcare: A Review. *International Journal of Telemedicine and Applications, 2020*, 1–18. DOI: 10.1155/2020/8830200 PMID: 33343657

Sharma, P., Moparthi, N. R., Namasudra, S., Shanmuganathan, V., & Hsu, C. (2022). Blockchain-based iot architecture to secure healthcare system using identity-based encryption. *Expert Systems: International Journal of Knowledge Engineering and Neural Networks, 39*(10). Advance online publication. DOI: 10.1111/exsy.12915

Shaw, S. K., & Dey, J. L. (2023). Emergence of IoT in Healthcare Industry: Towards Sustainable Digital Health Systems. In *Advances in Business Informatics empowered by AI & Intelligent Systems* (pp. 108–125). CSMFL Publications., DOI: 10.46679/978819573220308

Suherman, R., Nataraja, P. K., Pratama, A., & Kahfi, A. H. (2023). Electricity management system with technology internet of things. *Jurnal Techno Nusa Mandiri, 20*(2), 95–101. DOI: 10.33480/techno.v20i2.4520

Sunarno, S., Purwanto, P., & Suryono, S. (2020). The Monitoring System of Sulfur Dioxide Gas Using a Web-based Wireless Sensor. *Proceedings of the Proceedings of the 13th International Interdisciplinary Studies Seminar, IISS 2019,* 30-31 October 2019, Malang, Indonesia. https://doi.org/DOI: 10.4108/eai.23-10-2019.2293039

Tantum, L. K., Mahamane, E., Bauza, V., Mahamadou, K. O. B., Sanoussi, E. Y., Salzberg, A., & Anderson, D. M. (2024). Environmental Infrastructure Maintenance Bottlenecks in Healthcare Facilities and Coping Strategies Among Healthcare Workers in Niger. *Environmental Health Insights, 18*. Advance online publication. DOI: 10.1177/11786302241271554 PMID: 39148586

Tenepalli, D., & T M, N. (2024). A Systematic Review on IoT and Machine Learning Algorithms in E-Healthcare. *International Journal of Computing and Digital Systems, 15*(1), 279–294. DOI: 10.12785/ijcds/160122

Tundjungsari, V., Ernawati, K., & Mutia, N. (2020). *Public Health Surveillance to Promote Clean and Healthy Life Behaviours Using Big Data Approach (An Indonesian Case Study)*. Springer., DOI: 10.1007/978-3-030-23162-0_69

Udendhran, R., Sasikala, R., Nishanthi, R., & Vasanthi, J. (2023). Smart Energy Consumption Control in Commercial Buildings Using Machine Learning and IOT. *E3S Web of Conferences, 387*, 02003. https://doi.org/DOI: 10.1051/e3sconf/202338702003

Verdejo Espinosa, Á., Lopez Ruiz, J. L., Mata Mata, F., & Estevez, M. E. (2021). Application of IoT in Healthcare: Keys to Implementation of the Sustainable Development Goals. *Sensors (Basel), 21*(7), 2330. DOI: 10.3390/s21072330 PMID: 33810606

Visser, E. H., Brakema, E. A., Slootweg, I. A., Vos, H. M. M., & Adriaanse, M. A. (2024). *Patients' perspectives on ecologically sustainable healthcare in general practice*. https://doi.org/DOI: 10.1101/2024.10.18.24310602

Wafula, S. T., Musiime, J., & Oporia, F. (2019). Health care waste management among health workers and associated factors in primary health care facilities in Kampala City, Uganda: A cross-sectional study. *BMC Public Health, 19*(1), 203. DOI: 10.1186/s12889-019-6528-4 PMID: 30777034

Wassie, B., Gintamo, B., Mekuria, Z. N., & Gizaw, Z. (2022). Healthcare Waste Management Practices and Associated Factors in Private Clinics in Addis Ababa, Ethiopia. *Environmental Health Insights, 16*. Advance online publication. DOI: 10.1177/11786302211073383 PMID: 35095276

Wei, Y., Cui, M., Ye, Z., & Guo, Q. (2021). Environmental challenges from the increasing medical waste since SARS outbreak. *Journal of Cleaner Production, 291*, 125246. DOI: 10.1016/j.jclepro.2020.125246 PMID: 33250588

Wu, N. (2023). Research on the emissions of diesel engine and the selection of suitable diesel engine additives to reduce particulate emissions. *Journal of Physics: Conference Series, 2608*(1), 012053. DOI: 10.1088/1742-6596/2608/1/012053

Yang, J., He, M., Zhang, X., Ning, Q., Chen, Y., & Mazinan, M. A.-S. Z. (2025). *Climate-Adaptive Energy Efficiency Modeling: A Generalized Additive Approach for Optimizing Building Performance Across Chinese Climate Zones*. https://doi.org/DOI: 10.21203/rs.3.rs-6152814/v1

Yassaie, R., & Brooks, L. (2025). Reassessing 'good' medical practice and the climate crisis. *Journal of Medical Ethics, 51*(6), 365–370. DOI: 10.1136/jme-2023-109713 PMID: 38871401

Zbyrad, B., Zaborniak, M., Kochmański, Ł., Jasik, K., Kluczyński, J., Budzik, G., & Turek, P. (2025). Evaluation of High-Temperature Sterilization Processes: Their Influence on the Mechanical Integrity of Additively Manufactured Polymeric Biomaterials. *Materials (Basel), 18*(6), 1356. DOI: 10.3390/ma18061356 PMID: 40141640

Zengyu, C., Luqi, W., Yuan, F., & Jianwei, Z. (2021). Research and Progress on Data Security Based on Medical Information System. *Proceedings of 2021 The 11th International Workshop on Computer Science and Engineering*, 1–5. https://doi.org/DOI: 10.18178/wcse.2021.06.001

Zhang, M., Shao, F., Zheng, R., Liu, M., & Ji, Z. (2023). An Efficient Encryption Scheme with Fully Hidden Access Policy for Medical Data. *Electronics (Basel), 12*(13), 2930. DOI: 10.3390/electronics12132930

Zhou, H., Wang, T., Zhou, F., Liu, Y., Zhao, W., Wang, X., Chen, H., & Cui, Y. (2019). Ambient Air Pollution and Daily Hospital Admissions for Respiratory Disease in Children in Guiyang, China. *Frontiers in Pediatrics, 7*. Advance online publication. DOI: 10.3389/fped.2019.00400 PMID: 31681705

Zlateva, P., Ivanov, M., & Terziev, A. (2024). Analyses of the energy efficiency enhancement in Bulgarian health care premises. *E3S Web of Conferences, 551*, 01002. https://doi.org/DOI: 10.1051/e3sconf/202455101002

Chapter 3
An Agentic Approach to Sustainable Environmental Monitoring Systems in Healthcare

Cristina Elena Turcu
Ştefan cel Mare University of Suceava, Romania

Corneliu Octavian Turcu
https://orcid.org/0000-0002-3134-8769
tefan cel Mare University of Suceava, Romania

ABSTRACT

This chapter explores the transformative role of agentic AI in sustainable environmental monitoring for healthcare. The need for this shift arises from the sector's considerable environmental footprint and the challenge of ensuring contaminant-free spaces vital for patient safety and preventing Healthcare-Associated Infections (HAIs). The chapter introduces the theoretical foundations, architecture, and capabilities of AI agents, highlighting their contribution to "smart healthcare". A conceptual multi-agent system is then proposed to integrate intelligent agents into sustainable monitoring. The model covers functional requirements such as real-time monitoring and predictive analysis, as well as non-functional ones like scalability, security, and adherence to sustainability principles. The discussion concludes by addressing key technical, ethical, and regulatory challenges that must be overcome to fully harness agentic AI's potential in building proactive, personalized, and environmentally sustainable healthcare ecosystems.

DOI: 10.4018/979-8-3373-5636-5.ch003

INTRODUCTION

The adverse impact of pollution and environmental change on health is now widely recognized (Landrigan et al., 2018; Watts et al., 2018), yet the health sector's own environmental impact has been less explored (Lenzen et al., 2020). Performance assessment in healthcare traditionally focuses on clinical outcomes and financial costs. However, providing healthcare services generates a wide range of air, water, and soil pollutants, with indirect and negative effects on health. Researchers estimate that healthcare is a major contributor to environmental degradation, generating between 4.4% and 5.2% of total global greenhouse-gas emissions (Pichler et al., 2019). Consequently, all stakeholders must be aware of these effects and assume the practical and ethical responsibility to integrate sustainability principles into performance evaluation and the management of healthcare organizations (Dolcini et al., 2025).

Healthcare - an inherently complex sector - faces significant challenges in delivering high-quality care under resource constraints (D. Sharma & Cotton, 2023; Holmér et al., 2023). For example, maintaining safe, contaminant-free environments in healthcare settings represents a significant, ongoing challenge for professionals. From operating rooms to blood banks and pharmacies, precise monitoring and control of parameters such as temperature, humidity, and air pressure are essential for patient safety and compliance with strict regulations (Montuori et al., 2024; Sehulster et al., 2003). Hospital environments - especially enclosed spaces frequently used by patients, staff, and visitors - can become both vectors for pathogen transmission and factors that affect clinical care quality (Tsang et al., 2024; Fonseca et al., 2022). For example, it is estimated that 1 in every 31 inpatients in United States (US) hospitals is expected to contract a Healthcare-Associated Infection (HAI). The US Centers for Disease Control and Prevention (CDC) reports nearly 2 million nosocomial infections and more than 90,000 deaths annually (Epicenters, 2024). According to the Agency for Healthcare Research and Quality, HAIs are the most common inpatient complications and rank among the top ten causes of death in the United States (Health Care-Associated Infections, n.d.). Globally, approximately 7% of inpatients in high-income countries and 10% in low- and middle-income countries acquire such infections (Danasekaran et al., 2014). Studies in high-income countries find that between 5% and 15% of inpatients develop HAI, while in intensive care units (ICUs), these infections can affect 9% to 37% of patients (Allegranzi et al., 2007; Vincent, 2003). In Europe, hospital-level HAI prevalence ranges from 4.6% to 9.3% (Haque et al., 2018).

Environmental monitoring contributes substantially to compliance with national and international hygiene and health-safety standards. Guidelines from organizations such as World Health Organization (WHO) and the CDC highlight the need for continuous surveillance of environmental parameters to prevent health risks. Non-compliance can lead to serious legal and administrative consequences, affecting institutional operations and patient trust.

Integrating environmental sensors (for temperature, air quality, humidity, noise) and biosensors (for heart rate, oxygen saturation, etc.) enables a proactive approach aligned with the "smart healthcare" paradigm: digital, continuous, personalized, and predictive (Turner, 2021). Rapid advances in digitalization and artificial intelligence (AI) create opportunities to develop autonomous, intelligent, and sustainable systems dedicated to environmental and health monitoring. In a context where healthcare systems face unprecedented pressures - from aging populations and workforce shortages to the impacts of climate change - the integration of intelligent agents represents an essential strategic direction for the sustainable digitalization of healthcare. These agents can process complex, heterogeneous data (physiological signals, environmental data), learn and adapt in real time, and generate personalized responses, suggestions, and alerts. In doing so, they can contribute not only to improved clinical efficiency but also to maintaining a balanced relationship between people, technology, and the environment.

But AI is a power-hungry technology (O'Donnell & Crownhart, 2025). Few reports quantify the scale of this appetite, how much it may grow, where the power will come from, and who will pay for it. Monitoring AI's energy and resource use is critical so that AI-based systems evolve responsibly and sustainably.

This chapter aims to present the potential of AI agents and agentic AI in transforming environmental monitoring in healthcare through their advanced capabilities for data collection, integration and predictive analysis. It also seeks to examine how intelligent agents can be integrated into sustainable environmental monitoring systems in healthcare.

Understanding the agent ecosystem is crucial for a holistic, sustainable approach to the development of agent-enabled systems in medicine. To achieve this goal, the first section addresses the theoretical foundations of AI agents and agentic artificial intelligence, their architecture, and core capabilities. We outline advantages and limitations, along with possible practical applications. Then, we present a conceptual model for integrating agents into a sustainable environmental monitoring system for healthcare. Addressing the inherent technical, ethical, and regulatory challenges is essential to unlocking the full potential of agents. The chapter ends with conclusions and future research directions.

BACKGROUND

Environmental monitoring in healthcare settings is essential for improving care quality, preventing infections, and facilitating patient recovery. Multiple studies suggest that real-time monitoring, combined with artificial intelligence, can significantly reduce carbon emissions in healthcare (Arya et al., 2024; Tseng & Lin, 2024). In the context of increasing pressure on healthcare sector and the need to provide personalized, safe, and energy-efficient care, modern environmental-monitoring systems have evolved considerably, integrating advanced technologies such as the Internet of Things (IoT), artificial intelligence (AI), edge computing, and intelligent wireless sensor networks (WSNs) (Fonseca et al., 2022; Sorouri et al., 2025).

The Internet Of Things And The Internet Of Medical Things

The Internet of Things (IoT) represents "the expansion of current Internet services to provide connectivity to each object of this world" (Noaman et al., 2022), enabling the development of a network of interconnected physical objects equipped with sensors and communication capabilities, able to collect, analyze, and send data over the Internet without direct human intervention (Hemalatha et al., 2022; Internet of Things (IoT), n.d.). IoT integrates embedded systems, wireless sensor networks, and AI to support real-time decision-making, turning ordinary spaces into smart ones, with diverse applications across domains such as transportation, industry, education, and healthcare.

IoT technology has been a disruptive innovation, bringing valuable contributions to healthcare. Its adoption has led to the development of innovative medical devices and new applications, such as patient presence monitoring, in-home emergency medical care, fall detection, and improved medical diagnosis. Thus, IoT has expanded into the Internet of Medical Things (IoMT). The Internet of Medical Things, also called Healthcare IoT, represents a paradigm shift in healthcare that combines the power of the internet and medical devices to improve patient care, increase efficiency, and support better health outcomes (Hemalatha et al., 2022; Khaled, 2022). By leveraging the power of interconnected medical devices, sensors, and advanced analytics - with a strong focus on security and privacy - IoMT enables remote patient monitoring, enhances patient engagement, streamlines healthcare delivery, and facilitates predictive analytics. (Rocha et al., 2024; Ozcelik et al., 2025). But in healthcare, sensors are used not only to directly monitor patients' physiological parameters, but also to monitor the environment surrounding the patient and medical equipment, especially within the context of smart health systems and IoMT, enabling continuous monitoring and context-aware clinical decision-making (Qadri et al., 2020; Senturk et al., 2022).

Artificial Intelligence, Agents, and Agentic AI

Artificial Intelligence is a continuously evolving field focused on developing systems capable of imitating human cognitive processes, such as learning, reasoning, and problem-solving (S. J. Russell & Norvig, 2021). Globally, AI has been adopted across various domains to increase efficiency and drive innovation - including manufacturing, transportation, agriculture, environmental management, healthcare, and education. Examples include image recognition, computer-assisted medical diagnosis, industrial process optimization, energy management, and predictive analytics in the financial sector (Holzinger et al., 2017). By automating processes, analyzing complex data, and enabling early risk detection, AI plays an important role in promoting sustainability and ecological resilience. In healthcare, AI supports clinical activity and improves environmental quality in healthcare settings (Esmaeilzadeh, 2024); predictive analytics helps manage patient flows and available resources more effectively (Lin et al., 2024). Artificial intelligence is proving to be an essential tool for analyzing the complex relationships between the healthcare domain and energy requirements, due to its efficiency in processing large amounts of data in a short time.

Researchers emphasize the need for an ethical and responsible approach to the development and use of AI technologies. Van Wynsberghe (2021) proposes the adoption of "Sustainable AI", re-shaping the entire AI lifecycle - from ideation, training, fine-tuning, and deployment to governance - toward ecological integrity and social justice. This approach transcends the mere application of AI for sustainable purposes, targeting the entire socio-technical AI system. Accordingly, two complementary dimensions are considered: *AI for sustainability and the sustainability of AI.* AI for sustainability focuses on applying AI to achieve sustainability goals (e.g., using AI for clean energy or resource management). The sustainability of AI - a less explored area - addresses the environmental impact of AI development and use, including carbon emissions and energy consumption associated with training and running AI models. This direction emphasizes using sustainable data sources, optimizing algorithms for energy efficiency, and deploying green infrastructure (e.g., data centers powered by renewable energy). (Tabbakh et al., 2024) extends the discussion by introducing the Green AI concept, which aims to optimize models to reduce energy consumption, develop and implement efficient algorithms and sustainable hardware, and build green data centers powered by renewable energy. Green AI aligns with global sustainability objectives and provides a practical framework for reducing AI's environmental footprint.

Achieving the full potential of Sustainable AI requires overcoming limitations identified in (van Wynsberghe, 2021). The authors emphasize the need for rigorous empirical validation of the ecological impact of different AI models and infrastructures to ground design decisions in concrete evidence. Interdisciplinary collaborations among engineers, ethicists, ecologists, and policymakers are essential for developing integrated and contextualized solutions. Furthermore, creating clear and applicable public policy guidelines would facilitate the widespread adoption of sustainable practices. Future research should explore emerging technologies, such as quantum computing, which promise a significant reduction in the energy footprint of AI. Last but not least, the scalability and accessibility of these practices must be prioritized to enable their adoption even in resource-constrained settings. It is imperative that researchers, developers, and decision-makers simultaneously address AI's potential to support sustainability and its environmental impact. Only by integrating both dimensions - AI for Sustainability and the Sustainability of AI - can we ensure responsible and durable technological development.

AI is growing and maturing day by day, with multiple applications across different domains. In recent months, *agentic AI* has been highlighted as a transformative paradigm for smarter healthcare systems, marking "the beginning of a new era in healthcare" (Farraher, 2025). Some authors argue that "we're entering a new era, where humans and agentic AI work side by side to redefine sustainability and energy impact together" (Collaborative Intelligence, 2025).

Analyses of global Google search trends indicates a notable increase in queries related to "AI Agents" and "Agentic AI" after ChatGPT's launch in November 2022 (Figure *1*).

Figure 1. Global Google search trends showing rising interest in "AI Agents" and "Agentic AI"

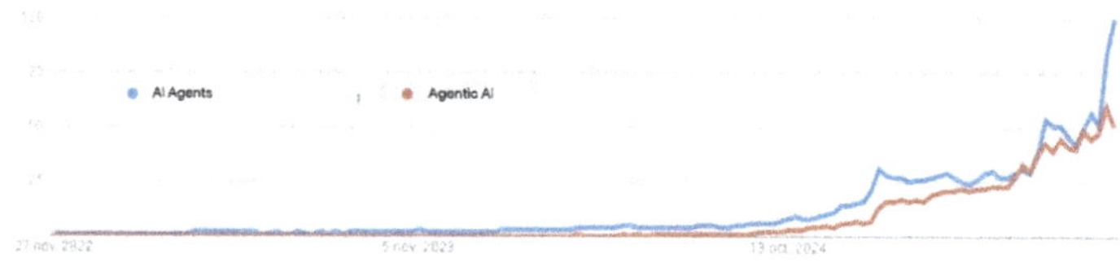

Multiple definitions for the term "agent" can be found in scientific literature. One of the most well-known definitions was provided by Russell and Norvig (S. Russell et al., 1995) - a fundamental definition widely used in academia to introduce the concept of an agent. According to (S. Russell et al., 1995), an agent is a system that perceives its environment through sensors and acts upon that environment through actuators. Another definition, from the perspective of software agents, focuses on their specific characteristics and is commonly found in scientific literature. According to (Wooldridge, 2002), an agent is an autonomous, proactive, reactive, and social software entity that operates in a complex environment to achieve specific goals.

With progress in deep learning and reinforcement learning, agent definitions have evolved to reflect enhanced capabilities. In this chapter, the term *AI agent* refers to an autonomous software entity that *perceives* (e.g., user queries, sensor data) and *acts* (e.g., API calls, messages, device commands) to fulfill specified goals - a goal-oriented system with continual learning that interacts with dynamic environments.

Although scientific literature includes various definitions - some technical, others unfortunately too vague - most agree on the following five essential traits of an agent:

1. **Autonomous execution** - performs tasks with minimal intervention.
2. **Goal-orientation** - works toward specific outcomes.
3. **Decision-making ability** - selects its own next step.
4. **Environmental awareness** - assesses context and responds accordingly.
5. **Tool use** - selects and applies tools, applications, or APIs as needed.

Agents are proactive - not merely reactive: they understand goals, plan steps, choose appropriate tools, and adapt as they proceed.

In healthcare, AI agents are reshaping care delivery, diagnosis, monitoring, operations management, and patient interaction. Unlike traditional software, these systems use advanced machine learning and natural language processing to perform tasks that previously relied on human judgment and reaction speed. Agents now play key roles in clinical reasoning, specialist assessment, and knowledge generation (Wang et al., 2025; Laymouna et al., 2024), evolving from automating administrative tasks to actively supporting complex clinical decision-making and optimizing end-to-end patient experience.

Over time, several types of agents have been developed in healthcare, including (K. Huang, 2025; Karunanayake, 2025):

- **Diagnostic agents** - improving diagnostic accuracy, workflow efficiency, and global accessibility.
- **Clinical decision-support agents** - analyzing electronic health records (EHR), imaging, and physiological signals; proposing likely diagnoses; prioritizing urgent cases; and recommending therapies.
- **Real-time monitoring/alert agents** - ingesting wearables/IoMT streams (Photoplethysmography - PPG, Electrocardiogram - ECG, temperature, air quality), detecting anomalies, triggering alerts, and recommending actions.
- **Virtual healthcare assistants/medical chatbots** - interacting with patients in natural language (natural-language triage, medication reminders, education), scheduling and reducing administrative burden.

- **Operational/RPA-like agents** - automating billing, medical coding, authorisations, document and report management, facilitating compliance and reducing human error.
- **Conversational therapeutic agents** - CBT-based interventions, anonymous support, and symptom monitoring, useful for triage and early intervention with appropriate clinical oversight.

Agent-development approaches increasingly integrate with IoT and the physical world - e.g., smart homes, offices, and cities where agents autonomously control devices. NVIDIA and GE HealthCare already collaborate on agentic robotic systems, where AI uses medical imaging to interact with the physical world (*NVIDIA and GE HealthCare Collaborate to Advance the Development of Autonomous Diagnostic Imaging With Physical AI*, n.d.). Within IoT/IoMT ecosystems, agents can acquire and process physiological and environmental data to support clinical decisions, generate real-time alerts, and optimize operations. This integration becomes essential in many applications, such as monitoring air quality in medical facilities, preventing nosocomial infections, and surveilling vulnerable patients in critical environments.

Although traditional AI agents represent substantial progress - especially by automating specialized tasks using reasoning tools - limitations remain, such as reduced scalability in complex, dynamic environments and limited collaboration capabilities. These limitations have led to the accelerated development of a more advanced paradigm: agentic artificial intelligence, concisely shortened to *agentic AI*. This new class of systems extends the functionality of traditional AI agents, enabling multiple intelligent entities to collaborate to achieve common objectives, facilitated by structured communication (Zhang et al., 2025; Miehling et al., 2025), shared memory (Xu et al., 2025; Riedl & De Cremer, 2025), dynamic task decomposition, and role allocation (Sapkota et al., 2025). According to (*Tech CEOs*, n.d.), "agentic AI systems are characterized by the ability to take actions that consistently contribute to achieving goals over an extended period, without behavior specified in advance". Gartner predicts that "by 2028, 15% of day-to-day work decisions will be made autonomously through agentic AI, up from 0% in 2024" (*Tech CEOs*, n.d.).

Agents are the building blocks of agentic AI systems. Unlike classic agents that merely respond to commands, an agentic AI system has a clearly defined objective and makes autonomous decisions to achieve it - analyzing possible paths and learning from experience. Agents can process huge volumes of data and perform research activities at a level beyond human capability. With the ability to act without direct human intervention, discover new information, and adapt over time, agents can become valuable collaborators across domains. Agentic AI systems extend this concept by integrating multiple specialized agents and relevant tools into a coherent, intelligent system (Chen, n.d.). Agentic AI plays an essential role in improving sustainability, optimizing resource management and enhancing quality of life for the population (Singh, 2025). Researchers view agentic AI as a transformative approach in medicine - beyond data analysis to collaborative, autonomous solutions - where specialized agents communicate and cooperate to manage complex tasks, improving efficiency and patient safety. For example, agentic AI offers collaborative support for medical decisions: rather than processing all information centrally, agentic AI systems distribute medical reasoning across specialized agents, each with a well-defined role.

This evolution of the AI landscape in recent years - from reactive tools to proactive collaborators - drives a paradigm shift that must be well understood to be applied. It also underscores the continuing evolution of the human–machine partnership, in which *agents should be a tool, not a replacement.* Implementing "human-in-the-loop" mechanisms is essential to ensure AI augments - not substitutes for - human judgment in critical scenarios.

By virtue of their advantages, adopting agentic AI in healthcare enables a transformation from a reactive model into a dynamic, self-learning ecosystem. Thus, integrating agentic AI represents a revolutionary leap in medical technology that narrows the gap between reactive and proactive models of healthcare. Agentic AI can learn and adapt continuously, becoming indispensable in addressing the ever-changing nature of the medical field (Hinostroza Fuentes et al., 2025).

Although artificial intelligence agents are more powerful, they also introduce new challenges related to orchestration, tool integration, and security; additionally, researchers emphasize the need for environmental responsibility. AI in general can be resource-intensive; training a single advanced model can consume as much energy as several households use in a year. As more autonomous agents are deployed, energy consumption increases. The environmental impact of AI systems is a major concern for researchers; an increasing number of studies in recent years attempt to quantify the energy, carbon and water costs associated with training and deploying large language models (LLMs) as well as running inference. Unlike training, which is done once or periodically, inference occurs daily at scale. Recent estimates suggest that inference may account for up to 90% of a model's total lifecycle energy consumption (O'Donnell & Crownhart, 2025). In this context, *Green Agentic AI* becomes critical to ensure that innovation in artificial intelligence and environmental responsibility support sustainable development. Green Agentic AI is an emerging framework for designing intelligent systems that balance performance with environmental responsibility. It sits at the intersection of agentic AI and sustainability, focusing on integrating sustainability considerations into independently operating AI agents. This autonomy implies a responsibility on the part of producers to guarantee that systems are not only intelligent and efficient but also compliant with sustainability principles. For example, GreenMetrica has developed an agent framework specialized in designing and building AI agents for sustainability-data tasks. This framework integrates with business functions and enables the building, testing, and iteration of agents and agentic systems (*AI Agents for Sustainable Enterprise*, n.d.). Next, we present a short review of environmental monitoring solutions in healthcare.

Environmental-Monitoring Solutions in Healthcare

Sustainable environmental monitoring systems are developed to track, evaluate and improve ecological performance within healthcare facilities. These systems cover a wide range of areas, including energy consumption, waste management, water consumption, greenhouse gas emissions and space sustainability. The aim is to minimize the ecological footprint of healthcare operations while maintaining - or even improving - clinical outcomes (Dolcini et al., 2025).

Air quality has a major impact on public health and the environment (Garcia et al., 2025). Over time, many studies link poor air quality to increased morbidity and mortality, with large urban populations exposed to air that does not meet health standards (Kelly & Fussell, 2015). This problem is amplified by climate change, which affects levels of key pollutants such as ozone, carbon dioxide (CO_2), nitrogen dioxide (NO_2), sulphur dioxide (SO_2), all with serious health implications (Hassan et al., 2015). Various studies have shown that air pollution is responsible for respiratory problems, including bronchitis, pneumonia, emphysema, asthma and lung cancer (Sunyer et al., 2006; Sarnat & Holguin, 2007; Mattjus, 2020; Buonanno et al., 2017; Kravchenko et al., 2014). Several papers have identified significant issues with indoor air quality in medical facilities, the most frequent being non-compliance with WHO guidelines on indoor air quality - even in sensitive clinical contexts - potentially compromising the safety of patients and staff (Fonseca et al., 2022; Sorouri et al., 2025). To mitigate the adverse effects of poor indoor air quality on human health, various AI-, big-data- and IoT-based applications for indoor air-quality monitoring and control have been implemented (Fonseca et al., 2022; Sorouri et al., 2025).

Distributed sensors and IoT networks enable continuous, real-time acquisition of environmental data (air quality, humidity, pollutants) with a direct impact on population health. A key pillar of modern environmental monitoring systems is the integration of medical IoT. Connected devices enable continuous collection of data on environmental parameters such as temperature, humidity, CO_2 levels, air quality, and noise levels, which directly influence the condition of patients, particularly the vulnerable (Zhou et al., 2023). IoT enables automated reactions to environmental changes. For example, in intensive care rooms, systems can automatically adjust ventilation or temperature to maintain optimal recovery conditions (Mao et al., 2023). Continuous monitoring of environmental parameters can prevent symptom exacerbation in patients with chronic respiratory diseases. Some researchers developed an IoT prototype that combines air monitoring with air purification (Anitha &

Kumar, 2023). Over time, many scientific papers have presented IoT-based solutions for real-time monitoring of health and environment (Sreejith et al., 2025; Jo et al., 2020) that are secure and energy-efficient (M. Sharma et al., 2019). Other studies and projects have also integrated IoT sensors and AI algorithms to monitor air quality in real time, offering personalised exposure assessments and health recommendations (Omidvarborna et al., 2021; Tanveer et al., 2024).

AI has been successfully integrated into indoor and outdoor environmental-monitoring systems, bringing gains in efficiency, accuracy, and responsiveness (Alotaibi & Nassif, 2024; Wani et al., 2024; Islam et al., 2020). In healthcare, AI is used to develop intelligent systems capable of monitoring environmental parameters and risk factors that influence patient status. Numerous studies have shown that AI technologies improve environmental monitoring by enabling better understanding, prediction and mitigation of environmental risks (Olawade, Wada, Ige, et al., 2024). For example, Fonseca et al. (2022) propose monitoring air quality in medical facilities by integrating IoT sensors for real-time identification of pollutants, spores, or harmful particles. Predictive analysis of correlations between environmental conditions and the progression of certain chronic or infectious diseases supports rapid clinical decisions (Sorouri et al., 2025). Thus, AI's ability to provide accurate predictions and real-time monitoring increases the efficiency and effectiveness of environmental management practices. Garcia et al. (2025) performed a systematic analysis of 147 studies exploring the use of IoT and AI in air-quality monitoring, proposing a taxonomy for AI techniques applied in five areas: data imputation, sensor calibration, anomaly detection, air-quality index estimation and short-term forecasting, with case studies in urban and industrial settings.

Much of today's hospital infrastructure reflects design paradigms from years past, making it inadequate to fully meet contemporary requirements (Karrouk et al., 2025). Healthcare institutions face increased pressure to maintain high standards of care amid significant challenges related to operational efficiency, competitiveness and sustainability. Patient expectations have also evolved considerably, requiring continuous adaptation. In this context, digital transformation has become a strategic imperative for modernizing hospitals. The emergence of smart-building technologies offers innovative solutions to optimize workflows, increase operational flexibility and control costs. By integrating and analyzing data from IT, operational and medical systems, hospitals can streamline processes, maximize productivity and improve the patient experience (Maleki Varnosfaderani & Forouzanfar, 2024; Dangi et al., 2025; Garg et al., 2025; Bekbolatova et al., 2024; Karrouk et al., 2025). Numerous scientific papers have examined the opportunities offered by emerging technologies such as AI for sustainable healthcare development, while analyzing the major challenges global institutions face in delivering high-quality services (Tan et al., 2025). Machine learning (ML) and AI play a key role in interpreting large volumes of sensor data. AI models can identify patterns, anticipate risks and trigger automated alerts for clinical staff. A notable example is the use of convolutional neural networks (CNNs) to analyze thermal images in hospital rooms to detect early fever or heat stress (Lu et al., 2023). In addition, machine-learning algorithms are used to correlate environmental conditions with patient trajectories, contributing to personalized medicine. More recently, autonomous agents based on large generative models (LLMs) - so-called *GenAI agents* - are being adopted to translate complex data into clear, intelligible explanations for clinicians and patients (Dwivedi et al., 2023).

Environmental monitoring is now integral to the "smart hospital" concept - an interconnected digital ecosystem. Modern platforms integrate sensor feeds with EHRs, clinical-management apps, and alerting systems. In addition, the use of augmented reality (AR) technologies and AI-supported voice interfaces provides clinical staff with real-time access to contextual information about patients and the environment (Cao et al., 2023).

The concept of an *AI hospital* (agent hospital or virtual hospital) has emerged as a model in which multi-agent systems simulate real workflows in hospitals and laboratories. China's *Agentic Hospital* represents a revolutionary initiative redefining how AI can be applied in healthcare (Li et al., 2024; O'Sullivan-Dale, 2024). The project was created to provide a scalable, efficient platform for training future generations of AI physicians, with the potential to transform healthcare globally. Agent Hospital is a simulation in which patients, nurses and physicians are autonomous agents powered by large language models. The system simulates the entire disease-care cycle - from onset, triage and registration through consultation, investigations, diagnosis, prescribing and administration of medicines, convalescence and post-discharge follow-up. Forty-two AI doctors operate across 21 medical departments, including paediatrics, cardiology and neurology. These AI agents are not simple chatbots; they are entities capable of simulating the entire patient journey - from consultation, diagnosis and treatment to recovery and follow-up. At the core of the system is MedAgent-Zero, an AI framework developed by the Institute for AI Industry Research (AIR) at Tsinghua University. This agent self-optimizes through continuous interactions with virtual patients, without requiring real data, enabling rapid and safe learning, including in rare or complex cases (Li et al., 2024). Despite growing research interest in developing AI-based hospitals, existing studies remain fragmented and lack a unified framework that systematically connects different AI hospital simulations to real-world scenarios (Yao & Yu, 2025).

Realizing AI's full potential in health faces obstacles such as the limited AI expertise in the environmental sector; challenges related to data access, control, and privacy. It is also important to recognize potential drawbacks associated with implementing AI technologies. A significant concern is the substantial energy burden of data centers, leading to higher greenhouse gas emissions (Olawade, Wada,

David-Olawade, et al., 2024). Globally, data centers consumed approximately 1.5% of electricity in 2024. A hyperscale data center specialized for AI can have a capacity of 100 MW or more - equivalent of the annual consumption of around 100,000 households. AI-focused data centers are increasing in size to host ever larger models and to cope with growing demand for AI services (Energy and AI, n.d.). Thus, the environmental impact of AI is dual: although it has the potential to significantly reduce greenhouse gas emissions globally, its implementation and use may also increase them (Tseng & Lin, 2024). Despite these challenges, the prospects for integrating AI into environmental monitoring are promising: advances in AI algorithms, data-collection techniques, and computing power are expected to further improve accuracy and efficiency in monitoring and managing environmental issues, contributing significantly to environmental protection, public health, and sustainable development (Olawade, Wada, Ige, et al., 2024).

In the following, an agentic approach to sustainable environmental monitoring in healthcare is considered.

A MULTI-AGENT SYSTEM FOR ENVIRONMENTAL MONITORING IN HEALTHCARE

Agentic artificial intelligence should not be viewed as a simple tool for automating healthcare processes. It represents a fundamental technological leap towards creating adaptive, self-improving systems that operate under ethical principles, with patient-care optimization as the central objective (Hinostroza Fuentes et al., 2025). In today's increasingly complex healthcare services, environmental monitoring within medical facilities will become an essential component of modern clinical practice and institutional management for delivering high-quality care. Monitoring critical environmental parameters - such as temperature, humidity, pressure, and air quality - is fundamental in healthcare for preventing infections and ensuring patient comfort and recovery. Through autonomy, proactivity, adaptive reasoning, and data integration, agentic AI supports the transformation of reactive environmental monitoring into proactive and predictive environmental management. This enables predictive maintenance, optimized resource allocation, and automated compliance, leading to improved clinical outcomes and significant operational efficiency.

System Requirements

As healthcare requirements become increasingly complex, integrating agentic AI into environmental monitoring systems offers a transformative opportunity that demands a holistic and sustainable approach.

As a case study, we consider a sustainable, agentic-AI-based environmental monitoring system in healthcare whose aim is to ensure optimal care environments while maintaining operational efficiency and sustainability. Integrating agentic intelligence into such a system requires a clear vision of the functional requirements - what the system should do - and the non-functional requirements - how the system should behave. Autonomous intelligent agents must not only be capable of making independent decisions; they must also be reliable, explainable, secure, and energy-efficient to support personalized, precise, and proactive care. The functional and non-functional requirements defined below aim to ensure efficiency, ethics, safety and scalability.

Functional Requirements

Real-time monitoring

- Collect real-time data from environmental sensors (temperature, humidity, air quality, noise, light intensity, toxic gases, radiation, etc.), biomedical sensors (e.g., heart rate), and IoT devices across medical infrastructure, with zone-specific monitoring.
- Provide long-term data storage.

Interoperability

- Support multi-directional communication with IoT ecosystems and healthcare information systems, ensuring secure data exchange.

Data processing and analytics

- Preprocess data (cleaning, validation, normalization, aggregation).
- Fuse heterogeneous sources for complete contextual views.
- Implement anomaly detection and environmental-pattern mining.
- Generate predictions for environmental quality and associated health risks.

Reasoning and decision-making

- Interpret data to assess environmental state and potential health impact.
- Identify health risks linked to environmental factors (e.g., higher risk for respiratory patients).
- Formulate action plans and recommendations (e.g., optimizing environmental conditions).
- Make autonomous, adaptive decisions.
- Orchestrate and coordinate other agents/modules to complete tasks.
- Interact proactively with staff (explanations and preventive suggestions).

Content generation and actions

- Generate automatic alerts/notifications (SMS, email, push) for relevant users (clinical and administrative staff).
- Produce tailored, concise reports for diverse stakeholders.
- Communicate with other systems (IoT ecosystems, health-IT platforms, public-health systems, emergency dispatch).
- Offer personalized health recommendations based on individual environmental exposure.

User interface and visualization

- Provide an interactive web dashboard for real-time environmental data, predictions, and alerts; responsive across device types.
- Enable user queries and exploration of historical data.

Device management

- Support adding, updating, or replacing sensors/devices without significant downtime.

Automated detection and prevention

- Detect anomalies and generate automatic alerts.
- Trigger alarms when critical thresholds are exceeded.

Non-Functional Requirements

Reliability and high availability

- 24/7 operation with minimal downtime; data integrity and consistency.
- Fault tolerance with automatic recovery from component failures.

Scalability

- Scale to growing devices, data volumes, and users without performance degradation.
- modular, horizontally scalable HW/SW designs for non-disruptive component addition/replacement.

Security and data protection

- Protect systems and sensitive patient data from unauthorized access, breaches, and cyberattacks.
- Encrypt medical data; restrict access to authorized users.
- Comply with General Data Protection Regulation/Health Insurance Portability and Accountability Act (GDPR/HIPAA); ensure full auditability of agent decisions.

Real-time performance

- Real-time processing for critical parameters.
- Generate critical decisions within hundreds of milliseconds of a critical event.

Explainability

- Justify agent decisions to users; ensure data traceability.

Portability and interoperability

- Support cloud/edge/mobile deployments and standard protocols (e.g., HL7, MQTT).

Usability

- Easy to learn and efficient to use; minimize user errors; use consistent medical terminology.
- Accessible voice/graphical interfaces for non-technical users.
- Conform to WCAG 2.2 for web interfaces.

Maintenance and support

- Provide complete documentation for admins and users.
- Enable remote diagnostics, maintenance, and troubleshooting.

Sustainability

- Include energy-efficient hardware.
- Provide dynamic, demand-aware energy management.
- Optimize compute via AI for efficient resource use.
- Track and report carbon footprint.

REGULATORY AND STANDARDS COMPLIANCE

- Comply with healthcare standards and data-protection regulations.

A robust environmental-monitoring system enables hospitals to track critical parameters across departments, ensuring users receive relevant data and alerts aligned with their responsibilities - supporting compliance, risk reduction, and operational efficiency across the medical institution. To achieve these objectives, we propose a holistic approach to integrating agents within the dynamic medical environment. The ability of agents to perceive, reason, plan and act autonomously enables real-time adaptation and proactive interventions - essential for building truly sustainable and resilient monitoring systems capable of anticipating and even mitigating problems, not merely signaling them.

We therefore propose an agent-based system for environmental monitoring in healthcare, covering aspects from sensor integration and advanced data analytics to the optimization of operational workflows. The synergy between GenAI and intelligent agents can be successfully harnessed in developing sustainable monitoring systems. The intrinsic ability of intelligent agents to act autonomously and learn from their environment complements GenAI's capacity to generate new information, formulate hypotheses and create predictive models. This combination goes beyond simple data processing, enabling systems not only to react to change but also to anticipate future states and generate optimal responses. Thus, truly adaptable and proactive monitoring systems can be achieved, directly contributing to sustainability by optimizing resource use and improving outcomes. Below, we present a general model for adopting agents in sustainable environmental monitoring (*Figure 2*).

Figure 2. The model of multi-agent system

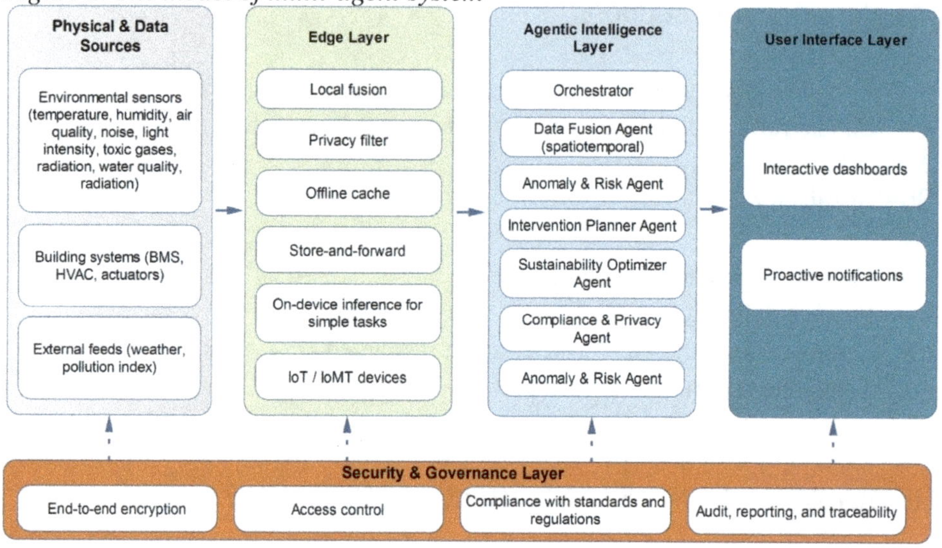

1. Physical & Data Sources Layer

This layer - comprising environmental sensors (IoT) and building-management systems (BMS/HVAC) - forms the foundation of the system. Including a wide range of sensors, from air quality to radiation, demonstrates a holistic approach to environmental monitoring. Integration with external data sources such as weather and pollution indices is crucial, providing the context needed for informed decisions.

2. Edge Layer

This layer adds a critical level of intelligence at the network edge. Capabilities such as privacy filtering, offline storage (store-and-forward) and local inference are essential. Pre-processing data at the edge reduces the volume transmitted centrally, lowering latency and bandwidth consumption. By filtering sensitive data locally, the edge layer reduces the risk of exposing confidential information, meeting privacy standards. Store-and-forward ensures the system continues to function during network interruptions by temporarily storing data and transmitting it later.

3. Agentic Intelligence Layer

This layer forms the core of the system, where its intelligence emerges. It employs a multi-agent architecture, with each agent assigned a specialized role, promoting both modularity and scalability.

- **Orchestrator.** Plans agent actions and evaluates performance to ensure optimal decisions.
- **Data-Fusion Agent.** Integrates spatiotemporal data from diverse sources to obtain a complete, contextualized environmental picture.
- **Anomaly & Risk Agent.** Rapidly detects potential problems, from dangerous CO_2 levels to HVAC faults, enabling prompt intervention.
- **Intervention Planner.** Translates detected anomalies into concrete actions, e.g., activating ventilation.
- **Sustainability Optimizer.** Ensures operations are efficient in terms of energy and resources, reducing the environmental footprint.
- **Compliance & Privacy Agent.** Ensures adherence to regulations such as HIPAA and GDPR - mandatory in the medical domain.
- **Explainability (XAI) Agent.** Provides transparency by explaining system decisions - vital for trust and regulatory requirements - allowing clinical staff to understand and validate system actions.

4. Security & Governance Layer

Placing security and governance in a dedicated layer underscores their importance. End-to-end encryption and access control are fundamental to protecting sensitive patient data. Audit and traceability ensure accountability and allow investigation of unexpected events - essential to defend system decisions before regulators or in litigation.

5. User Interface Layer

Through interactive dashboards and proactive notifications, this layer enables staff to interact efficiently with the system, providing a clear view of environmental status and actions taken by AI agents.

The integration of distributed sensors with IoT/IoMT networks enables the continuous, real-time acquisition of environmental parameters (e.g., air quality, humidity, pollutant levels) alongside patient-specific physiological data, both of which directly impact health outcomes. Agentic AI manages and integrates these data to anticipate environment-related health risks and to coordinate adaptive and personalized interventions, such as triggering alerts. Integrating agents into the system is important for ensuring easy scalability, flexible adaptation to infrastructure changes, parallel handling of large volumes of multi-source data, and proactive decision-making. The Orchestrator Agent governs the overall operation of the system, managing agent lifecycles, allocating computational resources, coordinating inter-agent communication, and maintaining global system state. It can dynamically instantiate or shutdown agents based on contextual demands. Individual agents are capable of autonomous operation, inter-agent collaboration, and adaptive learning from environmental and patient-derived data streams. These capabilities enable them to generate context-aware insights and initiate proactive responses tailored to specific scenarios. Through integration with IoMT systems and medical sensors, agents enable advanced automation of environmental monitoring and health-related processes. Their ability to process multidimensional data (e.g., time and space dimensions) supports real-time decision-making across diverse environmental contexts. For instance, the system can autonomously issue alerts in response to abnormal environmental parameter fluctuations and assist in the dynamic optimization of medical resource distribution. Incorporating large language model (LLM) agents further enhances system interaction by enabling natural language understanding and generation. This allows seamless integration into patient–staff–environment communication loops, improving usability and interpretability. A dedicated user interface supports proactive, real-time notifications (e.g., via SMS, email), ensuring timely user engagement. Additional agents can be added as needed to provide further functionality. Using multiple specialized agents in a dynamic environment such as healthcare can ensure greater flexibility and scalability, enabling more efficient resource allocation, parallel processing and robust problem-solving capacity for complex, domain-specific challenges.

MODEL COMPLIANCE WITH REQUIREMENTS

The proposed model satisfies the functional and non-functional requirements:

Functional Requirements

1. Real-Time Monitoring

- **Physical & Data Sources:** Provides the raw data from environmental sensors and IoT/IoMT devices to the Edge Layer.
- **Edge Layer:** Collects data from environmental, biomedical, and IoT devices. The offline cache and store-and-forward components ensure data isn't lost during network disruptions.
- **Agentic Intelligence Layer:** The *Data Fusion Agent* consolidates data for a comprehensive view. The *Sustainability Optimizer Agent* and *Intervention Planner Agent* monitor specific areas for optimization.
- **User Interface Layer:** Interactive dashboards.
- **Security & Governance Layer:** Audit, reporting, and traceability (for retained data).

2. Interoperability

- **Physical & Data Sources:** Integrates external feeds like weather and pollution indexes.
- **Edge Layer: IoT/IoMT devices** are the primary entry point for multi-directional communication. Ensures local fusion.
- **Agentic Intelligence Layer:** The *Orchestrator* coordinates communication and data exchange with external systems. *Compliance & Privacy Agent* is involved.
- **Security & Governance Layer:** Ensures secure data exchange through end-to-end encryption and access control. Compliance with standards/regulations.

3. Data Processing and Analysis

- **Physical & Data Sources:** Provides raw data (environmental sensors; BMS/HVAC; external feeds) for processing.
- **Edge Layer:** Performs on-device inference for simple tasks (pre-processing at edge), privacy filter and local fusion.
- **Agentic Intelligence Layer:** The *Data Fusion Agent* handles spatiotemporal data fusion. The *Anomaly & Risk Agent* implements algorithms for anomaly detection and pattern identification. *Sustainability Optimizer Agent* analyzes to develop predictive models. The *Orchestrator* manages data flow. *Compliance & Privacy Agent* assures governance over processing.
- **User Interface Layer:** Dashboards for analytics views.

- **Security & Governance Layer:** Ensures secure data. Compliance with standards/regulations.

4. Reasoning and Decision-Making

- **Edge Layer:** Performs on-device inference for simple tasks (simple local adaptations).
- **Agentic Intelligence Layer:** The *Orchestrator* is the core of this function, interpreting data, evaluating environmental states, and coordinating other agents. The *Intervention Planner Agent* formulates action plans and recommendations. The *Anomaly & Risk Agent* identifies specific risks. The *Explanation (XAI) Agent* ensures proactive, explanatory interactions with staff. *Sustainability Optimizer Agent* develops predictive models. *Compliance & Privacy Agen*t is involved in decision-making.
- **User Interface Layer:** Proactive notifications; UI messages with explanations.
- **Security & Governance Layer:** Access control (for actions); Audit/traceability (record decisions).

5. Content Generation and Actions

- **Agentic Intelligence Layer:** The *Intervention Planner Agent* and *Orchestrator* trigger actions, generate alerts and notifications. The *Explanation (XAI) Agent* and the *Intervention Planner Agent* create personalized recommendations and reports. *Data Fusion Agent* creates context; *Sustainability Optimizer Agent* makes recommendations.
- **User Interface Layer:** Proactive notifications (SMS/email) and interactive dashboards (for report delivery) are the direct output of this requirement.
- **Security & Governance Layer:** performs end-to-end encryption, access control, audit, reporting, and traceability; ensures that generated content is compliant.

6. User Interface and Visualization

- **User Interface Layer:** The interactive dashboards and proactive notifications directly address this requirement, providing real-time data visualization and historical data exploration.
- **Security & Governance Layer:** Access control (for actions); Audit, reporting and traceability (historical data access).

7. Device Management

- **Physical & Data Sources:** This layer is the source of the devices being managed, environmental sensors, BMS/HVAC.
- **Edge Layer:** The edge layer's design allows for adding, updating, or replacing sensors and devices without major disruptions.
- **Agentic Intelligence Layer:** *Orchestrator* coordinates onboarding flows; *Compliance & Privacy Agent* (policy for devices).
- **Security & Governance Layer:** Access control; Audit/traceability (asset changes).

8. Automatic Detection and Prevention

- **Edge Layer:** On-device inference can perform preliminary anomaly detection for faster response times; store-and-forward.
- **Agentic Intelligence Layer:** The *Anomaly & Risk Agent* is specifically designed to identify data anomalies and trigger alerts. The *Intervention Planner Agent* generates automated alarms based on critical thresholds. The *Orchestrator* is coordinating the agents.
- **User Interface Layer:** Proactive notifications display these alerts and alarms.

Non-Functional Requirements

9. High Reliability and Availability

- **Physical & Data Sources:** Redundant sensors/feeds as applicable.
- **Edge Layer:** The offline cache and store-and-forward capabilities ensure data integrity and system resilience against temporary disconnections.
- **Agentic Intelligence Layer:** The *Orchestrator*'s critical function is to manage and coordinate system components, enabling self-healing and error tolerance.
- **Security & Governance Layer:** Audit and traceability assure consistency checks.

10. Scalability

- **Physical & Data Sources:** Distributed sensors; BMS/HVAC across zones.
- **Edge Layer:** A distributed network of IoT/IoMT devices at the edge allows horizontal scaling.

- **Agentic Intelligence Layer:** Agents are separable by role. The modular, agent-based design ensures that new agents or modules can be added to handle increased data and user load.
- **Security & Governance Layer:** A scalable security model with robust access control is essential for managing a growing number of devices and users.
- **User Interface Layer:** Dashboards scale by role.

11. Security and Data Protection

- **Edge Layer:** The privacy filter is a critical component for initial data protection.
- **Agentic Intelligence Layer:** *Compliance & Privacy Agent* assures policy enforcement.
- **Security & Governance Layer:** This layer is purpose-built for this requirement, implementing end-to-end encryption, robust access control, and ensuring compliance with standards and regulations (e.g., GDPR/HIPAA). It also provides audit, reporting, and traceability.

12. Real-Time Performance

- **Edge Layer:** On-device inference and local fusion enable rapid processing of critical parameters.
- **Agentic Intelligence Layer:** The *Orchestrator, Anomaly & Risk Agent* and *Intervention Planner Agent* must be highly efficient to generate critical decisions within a few hundred milliseconds.
- **User Interface Layer:** Proactive notifications.

13. Explainability

- **Agentic Intelligence Layer:** The *Explanation (XAI) Agent* is the core component for justifying and explaining agent decisions to users.
- **Security & Governance Layer:** Audit, reporting, and traceability provide the necessary trail to ensure data and decision traceability.
- **User Interface Layer:** Provide dashboards for explanations.

14. Portability and Interoperability

- **Physical & Data Sources:** Provides raw data from environmental sensors and external feeds, standards-based.

- **Edge Layer:** The use of IoT/IoMT devices and standard protocols allows for compatibility with various infrastructures.
- **Agentic Intelligence Layer:** The agentic design and *Orchestrator* facilitate integration with different systems and data formats (e.g., HL7, MQTT). *Data Fusion Agent* processes heterogeneous inputs.
- **User Interface Layer:** Dashboards responsive across devices.
- **Security & Governance Layer:** Compliance with standards/regulations.

15. Usability

- **Agentic Intelligence Layer:** The *Explanation (XAI) Agent* clarifies concepts for non-technical users.
- **User Interface Layer:** The interactive dashboards are designed to be intuitive and accessible to a wide range of users, minimizing errors and ensuring consistent terminology. Enables proactive notifications, WCAG-conformant UI.

16. Maintenance and Support

- **Edge Layer:** Enables remote management of IoT/IoMT devices, supports operations such as offline cache/store-and-forward.
- **Agentic Intelligence Layer:** The *Orchestrator* assists workflows; *XAI Agent* enables human-readable summaries.
- **User Interface Layer:** Dashboards for admin & support views.
- **Security & Governance Layer:** Audit and reporting enable operational logs for troubleshooting.

17. Sustainability

- **Physical & Data Sources:** Utilizing energy-efficient hardware from the start contributes to this requirement.
- **Edge Layer:** Performs on-device inference for efficient computing at edge.
- **Agentic Intelligence Layer:** The *Sustainability Optimizer Agent* is specifically designed to manage dynamic energy use and optimize computational resources. It can also track and report on the carbon footprint. *Data Fusion Agent* and *Orchestrator* are also involved.
- **User Interface Layer:** Dashboards for sustainability views.
- **Security & Governance Layer:** Audit and reporting carbon footprint traces.

18. Regulatory and Compliance Requirements

- **Agentic Intelligence Layer:** The *Compliance & Privacy Agent* works within the agentic system to ensure all actions and data handling adhere to regulations.
- **Security & Governance Layer:** This layer is a cornerstone for meeting this requirement, ensuring compliance with standards and regulations and protecting patient data. Ensures audit/traceability, access control, end-to-end encryption.

In the design of this model, particular attention was devoted to integrating sustainability principles. Several key considerations can be emphasized:

- Modular design, enabling easy upgrades and replacements of components without affecting the entire system, thereby extending its operational lifespan.
- Scalability, as the system's architecture allows efficient scaling, facilitating adoption in diverse environments of varying complexity and adaptation to specific budgetary constraints.
- Energy efficiency, ensured through the optimization of algorithms and hardware infrastructure to reduce energy consumption. This includes the implementation of adaptive logic tailored to specific operating conditions, such as reducing or shutting down the activity of certain components depending on requirements.

Such a comprehensive approach enables the system to operate as an intelligent and proactive entity, capable of addressing the multifaceted challenges of environmental monitoring in healthcare, while making a significant contribution to sustainability objectives.

The proposed model offers a range of advantages, including:

- **Enhanced data collection and analysis**: the agentic AI can autonomously gather and interpret large volumes of environmental data, leading to more comprehensive monitoring.
- **Real-time responsiveness**: enables immediate detection of and reaction to environmental changes or hazards, thereby improving medical care.
- **Improved accuracy and precision**: reduces human error in environmental assessments, ensuring more reliable data to support evidence-based decision-making.

- **Scalability and coverage**: can be efficiently scaled to monitor extensive areas and diverse environmental parameters, in some cases without significantly increasing resource requirements.
- **Continuous operation**: capable of functioning 24/7, providing constant environmental surveillance without the limitations of human fatigue.
- **Proactive intervention**: facilitates early warning systems and preventive measures to mitigate environmental threats impacting health.
- **Cost efficiency**: automation of monitoring tasks may reduce labor and long-term operational expenses.
- **Decision-making support**: provides healthcare providers and policymakers with actionable insights derived from reliable environmental data.
- **Adaptability and learning**: able to improve monitoring strategies over time through machine learning, remaining effective under changing conditions.

CHALLENGES AND LIMITS OF AGENT ADOPTION

As research in the field of agents and agentic AI continues to advance, a significant expansion of these systems' capabilities is anticipated, which will foster their widespread adoption (Moritz et al., 2025). However, the integration of agentic AI into environmental monitoring systems in healthcare, while promising, also entails a series of emerging and complex challenges that extend beyond purely technical aspects into ethical, social, economic, and governance dimensions. Outlined below are key obstacles that must be addressed to responsibly unlock the full potential of agentic artificial intelligence, ensuring both its long-term acceptance and sustainable integration.

Environmental and patient monitoring systems generate vast volumes of data, often heterogeneous (text, numerical values, images, spatial and temporal data). Ensuring data quality (accuracy, completeness, consistency), efficient preprocessing, and the integration of data from multiple sources (sensors, medical records, public databases) represent major challenges. Moreover, it should be noted that the existing infrastructure for environmental monitoring in healthcare is frequently fragmented. The integration of AI agents into such legacy or disparate systems - while ensuring data and workflow interoperability, consistent performance across diverse environments, and sustainable long-term maintenance - can be both complex and costly.

Ensuring robustness, reliability, transparency, and explainability of AI agents in medical applications is essential for both patient safety and user trust. The autonomy of AI systems must be carefully balanced with mechanisms for validation and human oversight, through a "human-in-the-loop" approach, in order to prevent erroneous or unethical decisions in critical situations (Alotaibi & Nassif, 2024). The deployment of such agents also raises ethical dilemmas regarding autonomy and accountability. Furthermore, there is a risk of excessive dependence on AI, which may reduce human oversight. It should also be noted that their use may lead to a potential reduction in employment opportunities for human healthcare staff.

Healthcare information systems manage sensitive and personal patient data, which must be safeguarded from unauthorized access and misuse. Data security and confidentiality represent major concerns in the development of such systems, requiring the implementation of rigorous privacy and security measures to reduce risks and ensure compliance with relevant regulations. Frameworks such as HIPAA (Health Insurance Portability and Accountability Act) in the United States and GDPR (General Data Protection Regulation) in the European Union impose strict obligations on organizations to appropriately manage, store, and protect users' personal data. Yet, in some regions, regulatory frameworks governing the use of agentic AI remain insufficient, creating risks related to accountability, confidentiality, and security. Furthermore, AI systems must align with sustainability policies and the Sustainable Development Goals (SDGs), avoiding technological solutions that, while efficient in the short term, may have negative impacts on the environment or social equity (Gohr et al., 2025; van Wynsberghe, 2021).

One of the greatest challenges is the limited adaptability of AI models to local geographical, climatic, and socio-demographic conditions. Models trained on global datasets may fail to capture local realities, potentially leading to inadequate decisions in public health or environmental protection contexts (Alotaibi & Nassif, 2024). In addition, the uneven distribution of digital infrastructure hinders effective implementation in rural or underdeveloped regions (Gohr et al., 2025). The high costs associated with developing, deploying, and maintaining agentic AI systems may exacerbate existing inequalities, excluding regions with limited resources. Moreover, the digital divide affects the ability of communities to benefit equally from these technologies (Gohr et al., 2025).

Another significant challenge lies in the fact that training and operating large-scale AI models require significant computational and energy resources (van Wynsberghe, 2021), which, to some extent, contradicts sustainability principles. Therefore, it is important to evaluate not only how agentic AI can be used for sustainable healthcare, but also how AI models themselves can be developed in a sustainable manner. For instance, programming AI agents can take into account the ecological cost of their operations. A cloud-based AI system, for example, could prioritize task processing in regions powered by renewable energy or schedule non-urgent tasks during periods of lower energy demand. This type of dynamic adaptability can ensure efficiency without compromising sustainability.

AI agents can optimize resource consumption through the use of energy-efficient algorithms and smaller models that reduce computational demands. Thus, for simple tasks, instead of deploying large language models, agents may employ smaller, specialized models that are more energy efficient. Moreover, dynamic scaling enables agents to consume resources only when necessary, shutting down during idle periods to conserve energy. Ideally, AI agents should be designed to operate efficiently on energy-optimized hardware, including edge devices and servers powered by renewable sources, thus reducing reliance on resource-intensive infrastructures.

Sustainability, however, does not end at the stage of system implementation. Regular monitoring of an agent's energy consumption, combined with tools for measuring its carbon footprint, provides essential insights for minimizing long-term environmental impact. In multi-agent systems, tasks can be distributed strategically to minimize redundancy and maximize efficiency. In conclusion, it is essential that sustainability principles be applied throughout all stages of the agentic AI lifecycle, including design, development, deployment, and maintenance.

FUTURE RESEARCH DIRECTIONS

This chapter explores the transformative role of agentic AI in developing sustainable environmental monitoring systems for healthcare.

As many specialists anticipate, "embracing multi-agent architectures is what will truly reshape industries, as agents gain the ability to communicate with each other… The future will be about companies having agents in their devices and applications that can address needs and interact with other agents. These agents will work across entire businesses to assist humans in every role, from HR and finance to marketing and sales", including in healthcare and sustainability domains (*AI Agents in 2025*, 2025; *Building and Managing an Agentic AI Workforce | McKinsey*, n.d.; *Gartner's Top 10 Strategic Technology Trends for 2025*, n.d.). The powerful synergy between human expertise and agentic AI as a form of collaborative intelligence can accelerate innovation, increase efficiency, and enable organizations to deliver measurable sustainability at scale (*Collaborative Intelligence*, 2025).

Future developments across multiple sectors, including healthcare, will be strongly influenced by ongoing advances in artificial intelligence, particularly agentic AI. Given the significant advantages of agents, new perspectives are emerging for developing hybrid systems, complex modeling approaches, and proactive, personalized, and sustainable strategies in healthcare.

By integrating these agents into sustainable systems, healthcare institutions can become more intelligent and efficient while simultaneously ensuring more natural user interactions. This approach also opens new avenues of research in intelligent agents, complex adaptive systems modeling, human–machine interaction, AI ethics, and digitally augmented medicine, with the ultimate goal of developing a proactive, personalized, and sustainable healthcare ecosystem. Agentic AI, with its capacity to process large volumes of heterogeneous data and integrate external data sources, could incorporate localized environmental indicators - such as air quality metrics or water contamination alerts - to provide a holistic assessment of patient health. In the future, healthcare environmental monitoring systems may thus provide personalized health recommendations or issue warnings based on a patient's geographical location and environmental exposures, thereby advancing toward a strategy of healthcare that is truly both "person-centered" and "environment-centered".

Future research should also prioritize the accessibility of AI in a wide range of healthcare facilities, including those with limited resources. Low-cost, scalable, and ethically designed AI models are essential for ensuring equitable global adoption. While traditional AI has already produced notable improvements to healthcare management, agentic AI has the potential to become the backbone of a system that not only responds to change but anticipates and shapes it for the benefit of all. The adoption of agentic AI promises a learning, adaptive, and continuously evolving healthcare ecosystem, capable of addressing both current and future challenges (Hinostroza Fuentes et al., 2025).

Integrating agents as emerging actors into the dynamic and complex healthcare system requires a rethinking of digital architectures, decision-making processes, and mechanisms for human–machine collaboration. Such integration also necessitates the development of clear ethical and regulatory frameworks, as well as the strengthening of organizational capacities to ensure safe, efficient, and patient-centered care.

In parallel, rigorous quantification of the energy and carbon impacts of agentic solutions is necessary. Future research should propose robust methodologies for measurement (e.g., energy consumption per inference, carbon intensity) and operational strategies (e.g., carbon-aware scheduling, edge execution) to align technical performance with sustainability objectives.

CONCLUSIONS

Continuous environmental monitoring in healthcare facilities is not merely a technical or administrative obligation; it represents a fundamental pillar in ensuring the quality of medical services, protecting public health, and strengthening a sustainable and prevention-oriented healthcare system. Achieving this, however, requires the effective, energy-efficient, and ethical use of modern digital technologies such as IoT, edge computing, and artificial intelligence - implemented in an ethically responsible manner.

The purpose of this chapter has been to support the healthcare system in addressing current sustainability challenges by highlighting the potential of agentic AI in a holistic and coherent manner. Agentic AI refers to artificial intelligence systems capable of acting autonomously and making decisions based on contextual analysis and available information. These systems not only process and analyze data but also implement actions or solutions derived from their conclusions. Intelligent agents thus represent a viable pathway toward the sustainable digitalization of environmental monitoring in healthcare.

Real-world and medical data are inherently heterogeneous, often presented in diverse, unstructured, or semi-structured formats (e.g., sensor readings, clinical notes, images, environmental reports). Agents can process and integrate such complex, multimodal data, which justifies their integration into the development of a comprehensive and sustainable monitoring system capable of delivering a holistic and precise foundation for analysis and decision-making. The capacity of agents to perceive, learn, reason, and communicate in an adaptive and even empathic manner provides genuine potential for transforming environmental monitoring in healthcare. These agents can be integrated into IoT and IoMT ecosystems to acquire and process physiological data and environmental parameters, thereby supporting clinical decision-making, generating real-time alerts, and optimizing medical operations. The integration of agentic AI also enables resource optimization and energy efficiency in healthcare facilities through continuous monitoring and operational processes aimed at minimizing energy consumption and emissions, thereby advancing sustainable medical practices. This chapter considered aspects related to software sustainability (often referred to as *software sustainability* or *sustainability in software*), particularly in the context of AI agents, as well as the perspective of *sustainability by software*, which underscores the role of software as an active tool in achieving environmental goals.

The integration of agentic AI into sustainable environmental monitoring systems for healthcare offers numerous advantages, among which a few may be highlighted: it enables process automation, facilitates the comprehensive real-time collection and analysis of data, and supports proactive decision-making that can improve both health outcomes and environmental sustainability. Nevertheless, challenges such as data security and privacy, explainability, and high implementation costs must be carefully managed. The success of integrating AI agents into environmental monitoring systems for healthcare depends not only on technological innovation but also on the identification of risks and the development of solutions to address specific challenges, some of which are presented in this chapter. Addressing these challenges requires a multidisciplinary approach and a long-term vision.

Despite the challenges, the potential of agentic AI to enhance sustainability practices in healthcare is undeniable. By aligning the development of agents and agentic AI with global sustainability goals, innovations in this field can be ensured to be not only technologically advanced but also environmentally and socially responsible.

As organizations worldwide continue to focus on reducing their carbon footprint and improving resource efficiency, agents and agentic AI will play a pivotal role in achieving these objectives.

REFERENCES

AI Agents for Sustainable Enterprise: A Leader's Guide. (n.d.). GreenMetrica. https://www.greenmetrica.com/ai-agents

Allegranzi, B., Storr, J., Dziekan, G., Leotsakos, A., Donaldson, L., & Pittet, D. (2007). The first global patient safety challenge "clean care is safer care": From launch to current progress and achievements. *The Journal of Hospital Infection*, *65*, 115–123.

Alotaibi, E., & Nassif, N. (2024). Artificial intelligence in environmental monitoring: In-depth analysis. *Discover Artificial Intelligence*, *4*(1), 84. DOI: 10.1007/s44163-024-00198-1

Anitha, M., & Kumar, L. S. (2023). Development of an IoT-enabled air pollution monitoring and air purifier system. *MAPAN*, *38*(3), 669–688.

Arya, A., Bachheti, A., Bachheti, R. K., Singh, M., & Chandel, A. K. (2024). Role of artificial intelligence in minimizing carbon footprint: A systematic review of recent insights. *Biorefinery and Industry 4.0: Empowering Sustainability*, 365–386.

Bekbolatova, M., Mayer, J., Ong, C. W., & Toma, M. (2024). Transformative potential of AI in healthcare: Definitions, applications, and navigating the ethical landscape and public perspectives. *Health Care*, *12*(2), 125.

Building and managing an agentic AI workforce | McKinsey. (n.d.). Retrieved August 2, 2025, from https://www.mckinsey.com/capabilities/people-and-organizational-performance/our-insights/the-future-of-work-is-agentic

Buonanno, G., Stabile, L., Morawska, L., Giovinco, G., & Querol, X. (2017). Do air quality targets really represent safe limits for lung cancer risk? *The Science of the Total Environment*, *580*, 74–82.

Chen, M. (n.d.). *Agentic AI: The Next Big Thing in Artificial Intelligence*. Retrieved August 2, 2025, from https://www.oracle.com/ro/artificial-intelligence/agentic-ai/

Collaborative Intelligence: AI + Human Expertise for Sustainability. (2025, May 27). https://perspectives.se.com/blog-stream/collaborative-intelligence-ai-human-expertise-for-sustainability

Danasekaran, R., Mani, G., & Annadurai, K. (2014). Prevention of healthcare-associated infections: Protecting patients, saving lives. *International Journal of Community Medicine and Public Health*, *1*(1), 67–68.

Dangi, R. R., Sharma, A., & Vageriya, V. (2025). Transforming healthcare in low-resource settings with artificial intelligence: Recent developments and outcomes. *Public Health Nursing (Boston, Mass.)*, *42*(2), 1017–1030.

Dolcini, M., Ferrè, F., Brambilla, A., & Capolongo, S. (2025). Integrating environmental sustainability into hospitals performance management systems: A scoping review. *BMC Health Services Research*, *25*(1), 764.

Energy and AI. (n.d.). International Energy Agency (IEA): New Report on Energy and AI | BUILD UP. Retrieved August 21, 2025, from https://build-up.ec.europa.eu/en/resources-and-tools/publications/international-energy-agency-iea-new-report-energy-and-ai

Epicenters, P. (2024). *Healthcare-associated infections (HAIs): Reports and Data*. https://www.cdc.gov/healthcare-associated-infections/php/data/index.html

Esmaeilzadeh, P. (2024). Challenges and strategies for wide-scale artificial intelligence (AI) deployment in healthcare practices: A perspective for healthcare organizations. *Artificial Intelligence in Medicine*, *151*, 102861.

Farraher, S. G. (2025, July 23). Agentic AI In Healthcare: A New Era Of Intelligent Automation. *Forrester*. https://www.forrester.com/blogs/agentic-ai-in-healthcare-a-new-era-of-intelligent-automation/

Fonseca, A., Abreu, I., Guerreiro, M. J., & Barros, N. (2022). Indoor air quality in healthcare units—A systematic literature review focusing recent research. *Sustainability*, *14*(2), 967.

Garcia, A., Saez, Y., Harris, I., Huang, X., & Collado, E. (2025). Advancements in air quality monitoring: A systematic review of IoT-based air quality monitoring and AI technologies. *Artificial Intelligence Review*, *58*(9), 275. DOI: 10.1007/s10462-025-11277-9

Garg, P. P., Jayashree, J., & Vijayashree, J. (2025). Revolutionizing healthcare: The transformative role of artificial intelligence. In *Responsible and Explainable Artificial Intelligence in Healthcare* (pp. 1–23). Elsevier.

Gartner's Top 10 Strategic Technology Trends for 2025. (n.d.). Gartner. Retrieved August 2, 2025, from https://www.gartner.com/en/articles/top-technology-trends-2025

Gohr, C., Rodríguez, G., Belomestnykh, S., Berg-Moelleken, D., Chauhan, N., Engler, J.-O., Heydebreck, L. V., Hintz, M. J., Kretschmer, M., Krügermeier, C., Meinberg, J., Rau, A.-L., Schwenck, C., Aoulkadi, I., Poll, S., Frank, E., Creutzig, F., Lemke, O., Maushart, M., & von Wehrden, H. (2025). Artificial intelligence in sustainable development research. *Nature Sustainability*, •••, 1–9. DOI: 10.1038/s41893-025-01598-6

Haque, M., Sartelli, M., McKimm, J., & Bakar, M. A. (2018). Health care-associated infections–an overview. *Infection and Drug Resistance*, •••, 2321–2333.

Hassan, N. A., Hashim, Z., & Hashim, J. H. (2015). *Impact of Climate Change on Air Quality and Public Health in Urban Areas*. https://journals.sagepub.com/doi/10.1177/1010539515592951

Health Care-Associated Infections. (n.d.). Retrieved June 20, 2025, from https://www.ahrq.gov/professionals/quality-patient-safety/patient-safety-resources/resources/hais/index.html

Hemalatha, R. J., Akila, D., Balaganesh, D., & Paul, A. (2022). *The internet of medical things (IoMT): Healthcare transformation*. John Wiley & Sons.

Hinostroza Fuentes, V. G., Karim, H. A., Tan, M. J. T., & AlDahoul, N. (2025). AI with agency: A vision for adaptive, efficient, and ethical healthcare. *Frontiers in Digital Health*, *7*, 1600216.

Holmér, S., Nedlund, A.-C., Thomas, K., & Krevers, B. (2023). How health care professionals handle limited resources in primary care–an interview study. *BMC Health Services Research*, *23*(1), 6.

Holzinger, A., Biemann, C., Pattichis, C. S., & Kell, D. B. (2017). What do we need to build explainable AI systems for the medical domain? *arXiv Preprint arXiv:1712.09923*.

Huang, K. (2025). AI Agents in Healthcare. In *Agentic AI: Theories and Practices* (pp. 303–321). Springer.

Internet of Things (IoT). (n.d.). 2021 Edition - IEEE Electronics Packaging Society. Retrieved August 9, 2025, from https://eps.ieee.org/technology/heterogeneous-integration-roadmap/2021-edition.html

Islam, M. M., Rahaman, A., & Islam, M. R. (2020). Development of smart healthcare monitoring system in IoT environment. *SN Computer Science*, *1*(3), 185.

Jo, J., Jo, B., Kim, J., Kim, S., & Han, W. (2020). Development of an IoT-based indoor air quality monitoring platform. *Journal of Sensors*, *2020*(1), 8749764.

Karrouk, Y., Debasa, F., & Sanchez, L. M. F. (2025). The Digital Transformation of Smart Hospitals: Challenges and Opportunities. *Utilizing AI of Medical Things for Healthcare Security and Sustainability*, 1–54.

Karunanayake, N. (2025). Next-generation agentic AI for transforming healthcare. *Informatics and Health*, *2*(2), 73–83.

Kelly, F. J., & Fussell, J. C. (2015). Air pollution and public health: Emerging hazards and improved understanding of risk. *Environmental Geochemistry and Health*, *37*(4), 631–649. DOI: 10.1007/s10653-015-9720-1

Khaled, A. E. (2022). Internet of medical things (iomt): Overview, taxonomies, and classifications. *Journal of Computer and Communications*, *10*(8), 64–89.

Kravchenko, J., Akushevich, I., Abernethy, A. P., Holman, S., Ross, W. G.Jr, & Lyerly, H. K. (2014). Long-term dynamics of death rates of emphysema, asthma, and pneumonia and improving air quality. *International Journal of Chronic Obstructive Pulmonary Disease*, •••, 613–627.

Landrigan, P. J., Fuller, R., Acosta, N. J., Adeyi, O., Arnold, R., Baldé, A. B., Bertollini, R., Bose-O'Reilly, S., Boufford, J. I., & Breysse, P. N. (2018). The Lancet Commission on pollution and health. *Lancet*, *391*(10119), 462–512.

Lenzen, M., Malik, A., Li, M., Fry, J., Weisz, H., Pichler, P.-P., Chaves, L. S. M., Capon, A., & Pencheon, D. (2020). The environmental footprint of health care: A global assessment. *The Lancet. Planetary Health*, *4*(7), e271–e279.

Li, J., Lai, Y., Li, W., Ren, J., Zhang, M., Kang, X., Wang, S., Li, P., Zhang, Y.-Q., Ma, W., & Associates. (2024). Agent hospital: A simulacrum of hospital with evolvable medical agents. *arXiv Preprint arXiv:2405.02957.*

Lin, N., Paul, R., Guerra, S., Liu, Y., Doulgeris, J., Shi, M., Lin, M., Engeberg, E. D., Hashemi, J., & Vrionis, F. D. (2024). The frontiers of smart healthcare systems. *Health Care*, *12*(23), 2330.

Maleki Varnosfaderani, S., & Forouzanfar, M. (2024). The role of AI in hospitals and clinics: Transforming healthcare in the 21st century. *Bioengineering (Basel, Switzerland)*, *11*(4), 337.

Mao, Z., Liu, C., Li, Q., Cui, Y., & Zhou, F. (2023). Intelligent intensive care unit: Current and future trends. *Intensive Care Research*, *3*(2), 182–188.

Mattjus, C. (2020). *Indoor air quality in various healthcare facilities and potential solutions for improving air quality.: A scoping review.*

Miehling, E., Ramamurthy, K. N., Varshney, K. R., Riemer, M., Bouneffouf, D., Richards, J. T., Dhurandhar, A., Daly, E. M., Hind, M., & Sattigeri, P. (2025). Agentic ai needs a systems theory. *arXiv Preprint arXiv:2503.00237.*

Montuori, P., Russo, I., De Rosa, E., Di Duca, F., De Simone, B., & Triassi, M. (2024). Air Monitoring in Operating Rooms: Results from a Comprehensive Study in the Campania Region. *Atmosphere*, *15*(7), 859.

Moritz, M., Topol, E., & Rajpurkar, P. (2025). Coordinated AI agents for advancing healthcare. *Nature Biomedical Engineering*, •••, 1–7.

Noaman, M., Khan, M. S., Abrar, M. F., Ali, S., Alvi, A., & Saleem, M. A. (2022). Challenges in integration of heterogeneous internet of things. *Scientific Programming*, *2022*(1), 8626882.

NVIDIA and GE HealthCare Collaborate to Advance the Development of Autonomous Diagnostic Imaging With Physical AI. (n.d.). NVIDIA Newsroom. Retrieved August 9, 2025, from https://nvidianews.nvidia.com/news/nvidia-and-ge-healthcare-collaborate-to-advance-the-development-of-autonomous-diagnostic-imaging-with-physical-ai

O'Donnell, J., & Crownhart, C. (2025, May). We did the math on AI's energy footprint. Here's the story you haven't heard. *MIT Technology Review.*

O'Sullivan-Dale, U. (2024, May 30). *'World's first' AI hospital with virtual doctors opens in China.* https://www.roboticsandautomationmagazine.co.uk/news/healthcare/worlds-first-ai-hospital-with-virtual-doctors-opens-in-china.html

Olawade, D. B., Wada, O. Z., David-Olawade, A. C., Fapohunda, O., Ige, A. O., & Ling, J. (2024). Artificial intelligence potential for net zero sustainability: Current evidence and prospects. *Next Sustainability*, *4*, 100041.

Olawade, D. B., Wada, O. Z., Ige, A. O., Egbewole, B. I., Olojo, A., & Oladapo, B. I. (2024). Artificial intelligence in environmental monitoring: Advancements, challenges, and future directions. *Hygiene and Environmental Health Advances*, *12*, 100114.

Omidvarborna, H., Kumar, P., Hayward, J., Gupta, M., & Nascimento, E. G. S. (2021). Low-cost air quality sensing towards smart homes. *Atmosphere*, *12*(4), 453.

Ozcelik, M. M., Kok, I., & Ozdemir, S. (2025). A Survey on Internet of Medical Things (IoMT): Enabling Technologies, Security and Explainability Issues, Challenges, and Future Directions. *Expert Systems: International Journal of Knowledge Engineering and Neural Networks*, *42*(5), e70010.

Pichler, P.-P., Jaccard, I. S., Weisz, U., & Weisz, H. (2019). International comparison of health care carbon footprints. *Environmental Research Letters*, *14*(6), 064004.

Qadri, Y. A., Nauman, A., Zikria, Y. B., Vasilakos, A. V., & Kim, S. W. (2020). The future of healthcare internet of things: A survey of emerging technologies. *IEEE Communications Surveys and Tutorials*, *22*(2), 1121–1167.

Riedl, C., & De Cremer, D. (2025). AI for collective intelligence. *Collective Intelligence*, *4*(2), 26339137251328909.

Rocha, A., Monteiro, M., Mattos, C., Dias, M., Soares, J., Magalhaes, R., & Macedo, J. (2024). Edge AI for Internet of Medical Things: A literature review. *Computers & Electrical Engineering*, *116*, 109202.

Russell, S., Norvig, P., & Intelligence, A. (1995). A modern approach. *Artificial Intelligence. Prentice-Hall. Egnlewood Cliffs*, *25*(27), 79–80.

Russell, S. J., & Norvig, P. (2021). *Artificial Intelligence: A Modern Approach* (Global Edition 4e).

Sapkota, R., Roumeliotis, K. I., & Karkee, M. (2025). Ai agents vs. Agentic ai: A conceptual taxonomy, applications and challenges. *arXiv Preprint arXiv:2505.10468.*

Sarnat, J. A., & Holguin, F. (2007). Asthma and air quality. *Current Opinion in Pulmonary Medicine*, *13*(1), 63–66.

Sehulster, L., Chinn, R. Y., Arduino, M. J., Carpenter, J., Donlan, R., Ashford, D., Besser, R., Fields, B., McNeil, M. M., & Whitney, C. (2003). Guidelines for environmental infection control in health-care facilities. *Morbidity and Mortality Weekly Report Recommendations and Reports RR, 52*(10).

Senturk, S., Kok, I., & Senturk, F. (2022). Internet of nano, bio-nano, biodegradable and ingestible things: A survey. *arXiv Preprint arXiv:2202.12409.*

Sharma, D., & Cotton, M. (2023). Overcoming the barriers between resource constraints and healthcare quality. [). SAGE Publications Sage UK: London, England.]. *Tropical Doctor*, *53*(3), 341–343.

Sharma, M. Samriti, & Singh, G. (2019). Need and design of smart and secure energy-efficient IoT-based healthcare framework. In *Energy Conservation for IoT Devices: Concepts, Paradigms and Solutions* (pp. 259–281). Springer.

Singh, D. P. (2025, April 3). Agentic AI: A Catalyst for Achieving Sustainability Goals. *Daily Host News*. https://www.dailyhostnews.com/agentic-ai-a-catalyst-for-achieving-sustainability-goals

Sorouri, S., Ahmari Tehran, H., Parhoon, M., & Saeidi, M. (2025). Air Pollution in Hospitals: A Critical Public Health Emergency and Strategies for Improving Indoor Air Quality and Patient Safety. *Health Providers*, *5*(1), 15–34.

Sreejith, S., Panigrahy, A. K., Ajayan, J., Radhika, J. M., Reddy, N. V. R., Reddy, N. V. U., & Umamaheswaran, S. (2025). IoT sensor-based systems in real-time monitoring of health and environment: A review. *Journal of the Korean Physical Society*, *87*(1), 1–27. DOI: 10.1007/s40042-025-01378-7

Sudarvizhi, T., Chandran, A. A., Gowtham, L., & Poomainthan, M. (2025). Smart Air Quality Monitoring With Model Context Protocol for Environmental Safety Technology. *2025 3rd International Conference on Inventive Computing and Informatics (ICICI)*, 01–07. https://doi.org/DOI: 10.1109/ICICI65870.2025.11069802

Sunyer, J., Jarvis, D., Gotschi, T., Garcia-Esteban, R., Jacquemin, B., Aguilera, I., Ackerman, U., de Marco, R., Forsberg, B., & Gislason, T. (2006). Chronic bronchitis and urban air pollution in an international study. *Occupational and Environmental Medicine*, *63*(12), 836–843.

Tabbakh, A., Al Amin, L., Islam, M., Mahmud, G. I., Chowdhury, I. K., & Mukta, M. S. H. (2024). Towards sustainable AI: A comprehensive framework for Green AI. *Discover Sustainability*, *5*(1), 408.

Tan, L., Singi, A., & Cross, A. (2025). AI-Driven Innovation For A Sustainable Future: Transforming Healthcare. *Metallurgical and Materials Engineering*, 1432–1439.

Tanveer, S., Ahmad, M. I., & Khan, T. (2024). Technological progression associated with monitoring and management of indoor air pollution and associated health risks: A comprehensive review. *Environmental Quality Management*, *34*(1), e22236.

Tech CEOs: Grab the Competitive Advantage with Agentic AI | Gartner Webinars. (n.d.). Gartner. Retrieved July 28, 2025, from https://www.gartner.com/en/webinar/721397/1619143

Topol, E. (2018). *Deep Medicine*. https://www.hachettebookgroup.com/titles/eric-topol/deep-medicine/9781541644649/?lens=basic-books

Tsang, T. W., Wong, L. T., & Mui, K. W. (2024). Experimental studies on airborne transmission in hospitals: A systematic review. *Indoor and Built Environment*, *33*(4), 608–640.

Tseng, C.-J., & Lin, S.-Y. (2024). Role of artificial intelligence in carbon cost reduction of firms. *Journal of Cleaner Production*, *447*, 141413.

Turner, S. (2021). The Role of Iot In Smart Healthcare Facilities: Improving Operational Efficiency. *American Journal Of Internet Of Things*, *2*(5), 1–7.

van Wynsberghe, A. (2021). Sustainable AI: AI for sustainability and the sustainability of AI. *AI and Ethics*, *1*(3), 213–218. DOI: 10.1007/s43681-021-00043-6

Vincent, J.-L. (2003). Nosocomial infections in adult intensive-care units. *Lancet*, *361*(9374), 2068–2077.

Wani, A. K., Rahayu, F., Ben Amor, I., Quadir, M., Murianingrum, M., Parnidi, P., Ayub, A., Supriyadi, S., Sakiroh, S., & Saefudin, S. (2024). Environmental resilience through artificial intelligence: Innovations in monitoring and management. *Environmental Science and Pollution Research International*, *31*(12), 18379–18395.

Watts, N., Amann, M., Arnell, N., Ayeb-Karlsson, S., Belesova, K., Berry, H., Bouley, T., Boykoff, M., Byass, P., & Cai, W. (2018). The 2018 report of the Lancet Countdown on health and climate change: Shaping the health of nations for centuries to come. *Lancet*, *392*(10163), 2479–2514.

Wooldridge, M. (2002). *An Introduction to Multi-Agent System*. John Wiley & Sons. LTD.

Xu, W., Mei, K., Gao, H., Tan, J., Liang, Z., & Zhang, Y. (2025). A-mem: Agentic memory for llm agents. *arXiv Preprint arXiv:2502.12110*.

Yao, Z., & Yu, H. (2025). *A survey on LLM-based multi-agent ai hospital*. OSF.

Zhang, R., Tang, S., Liu, Y., Niyato, D., Xiong, Z., Sun, S., Mao, S., & Han, Z. (2025). Toward agentic ai: Generative information retrieval inspired intelligent communications and networking. *arXiv Preprint arXiv:2502.16866*.

Chapter 4
AI-Driven Environmental Monitoring Systems in Smart Hospitals: Enhancing Patient Outcomes and Sustainable Care

Muhammad Usman Tariq
https://orcid.org/0000-0002-7605-3040
Abu Dhabi University, UAE & University College Cork, Ireland

ABSTRACT

The convergence of artificial intelligence (AI), the Internet of Medical Things (IoMT), and advanced environmental surveillance in intelligent hospitals represents a transformative leap in healthcare. Continuing analysis of data on air quality, temperature, humidity, particle levels, and energy consumption optimizes KI-controlled environmental monitoring systems to support sustainable care. These intelligent systems actively identify deviations from optimal environmental conditions, reducing the risk of infection, improving patient comfort and recovery rates, and minimizing energy consumption and waste. Hospitals can utilize real-time views, adaptive controls, and predictions to deliver safer, greener, more cost-effective, and more effective services. This chapter examines key technologies, integration issues, regulatory considerations, and practical implementations worldwide that support these systems. Future discussions on in-depth research and analysis outline the path to an intelligent hospital ecosystem that prioritizes both patient outcomes and environmental responsibility.

DOI: 10.4018/979-8-3373-5636-5.ch004

INTRODUCTION

The global healthcare ecosystem is located at a central intersection. The increasing demand for care among aging groups and those with chronic diseases, rising capital costs, and more stringent environmental standards have put hospitals under multifaceted pressure. The hospital is consistently one of the most intense buildings of energy and resources. The extensive HLK network, lighting systems, sterilization processes, water consumption, and waste flows collectively contribute to a significant ecological footprint. Hospitals face these challenges and traditionally operate as a new system of clinical care, management, and administrative functions, with responsiveness that often requires independent action. The result is optimal use of resources, environmental pollution, and gaps in how the built environment supports patient outcomes (Pariso et al., 2025). In this regard, it has become increasingly clear that hospitals must evolve into intelligent and adaptive entities to monitor themselves, optimize their operations, and coordinate responses across clinical and environmental fields. Smart Hospital Sensor Network, Connectivity, Analytics, and Automation create real-time, dynamically adaptable environments. Air conditions, including internal air quality, temperature, lighting, humidity, and occupancy patterns, are continuously monitored using IOMT devices, which range from simple air quality sensors to sophisticated HLK performance measurement devices. In combination with AI algorithms, such data allows the system to recognize patterns, predict anomalies, and implement preventive controls. The air-absorbing unit in the ward may increase filtration before the microbial count increases. Lighting may be weakened to support the patient's sleep cycle. Heating and cooling can be adjusted to meet the occupancy level, thereby reducing waste without compromising comfort. This intelligent orchestration bridges two historical orders. It promotes optimal patient care and sustainable operation. Numerous studies have demonstrated that air quality, temperature stability, and lighting conditions have a significant impact on infection rates, medication errors, recovery time, and patient well-being. For example, inadequate ventilation can contribute to the spread of pathogens in the air. However, lighting and fluctuating lighting can interfere with circadian rhythms and stress responses. The psychological effects of environmental complaints, such as noise, air pollution, and heat stress, extend to both patients and staff, impairing healing and productivity (Maleki Varnosfaderani & Forouzanfar, 2024). In this sense, the design of intelligent hospitals transcends energy savings. It becomes the center of a healing environment that prioritizes human experiences at all levels.

Connective tissue provides the medical internet for these functions. IOMT includes devices that collect, transfer, and sometimes act on environmental and physiological data. Air quality monitors track the presence of fleeting organic compounds (VOCs), particulate matter, and humidity, specific to the smart Thermostat Control

Zone of the HVAC system. Sensors manage lighting and ventilation based on the presence of people (Ueda et al., 2024). These devices assess the detailed visibility required for evaluating AI systems, how variables interact, and how they lead to hospital ecosystem interventions. In intensive care units, where infection control is crucial, this level of ecological accuracy is a matter of life and death for neonates, as microclimate affects vulnerable patients. Artificial intelligence functions as an orchestra director. By analyzing historical performance data, clinical schedules, weather forecasts, supply chain structures, and sensor inputs, the AI platform generates actionable insights. For example, the predictive model can predict peaks in particle concentration in the air and initiate calculations for filter changes or adjustments to air flow. Learning reinforcement allows you to optimize the H-solloll value by the minute to maintain comfort, and at the same time, minimize energy stress. Combined with a failure prediction model, AI can assemble maintenance teams with awareness of future equipment failures, enabling preventive maintenance rather than costly reactive repairs. As a result, it is a hospital that behaves like a vibrant, living organism, continuously adapting to provide services for both human and ecosystem health. Regulators, accreditation points, and payers are increasingly highlighting the value of patient outcomes per unit of spending and social impact. Therefore, hospitals are seeking strategies to reduce both costs and carbon emissions. Innovative environmental systems support this dual goal by blocking energy savings and resource efficiency, while simultaneously providing concrete clinical benefits. In the meantime, socially responsible investors, patients, and employees will consider institutions that demonstrate ecological accountability. Hospitals that can report reduced emissions, water protection, and green building certifications can enhance community resilience and attract individuals and partners seeking sustainable value. The hospital's infrastructure is complex, with some buildings functioning without digital networks or standardized control architectures. After modification, hardware upgrades, network security protection, and departmental adjustments are required. Data privacy is less sensitive to surrounding contexts. However, it still requires careful government oversight, especially when occupancy patterns can correlate with patient presence (Ueda et al., 2024). The AI model should be carefully examined to avoid false alarms and control errors that may interfere with the clinical workflow. Staff need to be trained to use these systems, as well as interpret AI recommendations and respond more. Therefore, methods for completing digital maturation include technical, organizational, and cultural changes. To examine this evolving landscape, this chapter first examines the promotion of intellectual and sustainable hospitals, ecological orders, economic pressures, regulatory expectations, and research work in the field of health. It then explores a technology ecosystem based on AI-controlled environmental monitoring, introducing the core components of sensor networks, connection levels, data platforms, machine learning systems, and control aspects (Jain & Mitra, 2025).

BACKGROUND AND THEORETICAL FRAMEWORK

Natural determinants of health, such as quality, comfort, temperature, humidity, and lighting, play a fundamental role in quiet recovery and overall well-being. Excessive discussion and high levels can increase push and respiratory issues, whereas poor lighting and temperature disturb rest and recuperation. These stressors, conversely, affect recovery times and overall well-being. Green healthcare emphasizes reducing environmental harm through energy-efficient frameworks, non-toxic materials, and the preservation of resources (Rajput et al., 2024). An economical clinic plan consolidates these standards by creating recovery situations that support physical and mental well-being while minimizing environmental impacts. This hypothetical system adjusts natural quality with patient-centered, maintainable care.

Environmental Sensing Technologies in Medical Settings

In present-day restorative situations, the role of natural detection innovations has evolved significantly, moving beyond straightforward system management into the realm of enhancing patient outcomes and staff well-being. These sensors, which were once primarily used for maintaining HVAC systems or improving lighting efficiency, now provide crucial information that directly impacts disease control, quiet comfort, and even clinical decision-making. A wide assortment of sensors is utilized in clinics and clinical care offices, each designed to monitor specific aspects of the environment. Among the most common are temperature and stickiness sensors. These are fundamental not only for maintaining comfort but also for preventing the development of bacteria and microbes, which can pose significant health risks, particularly in immunocompromised patients (Rangarajan et al., 2025). Accurate temperature control is also significant in areas such as operating rooms and neonatal units, where even minor variations can affect critical outcomes or the operation of delicate medical equipment.

Humidity levels, when not maintained within satisfactory ranges, can facilitate microbial growth or lead to the drying of mucous layers in patients and staff, thereby increasing susceptibility to diseases. Carbon dioxide (CO2) sensors are also widely used in healthcare settings to monitor air quality and ensure adequate ventilation. Raised CO2 levels are frequently a sign of stagnant wind streams, which can increase the risk of airborne disease transmission a significant consideration in a post-pandemic world. Nearby CO2 sensors for unstable natural compounds (VOCs) are crucial for detecting hazardous chemical buildups within the discussion, especially in areas where solid disinfectants or medical-grade cleaning products are frequently used. Determined introduction to high VOC levels has been connected to cerebral pains, respiratory issues, and long-term wellbeing complications for healthcare specialists and patients alike. Particulate matter sensors provide an additional layer of knowledge by identifying airborne particles such as dust, dander, or pathogens. These are especially vital in sterile situations, such as surgical suites or intensive care units, where any outside particles can compromise ongoing security. Such sensors are regularly part of a broader discussion on filtration and monitoring frameworks that ensure the continued viability of high-efficiency particulate air (HEPA) filters and ventilation systems (Adibi et al., 2024). Sound and light sensors, although perhaps less self-evident in their significance, are also increasingly utilized in quiet care areas. Chronic presentation to high noise levels in clinics has been shown to extend duration and adversely affect recovery. Sound sensors can help offices monitor decibel levels and direct noise-reduction activities. Essentially, light sensors help regulate circadian lighting systems that mimic natural day-night cycles, which have been shown to improve sleep quality, mood, and recovery times in both patients and staff.

One of the most transformative improvements in healthcare detection is the integration of wearable and comprehensive sensors within understanding care ranges. Wearable sensors such as patches that track heart rate, oxygen saturation, and skin temperature allow continuous, non-invasive monitoring of patients without limiting their portability (Asiri et al., 2024). These gadgets are especially beneficial for patients with persistent conditions or those recovering from surgery, where early detection of changes in vital signs can lead to prompt medical interventions. Surrounding sensors, inserted into the environment whether in ceilings, dividers, or furniture monitor broader natural conditions and persistent behavioral patterns. For instance, movement detectors and weight sensors can be utilized to track a patient's development, allowing for the anticipation of falls or identifying changes in activity that will flag health deterioration. The combination of information from both wearable and surrounding sensors allows for a more comprehensive understanding of a patient's condition. This coordinated approach is foundational to the concept of savvy understanding rooms spaces planned to adapt in real-time to the requirements of patients and caregivers. For example, suppose a wearable sensor detects elevated blood pressure levels. In that case, the surrounding environment might adjust the lighting and temperature or trigger a calming sound to help relieve the patient. In serious care units, combining environmental data with physiological readings can offer assistance in distinguishing between natural causes of distress such as poor air quality or excessive noise and genuine medical emergencies (Kumar et al., 2025). The objective isn't to supplant clinical judgment, but to supply clinicians with richer, context-aware information that informs superior care decisions.

However, executing such a sensor-rich environment comes with its own set of challenges, particularly concerning energy utilization and maintenance. Healing centers operate 24/7 and are energy-intensive facilities, equipped with thousands of sensors, which can significantly increase their control requests unless energy-efficient methodologies are employed. To address this, present-day sensor systems are progressively designed to be ultra-low-power. Many of today's sensors utilize advanced communication protocols, such as Bluetooth Low Energy (BLE), Zigbee, or LoRaWAN, which enable them to transmit data with minimal power. A few sensors are indeed capable of collecting energy from surrounding sources, such as solar, thermal, or motor sources, making them successfully self-powered. It not only diminishes operational costs but also makes it less demanding to send sensors in hard-to-reach or high-risk zones without requiring frequent battery replacements.

A low-maintenance plan is another basic figure for healing center settings, where downtime or steady mediation is essentially not feasible. Present-day natural sensors are designed with a lifespan and self-diagnostics in mind. They can alert support staff when calibration is required or when a breakdown is identified; this has become a frequent issue recently. Remote, plug-and-play sensor hubs can be effectively swapped out or overhauled without disturbing existing care or tearing apart the foundation. Cloud-based administration platforms enable centralized monitoring of thousands of devices, allowing for predictive support and real-time analytics that enhance operational efficiency and effectiveness (Pariso et al., 2025). These stages often incorporate dashboards that highlight patterns, inconsistencies, and potential risks, providing office directors and clinical teams with valuable insights. Beyond specialized productivity, sensor systems must also be secure and compliant with healthcare controls. Information gathered from natural and wearable sensors can be sensitive, especially when combined with patient data. In this way, these frameworks must utilize robust encryption and secure communication conventions to protect confidentiality and integrity (Elendu et al., 2024). Compliance with guidelines such as HIPAA within the United States or GDPR within the European Union isn't just a legal requirement it is a fundamental component of understanding business. Ensuring that these advances are both compelling and morally conveyed is crucial to their long-term success and recognition.

System Design and Sustainable Architecture

Within the rapidly advancing field of framework planning and economic engineering, the integration of cutting-edge computing innovations with natural considerations has become increasingly imperative. Among the most transformative developments in this space is the shift from centralized cloud computing to decentralized edge computing, particularly for applications that require real-time data processing, such as natural language processing. Conventional cloud computing relies on transmitting information to remote servers, where computation and analysis occur, and then returning the results to the local system. It demonstrates that, although effective and adaptable, it is inactive and requires a considerable amount of bandwidth. These factors can be inconvenient in scenarios requiring immediate action, such as discussing quality monitoring in urban areas or issuing water pollution warnings in remote locations (Dewasiri et al., 2025). Edge computing, by definition, forms information at or close to the source of collection. It radically diminishes idleness, moderates transfer speed, and improves the responsiveness of observing frameworks. Moreover, since basic information is transmitted to the cloud, overall energy consumption related to data exchange is reduced, which positively contributes to environmental sustainability.

Edge computing also presents focal points in terms of framework versatility. In locales with unstable web networks, edge devices can continue to operate and make critical decisions without relying on a consistent connection to a central server. Typically, sensor systems deployed in woodlands, seas, or high-altitude ranges must remain functional regardless of the network. Additionally, edge computing enhances information security, as sensitive data does not have to be transmitted across different systems, thereby reducing the likelihood of breaches. In any case, it's imperative to recognize that edge computing doesn't completely supplant cloud computing, or maybe, the two models are complementary. While edge gadgets handle prompt, localized tasks, cloud computing remains crucial for collecting data, conducting long-term investigations, and developing large-scale machine learning models that inform future decisions.

When we consider savvy healing centers, the significance of a measured and versatile framework design becomes clear. These healthcare offices must be able to adapt to changing patient volumes, evolving medical practices, and increasing demand for mechanical services. A secluded plan approach permits components, such as persistent monitoring frameworks, demonstrative tools, and data analytics platforms, to be included, updated, or replaced autonomously, without disrupting the entire system. This not only streamlines support and reduces costs but also accelerates the integration of modern advancements. For instance, amid the COVID-19 pandemic, healthcare centers with adaptable IT frameworks were able to rapidly implement contact tracing, further diagnostics, and telehealth services (Katal, 2024). Versatility ensures that as requests grow whether due to population increases, public health emergencies, or extended hospital services the system can adapt without requiring a complete overhaul. Cloud-native design, microservices, and containerization are advancements that support this kind of adaptability, enabling designers and healthcare directors to scale services evenly and maintain high availability even during peak usage.

The measured nature of a hospital's framework engineering upgrades persistent care by empowering consistent interoperability among diverse therapeutic devices and software platforms. A patient's vitals collected from bedside screens can be subsequently coordinated with their electronic health records (EHRs), which in turn can inform clinical decision-making systems. This interoperability ensures that healthcare experts have access to comprehensive, real-time data, ultimately leading to improved outcomes. Moreover, this design underpins data-driven personalization of medications (Nwokedi, 2025). With access to large-scale, quantitative information across departments and the teaching sector, AI calculations can identify designs and provide demonstrative or restorative proposals tailored to individual patients. The design must also support thorough information management and security protocols, particularly given the sensitivity of medical data. Versatility and seclusion don't compromise compliance with guidelines like HIPAA or GDPR, but rather planning frameworks that can implement these controls viably as they expand.

A regularly underappreciated perspective on maintainable architecture particularly in technology-heavy spaces such as natural observation and healthcare is the inherent maintainability of the equipment used. Equipment determination and arrangement play a crucial role in determining the energy efficiency, lifecycle costs, and e-waste impact of a system. Choosing energy-efficient processors, utilizing components that support low-power operation modes, and planning for longevity are all techniques that can significantly reduce the environmental impact of technology solutions. For instance, low-power microcontrollers are ideal for edge computing devices in remote natural observation frameworks, not only because they reduce the frequency of battery replacement but also because they generate less heat and require simpler cooling systems. In smart hospitals, selecting equipment that underpins virtualization and energy-efficient control management can decrease the total number of physical servers required, thereby reducing energy consumption and cooling requirements.

The sending technique of hardware also plays a significant role. Centralizing equipment in well-cooled, energy-efficient information centers may be more economical than dispersing capable computing units to each room in an office, particularly when the gadgets are not in constant use (Adel et al., 2024). In any case, this must be adjusted to meet execution needs some real-time applications require local control. Wherever feasible, equipment reuse should be integrated into the supply chain lifecycle. Secluded equipment plans permit components to be updated independently, extending the life of a framework and reducing waste. Joining forces with merchants who follow best sourcing practices and offer take-back or reuse programs also contributes to a more sustainable innovation lifecycle.

Furthermore, lifecycle evaluations (LCAs) should be a scheduled part of the design process for any framework engineering. These appraisals can assess the natural impact of equipment from generation to transfer and provide guidance to architects in making informed decisions. LCAs can uncover, for example, that two components with comparable upfront costs may have significantly different long-term impacts due to differences in control usage or recyclability (Pariso et al., 2025). Selecting equipment based on such knowledge empowers a shift away from a short-term cost-benefit analysis toward a more comprehensive, sustainability-focused approach. As more organizations commit to net-zero objectives, these considerations are not only morally sound they're also increasingly required by regulatory systems and customers alike. Eventually, planning frameworks that incorporate both specialized execution and maintainability require a shift in worldview on how we approach engineering. It's not just about what a framework can do, but how it does it. The combination of edge and cloud computing empowers optimized execution with minimal impact on natural resources. Measured and adaptable structures ensure versatility and flexibility in mission-critical situations, such as healthcare centers. And naturally, cognizant equipment choice and arrangement procedures decrease the biological impact of our increasingly advanced world. As innovation continues to permeate every aspect of society, framework planners and innovators bear a growing responsibility to ensure that development does not come at the expense of the planet. Planning with supportability as a central focus is no longer optional it is essential (Tariq, 2025).

AI AND DATA ANALYTICS FOR ENVIRONMENTAL INTELLIGENCE

AI and information analytics are progressively becoming essential tools in hospitals and healthcare settings, not only for diagnosis and treatment, but also for understanding and managing the biological factors that influence patient outcomes. As healthcare offices became more data-driven, the ability to analyze complex and high-volume information in real-time gave clinical and operational staff the knowledge that was previously unattainable. Machine learning, a central method in AI, plays a crucial role in inconsistency detection and natural language processing within healthcare systems. In a complex environment like a healthcare center, maintaining steady indoor conditions is crucial for both quiet security and infection control. Sensors inserted throughout the building continually monitor various factors, including temperature, humidity, dust weight, particulate matter, and CO2 levels. This information is collected continuously and in high volume, making it challenging for human administrators to identify subtle or emerging irregularities in real-time. Machine learning calculations, be that as it may, exceed expectations at distinguishing designs and deviations from the standard (Katal, 2024). These calculations can learn from chronicled natural information to characterize what "ordinary" conditions look like for each room or region, and then identify any information points that fall outside those expected ranges.

Anomaly location calculations can, for example, alert maintenance teams to unusual increases in humidity in a sterile surgical suite, which may indicate a malfunctioning HVAC system or a concealed water leak. Such early notices permit staff to initiate activity some time after conditions become risky for patients or compromise therapeutic methods. In a neonatal intensive care unit (NICU), where newborn children are susceptible to natural changes, even slight temperature changes can pose genuine dangers. AI frameworks can identify these minute changes more precisely than conventional observation strategies, informing staff promptly. Additionally, machine learning can help identify long-term natural patterns that may go unnoticed by the human eye, such as gradual increases in particulate levels over weeks, which may relate to regular changes or developmental movements near the clinic (Dewasiri et al., 2025). Understanding these designs enables healthcare centers to adjust their operations and proactively mitigate risks to patient health. Beyond recognizing and translating inconsistencies, AI also bolsters predictive modeling that connects natural variables with subtle results. It can be especially critical in scenarios where the physical clinic environment specifically influences wellbeing dangers, such as disease control. For instance, machine learning models can be prepared on combined datasets that incorporate quiet healthcare records, quality measurements, room occupancy rates, and cleaning plans to predict the probability of healthcare-associated infections (HAIs). These models can learn complex relationships that would be troublesome for people to deduce, for example, how a combination of destitute discussions about trade rates and high humidity levels might increase the risk of parasitic diseases in immunocompromised patients. Once prepared, these prescient models can provide early warnings or suggest adjustments to room assignments, ventilation settings, or cleaning protocols to reduce disease risks (Tariq, 2025).

Another application of prescient modeling is in foreseeing quiet reactions to natural conditions. A few patients, such as those with respiratory ailments like asthma or chronic obstructive pulmonary disease (COPD), are profoundly sensitive to indoor air quality. AI frameworks can analyze information from natural sensors and persistent monitoring devices to estimate exacerbations of symptoms based on changes in particulate levels or carbon dioxide concentrations. It empowers clinical groups to intervene at some point when a patient's condition declines, possibly avoiding crisis mediations or delayed clinic visits. Prescient analytics can also assist in optimizing quiet situations by suggesting rooms with ideal natural conditions tailored to each patient's needs, thereby enhancing comfort and improving recovery rates. In addition to backend examination and forecasting, the introduction of information in a readily accessible and meaningful format is key to the successful application of AI in natural insights. Visualization dashboards serve this purpose by providing clinical and office staff with a comprehensive view of natural information alongside key understanding data. These dashboards are frequently updated in real-time and can be customized to highlight the most critical metrics for each office (Rattal et al., 2025). For instance, contamination control groups might focus on discussing quality, surface contamination risks, and compliance with hand hygiene. In contrast, office administration may track temperature fluctuations, HVAC system performance, and energy usage. Well-designed dashboards utilize natural illustrations, color-coded alerts, and clear patterns to communicate complex information rapidly, empowering staff to make informed decisions without needing to translate raw data (Tariq, 2025).

Real-time choice back frameworks fueled by AI take this a step further by not only showing information but also providing valuable insights. These systems can issue warnings when certain thresholds are crossed or suggest interventions based on predictive analytics. For example, suppose an AI framework identifies a design that poses a higher risk of contamination in a specific ward. In that case, it may prompt nursing staff to increase the frequency of room sanitation or reassign patients to a different location. In crisis divisions, real-time dashboards can combine natural information with streaming measurements and insights to help prioritize assets and streamline understanding (Al-Balushi et al., 2025). This sort of situational mindfulness is invaluable in high-stakes, fast-paced clinical situations where time and precision are crucial.

Imperatively, AI and information analytics also contribute to long-term strategic planning in healthcare organizations. By analyzing natural and quantitative information over time, healing centers can identify areas where framework updates, arrangement changes, or operational improvements are required. For example, suppose information reveals that certain wards consistently experience temperature control issues or have higher rates of contamination. In that case, this may inform future HVAC overhauls or design updates (Jayachandran et al., 2025). Natural insights also bolster maintainability endeavors by enabling clinics to screen and optimize energy use, reduce waste, and lower their overall carbon footprint. The integration of natural information with clinical results empowers teachers to illustrate the unmistakable impact of green building activities on long-term health and well-being. One of the key qualities of AI in this setting is its ability to scale and adapt to the unique conditions of each healthcare facility. Each clinic has a distinctive format, hardware, understanding population, and external natural variables. AI models can be trained on localized information to ensure that proposals are context-specific and relevant to the user's specific needs. As more information becomes accessible through IoT devices and electronic health records, the precision and utility of these models will continue to improve. Besides, AI frameworks can learn from feedback. When staff act on an AI-generated proposal, the framework can observe the result and adjust future expectations accordingly, creating an ethical cycle of learning and refinement.

However, the success of AI and information analytics in generating natural insights ultimately depends on how well the innovation is integrated into clinical workflows. Suppose experiences are not conveyed at the correct time, in the proper manner, and to the right individuals. In that case, their potential impact may be lost (Al-Barazie & Mohamed, 2025). Collaboration between clinical staff, IT experts, and information researchers is essential to ensure that tools are user-friendly, relevant, and seamlessly integrated with clinical operations processes. Preparing and altering administration also plays a crucial role in cultivating trust in AI frameworks and facilitating their adoption (Pariso et al., 2025).

CYBERSECURITY AND PRIVACY IN HOSPITAL IOMT ENVIRONMENTS

In advanced clinics, the Internet of Medical Things (IoMT) has become a foundation of advanced healthcare delivery. This organization of associated devices, ranging from wearable health screens and combination pumps to intelligent HVAC systems and environmental sensors, enables continuous data collection and real-time monitoring, advancing the understanding of care and operational efficiency. In any case, this expanded network also presents noteworthy cybersecurity and security challenges (Bhambri & Khang, 2024). Securing understanding and natural information streams, guaranteeing secure information transmission, implementing robust access controls, and maintaining compliance with stringent regulations such as the General Data Protection Regulation (GDPR) and the Health Insurance Portability and Accountability Act (HIPAA) are now critical concerns within the hospital IoMT environment.

One of the primary data compression challenges is securing the endless streams of sensitive information that are constantly being produced, transmitted, and stored by IoMT devices. These information streams incorporate not only basic physiological data, such as heart rate, blood pressure, oxygen saturation, and medication administration, but also environmental parameters like room temperature, air quality, and humidity levels (Katal, 2024). When appropriately secured, this information helps ensure both personal privacy and security, as well as a safe clinical environment. Nevertheless, when taken offline, they become prime targets for cyberattacks. Aggressors may endeavor to capture or control this information to cause harm, blackmail, or essentially disrupt operations. For example, misrepresented persistent vitals may lead to inaccurate restorative choices. In contrast, controlled natural information may damage HVAC systems or contaminate working areas. To combat this, healthcare centers must implement robust information security measures at every stage of the information lifecycle, including collection, transmission, storage, and access (Tariq, 2025). Protecting information starts with the gadgets themselves. IoMT endpoints are frequently small, resource-constrained, and not initially designed with security in mind. As such, they may require fundamental defensive measures, such as firmware encryption, secure boot features, or standard security components. These restrictions make them especially vulnerable to abuse. Healing centers must hence prioritize the acquisition of gadgets that come with built-in security features and seller support for convenient maintenance (Maleki Varnosfaderani & Forouzanfar, 2024). Organizing division is another imperative methodology, wherein IoMT devices are isolated from other parts of the hospital's IT infrastructure to limit the scope of potential breaches. A compromised thermometer, for example, should not provide access to electronic medical records or authorized systems.

Once information is produced, secure transmission is pivotal. Information traveling over clinic systems or being sent to cloud capacity must be protected against interference and alteration. Secure information transmission protocols, such as HTTPS, SSL/TLS, and VPNs, ensure that information is encrypted during transmission, thereby maintaining its privacy and integrity. Moreover, end-to-end encryption can be utilized so that data remains unreadable even if it is intercepted (Hossain et al., 2025). It can be especially imperative in telemedicine and inaccessible observation scenarios, where information often travels over open or less secure networks. Without strong encryption conventions, sensitive data such as personal health records, medical regimens, or genetic information can be exposed to unauthorized parties. Access control is another fundamental component of IoMT cybersecurity. With hundreds or even thousands of associated gadgets in a healthcare center, it is essential to manage who can access what information and systems. Role-based access control (RBAC) is commonly utilized to ensure that individuals can only access data and systems essential for their specific job functions. For instance, a nurse may require access to persistent monitoring information on a specific floor. In contrast, an office supervisor requires access to natural control systems (Dewasiri et al., 2025). Implementing multifactor authentication (MFA) enhances access security by requiring multiple forms of authentication before granting entry. Past mechanical arrangements, staff preparation, and mindfulness are basic. Indeed, the most secure frameworks can be compromised by human error, such as weak passwords, phishing attacks, or unintentional information sharing. Regular preparation sessions and mimicked cyberattack exercises can help reinforce good cybersecurity hygiene among hospital staff.

A crucial consideration in this context is compliance with legal and administrative systems that oversee information security and protection. Two of the most prominent regulations are the General Data Protection Regulation (GDPR) in the European

Union and the Health Insurance Portability and Accountability Act (HIPAA) in the United States. Both force strict rules on how individual and well-being information must be handled, with severe penalties for non-compliance. Under GDPR, any information that can be used to identify a person, whether directly or indirectly, is considered personal data and must be protected in the same manner. Healing centers must obtain express consent from patients to gather and prepare their information, provide clear information on how the information will be used, and offer patients the right to access, modify, or delete their data (Kumar et al., 2025). Within the context of IoMT, this implies ensuring that devices and systems are designed with security-by-default and security-by-design principles in mind. Information minimization, anonymization, and straightforwardness must be integrated into each stage of framework development and deployment.

HIPAA, although comparative in nature, has specific arrangements tailored to healthcare within the U.S. It mandates the protection of Protected Health Information (PHI) through administrative, physical, and technical safeguards. For natural observation frameworks in hospitals, such as those monitoring room temperatures, discussing streams, or pathogen presence, HIPAA becomes significant when this information is linked to protected records or used to make medical decisions (Bala Dhandayuthapani, 2024). For illustration, if an HVAC system alters room airflow based on a patient's susceptibility to disease, the information it generates can be considered part of the patient's health data and must be protected under HIPAA. Ensuring HIPAA compliance involves encrypting information both at rest and in transit, maintaining accurate audit trails, and conducting regular risk assessments to ensure ongoing compliance. Beyond administrative compliance, the moral importance of understanding security cannot be overstated. Belief is foundational to the patient-caregiver relationship, and any breach of privacy, intentional or accidental, can significantly harm that belief. As healing centers adopt savvy innovations, they must be transparent with patients about what information is being collected, why it is essential, and how it'll be secured (Bhamidipaty et al., 2025). This straightforwardness cultivates a culture of responsibility and regards persistent independence. Advertising patients the capacity to opt in or out of certain types of information collection, wherever possible, engages them and aligns regulatory practices with broader moral standards.

As cyber threats continue to evolve, healthcare organizations must adopt a proactive and layered approach to cybersecurity. It incorporates customary security evaluations, entrance testing, and updates to security protocols based on the latest threat intelligence. Occurrence reaction plans must be well-defined and routinely practiced so that breaches can be rapidly contained and remediated (Ahmad, 2024). Cyber protection is also becoming an essential component of risk management, providing financial assurance in the event of an attack. Collaboration with cybersecurity specialists, healthcare consortia, and government organizations can provide clinics with assistance in staying informed about emerging threats and best practices.

CASE STUDIES AND APPLICATIONS

Intensive care units (ICUs) utilize environment-adaptive frameworks to adjust lighting, temperature, and noise levels based on real-time patient information, making strides in recovery and reducing stress (Katal, 2024). In pediatric wards, sensory-sensitive configurations such as dimmable lights, soundproofing, and hypoallergenic materials help create a calming, child-friendly environment that supports healing. Geriatric care settings prioritize warm comfort and high-quality discussion, attending to the decreased thermoregulation and respiratory sensitivity of older adults. These custom-fitted natural controls diminish dizziness, enhance comfort, and support better clinical results. Together, these case studies highlight how a versatile, patient-centered natural plan improves well-being across different clinic populations.

BENEFITS AND OUTCOMES

The integration of innovative solutions and data-driven frameworks into healthcare and organizational settings brings about a wide range of benefits and quantifiable results. These encompass patient-centric preferences that enhance well-being and accelerate recovery, as well as operational efficiencies that drive energy savings and maintenance optimization, and broader regulatory impacts that support sustainability objectives and environmental responsibility (Pradeep et al., 2024). As clinics, care offices, and healthcare organizations progressively adopt a brilliant foundation, the positive impacts are being observed across all levels of benefit delivery, service, and environmental performance. One of the most compelling results of these advancements is the enhancement in patient-centric care, where the focus shifts from standardized treatment to individualized encounters that promote healing and comfort. Savvy, persistent rooms equipped with flexible lighting, noise control, and personalized climate settings significantly contribute to enhancing patient comfort. These variables have a coordinate effect on physiological and mental well-being (Dewasiri et al., 2025). For illustration, energetic lighting frameworks that mimic natural sunlight can help regulate circadian rhythms, leading to improved sleep cycles. In a clinical context, good sleep isn't merely rest; it may be a fundamental factor that contributes to quicker recovery, shorter hospital stays, and improved immune function. It seems that patients who experience fewer disturbances during rest and are exposed to natural-like lighting recover more rapidly from surgery and report higher satisfaction with their care. Moreover, temperature control frameworks custom-made to individual preferences offer assistance in maintaining an ideal recovery environment. This individual's control over the room environment not only decreases pressure but also engages patients, which contributes to a general sense of comfort and well-being during their stay.

Furthermore, savvy advances encourage calmer situations by reducing unnecessary alerts and controlling noise levels in prolonged periods. Conventional clinics often feature caution warnings, where the steady beeping of screens and equipment can disturb rest and even desensitize staff to genuine crises. Keen frameworks mitigate this by prioritizing alarms, reducing false alarms, and enhancing sound coverage. It contributes to improving rest and mental well-being, particularly in seriously ill care units or long-term care settings (Verma et al., 2024). From a mental point of view, consolation and control are pivotal for patients who may be managing with instability, torment, or fear. The ability to personalize their environment provides a sense of well-being, which has been linked to improved clinical outcomes.

On the operational side, healthcare facilities benefit significantly from the integration of advanced frameworks, primarily through energy management and predictive support capabilities. One of the most notable operational gains is the decrease in energy consumption achieved through the intelligent control of heating, ventilation, and air conditioning (HVAC) systems (Ahmadi, 2024). Clinics are among the most energy-intensive buildings due to their 24/7 operations and the requirement for strict temperature and humidity control. Shrewd HVAC frameworks, equipped with sensors and analytics programs, monitor occupancy, discuss quality, and outside climate conditions in real-time, adjusting performance to match actual demand. For instance, when a well-insulated room is abandoned, the framework can consequently decrease wind flow and temperature control, preserving energy without compromising comfort or accessibility. These alterations, accumulated over a complete office, can lead to significant energy savings, reducing operating costs and the facility's environmental impact.

Predictive support is another transformative result driven by savvy innovation. Conventional maintenance often follows a reactive or planned approach, which can lead to wasteful aspects, unexpected equipment failures, and increased downtime (Pariso et al., 2025). Differentiated, prescient maintenance leverages real-time information from sensors embedded in core systems, such as HVAC units, medical equipment, or water systems, to optimize maintenance. To detect issues, office supervisors can analyze designs and irregularities in gear behavior, planning repairs before problems become serious. It not only minimizes disturbances to persistent care but also expands the life expectancy of costly equipment. Additionally, preventive maintenance diminishes the need for emergency repairs, which are often more expensive and time-consuming than scheduled interventions. It also bolsters a more secure environment, as well-maintained frameworks are less likely to cause mishaps, contamination, or service outages. The broader organizational impact of these innovations is most clearly seen within the space of natural maintainability and compliance with global benchmarks. Healthcare institutions, like other large organizations, are under increasing pressure to reduce their environmental impact and demonstrate responsible stewardship of shared resources. A solid foundation plays a pivotal role in making a difference, as certifications like LEED (Leadership in Energy and Environmental Design) or WELL Building Standard help ensure maintainability. These certifications not only verify the institution's natural execution but also enhance its reputation among patients, staff, and the broader community. Achieving them regularly requires a comprehensive approach that incorporates energy efficiency, water conservation, indoor air quality, and waste reduction all areas that specifically benefit from innovative building technologies.

Reducing the biological impact of healthcare offices has both moral and practical implications. Morally, healthcare professionals should "not harm," which can be expanded to encompass natural harm that contributes to public health emergencies, such as climate change, and address contamination (Kajornkasirat et al., 2025). By decreasing nursery gas emissions through energy-efficient systems and reducing waste through improved resource management, hospitals and clinics align their operations with their overarching mission to promote health and well-being. Essentially, budgetary investment funds from decreased vitality and asset utilization can be reinvested in persistent care, research, or staff development. These investment funds also promote regulatory flexibility by reducing reliance on unstable energy markets or strained public infrastructure.

Sustainability endeavors to improve staff resolve and understanding. Healthcare specialists are increasingly valuing working environments that reflect their values, including environmental responsibility. When they educate themselves to commit to supportability, they cultivate a sense of pride and reason among workers (Katal, 2024). Additionally, patients are becoming increasingly conscious of their needs and may select care providers who share their values. Straightforwardness in supportability, such as displaying energy usage insights or promoting green initiatives, reinforces the relationship between the institution and the communities it serves. Another critical result of these innovative and operational advancements is the ability to accumulate and analyze information for sustained improvement. Savvy frameworks generate vast amounts of information that can be utilized to refine operations, identify wasteful aspects, and support evidence-based decisions. For illustration, information on energy utilization designs can inform superior building plans, whereas support logs can guide acquisition methodologies. Understanding criticism on natural consolation can be coordinated into future remodels or arrangement upgrades. This persistent criticism circle ensures that educators stay informed and responsive to evolving needs.

In total, the benefits and results of integrating innovative advances into healthcare and organizational settings are both significant and wide-ranging. On a quiet level, these developments enhance comfort, promote rest, and accelerate recovery key components in achieving positive health outcomes. Operationally, keen frameworks drive vitality productivity and upkeep optimization, yielding lower investment funds and more dependable services (Pradeep et al., 2024). Foundations bolster natural sustainability, offer assistance in achieving universally recognized certifications, and strengthen the moral mission of care organizations. By embracing these innovations and integrating them into their operational models, healthcare educators can not only enhance the quality of care they provide but also position themselves as pioneers in economic and patient-centered development.

CHALLENGES AND FUTURE OPPORTUNITIES

The rapid advancement of computerized technologies has transformed numerous aspects of society, including healthcare, urban planning, manufacturing, and environmental monitoring. In any case, alongside these advancements come significant challenges and substantial opportunities. Among the essential specialized requirements that must be addressed are issues related to sensor calibration, information integration, and framework interoperability (Pariso et al., 2025). At the same time, moral and administrative concerns in algorithmic decision-making are gaining significance, particularly as artificial intelligence (AI) plays an increasingly central role in shaping decisions in both the public and private sectors. Looking ahead, future advancements such as computerized twins, generative plans, and closed-loop natural frameworks offer transformative possibilities, albeit they also come with their own set of challenges and considerations.

One of the foundational challenges in executing advanced frameworks lies in calibrating sensors. Sensors serve as the eyes and ears of cutting-edge frameworks, collecting crucial information from situations ranging from mechanical equipment and urban infrastructure to human bodies and rural areas. In any case, these sensors are prone to drift, corruption, and natural obstructions over time, leading to errors in the information they provide. In basic applications, such as restorative checking or quality evaluation, even minor calibration errors can result in critical misjudgments (Dewasiri et al., 2025). Currently, sensor calibration often requires manual intervention, specialized equipment, and a prepared workforce, which can be time-consuming and expensive, particularly when scaled up. Moreover, contrasts in plan and innovation among producers result in variations in sensor performance, complicating efforts to establish standardized calibration standards. The development of self-calibrating sensors and robotized calibration frameworks may be a promising direction, as it would enable continuous precision and reduce the need for human intervention. Standardizing calibration across businesses and advancing cross-platform compatibility will improve unwavering quality and encourage a broader selection of sensor-dependent technologies.

In parallel with sensor calibration issues, information integration presents another significant technical challenge. The volume, speed, and assortment of information being created nowadays are unprecedented; however, most organizations struggle to reach their full potential due to fragmented systems and siloed data sources. Information may exist in various formats, including structured, semi-structured, and unstructured. It may be stored in disconnected databases across various divisions or organizations. As a result, combining and analyzing these disparate datasets becomes a complex and resource-intensive endeavor. The need for a bound-together information system represses comprehensive investigation and decreases the value of other rich information streams. This challenge is especially intense in divisions such as healthcare, where the integration of electronic health records, imaging information, and real-time monitoring is crucial for advancing personalized medicine (Chirchi et al., 2024). Developing arrangements such as information lakes, which permit raw data to be stored in a centralized repository, and a more decentralized information architecture design, which emphasizes domain-oriented ownership and interoperability, are creating new pathways to address this issue. Moreover, semantic advances that empower frameworks to comprehend and contextualize information, rather than merely store it, are likely to play a pivotal role in facilitating effective information integration.

Closely connected to information integration is the challenge of interoperability, which refers to the ability of distinct frameworks, stages, and devices to communicate and work together seamlessly. Typically, especially in basic situations like smart cities, where frameworks for activity management, energy delivery, public security, and waste management are integrated, many of today's frameworks are built using proprietary advances that prioritize vendor lock-in over openness. As a result, coordinating unused advances with the bequest framework becomes both factually and financially overwhelming. Indeed, when frameworks are planned to be interoperable, inconsistent measures across districts or divisions can hinder their practical use. For example, distinct nations may have specific communication conventions or information groups for advanced network innovations, which can create obstacles to global collaboration (Pariso et al., 2025). The need for interoperability moreover poses genuine security and protection risks, as information shared over incompatible systems can be more vulnerable to breaches. Empowering the adoption of open benchmarks, advancing collaboration among innovation suppliers, and leveraging emerging innovations such as blockchain to oversee information judgment and gain control can help address these issues. Ultimately, achieving genuine interoperability will require both specialized development and streamlined implementation.

Beyond these specialized challenges, moral and administrative considerations in algorithmic decision-making have become increasingly noticeable. As AI frameworks become increasingly embedded in decision-making processes, from credit scoring and contracting to law enforcement and healthcare, the outcomes of algorithmic choices can have a profound impact on individuals' lives. One of the primary concerns regarding squeezing is the issue of bias in calculations. Machine learning models are trained on authentic data, which often reflects existing social inequalities. Without careful oversight, these predispositions can be duplicated or indeed intensified, leading to biased outcomes. For example, AI-driven enlistment tools may favor certain socioeconomics based on one-sided data, or prescient policing frameworks may excessively target marginalized communities. These results not only raise genuine moral concerns but also have the potential to undermine public trust in AI frameworks (Pradeep et al., 2024). To mitigate bias, it is essential to conduct regular reviews of algorithmic choices, utilize diverse and agent training datasets, and involve multidisciplinary teams, including ethicists and social scientists, in the development and evaluation of AI technologies.

Another fundamental moral issue is the need for transparency and explainability in many AI systems. Progressed machine learning models, especially profound neural systems, frequently work as black boxes, making it troublesome to understand how they arrive at particular choices (Katal, 2024). This mistiness poses noteworthy challenges in divisions where responsibility is pivotal, such as healthcare, criminal justice, and social equity. If an AI framework denies a credit application or recommends a medical treatment, individuals affected by these decisions have the right to understand the basis behind them. Logical AI (XAI) aims to address this by creating models that provide interpretable insights into their decision-making processes. In addition to specialized arrangements, administrative systems must evolve to promote transparency and accountability. For instance, the European Union's General Data Protection Regulation (GDPR) grants individuals the right to an explanation when subjected to automated decision-making, setting a crucial point of reference for algorithmic management.

Security and information assurance are also central to the ethical use of technology. With the expansion of data-driven services, tremendous amounts of personal data are being collected, stored, and analyzed. In any case, numerous clients are uninformed of how their information is being utilized or need the capacity to control its spread. The conventional display of educated assent is increasingly insufficient in the face of complex information environments. Besides, the use of reconnaissance advances such as facial recognition raises concerns about civil liberties and the potential for abuse by dictators. To address these concerns, privacy-by-design standards must be integrated into innovation advancement from the outset, ensuring that frameworks are secure and client information is handled with care. Clients should be able to engage with tools that allow them to manage their data, including options to view, edit, and delete their information. Policymakers also play a significant role in creating laws that strike a balance between personal protection and innovation (Tariq, 2025). Looking to the longer term, a few groundbreaking developments hold the promise of reshaping our interaction with innovation and the environment. Among these, advanced twins represent a transformative approach to modeling and managing complex systems (Rath et al., 2024). An advanced twin could be a virtual reproduction of a physical protest, handle, or framework that receives real-time information from its physical counterpart. It empowers persistent checking, reenactment, and optimization. In fabrication, computerized twins can be utilized to predict hardware failures and plan maintenance, thereby decreasing downtime and costs. In healthcare, patient-specific computer-generated twins may empower personalized treatment plans by simulating the effects of various treatments. In urban planning, city-wide advanced twins can help optimize activity streams, energy usage, and emergency responses. The challenge lies in creating accurate models and ensuring that the vast amounts of data required are collected, processed, and managed safely and efficiently. In any case, the potential benefits in terms of productivity, flexibility, and maintainability are substantial.

A generative plan is another promising development that leverages AI and computational control to produce plan arrangements based on specified parameters and constraints naturally. This approach imitates the way nature advances designs through iterative enhancement and adjustment. In design, a generative plan can create structures that are not only aesthetically pleasing but also optimized for materials, durability, and energy efficiency (Dewasiri et al., 2025). In designing, it can create lightweight yet solid components for aviation or automotive applications. Generative plans enable rapid prototyping and exploration of a wide range of plan outcomes that would be impractical using conventional methods. As computational control and algorithmic advancements increase, generative planning is likely to become a standard tool in various industries, enabling more creative and effective solutions.

Finally, the concept of closed-loop natural frameworks is gaining consideration as a fundamental technique for economic improvement. These frameworks aim to minimize waste and maximize resource utilization by recycling and reusing materials in a sustainable cycle. In contrast to the conventional direct demonstration of generation and consumption, closed-loop frameworks are propelled by natural biological systems, where waste from one process becomes input for another. In farming, for example, closed-loop frameworks coordinate livestock and animal production with waste reuse to improve soil health and reduce reliance on synthetic inputs (Pariso et al., 2025). In fabricating, circular economy standards direct the plan of items that are less demanding to repair, restore, or reuse. Advanced innovations, including sensors, blockchain, and AI, play a significant role in tracking fabric streams and optimizing asset utilization in these systems. Executing closed-loop frameworks at scale requires not only mechanical advancements but also innovative business models, operational systems, and social shifts in how value and waste are perceived.

In conclusion, the advancement of innovation is hindered by both imposing challenges and creating opportunities. Specialized considerations in sensor calibration, information integration, and interoperability must be addressed to enable dependable, adaptable, and intelligently designed frameworks. At the same time, moral and administrative considerations are fundamental to ensure that algorithmic decision-making is fair, transparent, and respectful of human rights (Pradeep et al., 2024). Looking ahead, developing innovations such as digital twins, generative plans, and closed-loop natural frameworks offer capable instruments for addressing complex societal issues and progressing toward a more sustainable and intelligent world. The key to realizing this future lies in a mindful plan, interdisciplinary collaboration, and a commitment to moral and comprehensive advancement.

CONCLUSION

As healthcare frameworks around the world struggle with rising costs, natural concerns, and ever-increasing demands for high-quality, long-term care, the adoption of AI-driven natural language processing frameworks in smart healthcare centers offers a practical approach to addressing these multifaceted challenges. Illustrated through various pilot programs and early-stage organizations, these frameworks have begun to yield essential enhancements in quantitative results, operational strength, and maintainability metrics. This conclusion synthesizes the transformative potential of these coordinated advances, reflecting on lessons learned, execution challenges, approach, and moral considerations, as well as future implications that can guide both suppliers and policymakers toward a versatile and impactful adoption. One of the most critical pieces of knowledge emerging from early usage is that intelligent natural controls directly relate to significantly better clinical results. Healing centers that provide real-time monitoring of discussion quality, ventilation rates, and humidity have seen significant reductions in hospital-acquired infection rates. Patients recovering from surgery or respiratory ailments, in particular, benefit from situations where particulate levels, CO concentrations, and pathogen proximity are effectively controlled through automated HVAC adjustments (Katal, 2024). The utilization of AI models to estimate unfavorable natural events, such as spikes in humidity or external pollution, enables preventive interventions that maintain stable conditions ideal for long-term health. This proactive natural stewardship not only improves personal recovery directions but also contributes to overall framework preparation, decreasing the likelihood of outbreak-driven convergences and asset strain.

The integration of IoMT sensor systems lies at the heart of this change. In present-day healthcare centers, a thick cluster of associated devices continuously streams information related to temperature, humidity, volatile organic compounds, airborne molecule checks, and energy utilization. These information streams converge at cloud or edge computing stages, where machine learning algorithms identify patterns and anomalies. One healing center, for instance, recently identified a malfunctioning air handling unit, which compromised natural conditions and prevented a week-long framework blackout that would have otherwise disrupted basic care units (Pradeep et al., 2024). This prescient maintenance capability, where AI detects subtle deviations in real-time sensor data, reduces downtime, cuts maintenance costs, and minimizes inefficient energy use.

Sustainability picks up is similarly compelling. Keen natural frameworks have demonstrated vitality investment funds of 10-30% in pilot arrangements, achieved by optimizing HVAC and lighting systems based on usage patterns, external climate data, and tenant comfort models. The budgetary benefits are evident, with significant reductions in monthly utility bills and concessionary capital expenditures through optimized resource life cycles (Pariso et al., 2025). More critically, decreased nursery gas emissions and water conservation contribute specifically to broader sustainability commitments. Clinics prepared with these frameworks can pursue certifications such as LEED (Leadership in Energy and Environmental Design) or WELL Building Standard, demonstrating an organization's commitment to environmentally friendly practices and providing reputational benefits to attract patients, staff, and partners who share environmental goals.

However, executing AI-driven natural observing at scale has uncovered noteworthy challenges. To begin with, this includes information interoperability (Dewasiri et al., 2025). Healing centers regularly work an interwoven system of building management systems (BMS), HVAC systems, and ventilation controls that require standardized integration. Retrofitting these frameworks with IoMT-compatible sensors and portals requires significant foundation work and coordination with office administration groups. To overcome interoperability gaps, some have adopted middleware stages and APIs that translate vendor-specific information into a unified schema, enabling cross-system analytics, albeit at an increased level of complexity. Privacy and cybersecurity concerns emerge when natural information converges with clinical operations. Although temperature and stickiness information are not inherently sensitive, the potential to infer occupancy patterns (e.g., when rooms are abandoned or heavily utilized) from sensor clusters raises concerns about persistent security and competitive office surveillance. More concerning is the plausibility of sensor spoofing or malicious control, which in ineffectively secured systems may inadvertently compromise data handling or trigger false alarms a rigorous cybersecurity framework, including end-to-end encryption, zero-trust architecture, and thorough device authentication, is necessary. Regulatory frameworks, such as HIPAA within the U.S., may apply when natural information can be connected to clinical workflows; healthcare centers must treat natural information with the same care as clinical data.

Workforce preparation and training administration also present challenges. Office staff and clinical groups may be new to AI-driven operations. Ensuring smooth selection requires joint preparation modules, easy-to-use dashboards, and clearer responsibility structures when digital systems issue alerts or recommendations (Katal, 2024). A few early arrangements revealed tension between clinical groups, who may override automated systems during perceived crises, and office directors who must justify the autonomy of AI controls. Building standardized acceleration methods and clarity around algorithmic choices is imperative for developing trust.

Pioneers can be propelled by fetched shirking, administrative compliance, reputation enhancement, and quiet satisfaction measures. The most grounded cases cite multi-year ROI projections; for instance, forthright investments in IoMT sensors and intelligent controls have yielded payback periods of one to three years in several clinics. Illustrating this financially viable possibility, nearby patient-care advancements have contributed to securing both capital funding and board-level sponsorship.

Standardization and administrative advancement will help shape future adaptability. As more healing centers emerge, third-party certification systems and interoperability benchmarks can provide assurances to buyers and patients. National and worldwide bodies are currently working toward benchmarks that indicate satisfactory levels of indoor discussion quality, sensor accuracy, data latency, and system interoperability. Meeting these benchmarks will decrease the arrangement contract and minimize the seller's lock-in risk (Pariso et al., 2025). Additionally, payers and accreditation organizations may tie repayment or certification status to quantifiable execution in natural quality, energy efficiency, and sustainability, further incentivizing hospitals to improve their systems (Dewasiri et al., 2025).

REFERENCES

Adel, H. M., Khaled, M., Yehya, M. A., Elsayed, R., Ali, R. S., & Ahmed, F. E. (2024). Nexus among artificial intelligence implementation, healthcare social innovation, and green image of hospitals' operations management in Egypt. *Cleaner Logistics and Supply Chain*, *11*, 100156.

Adibi, S., Rajabifard, A., Shojaei, D., & Wickramasinghe, N. (2024). Enhancing healthcare through sensor-enabled digital twins in smart environments: A comprehensive analysis. *Sensors (Basel)*, *24*(9), 2793. PMID: 38732899

Ahmad, A. (2024). Enhancing Hospital Efficiency through IoT and AI: A Smart Healthcare System. [JOSAPEN]. *Journal of Computer Science Application and Engineering*, *2*(2), 34–38.

Ahmadi, A. (2024). Artificial Intelligence Revolution: A Comprehensive Review of its Transformative Impact on Hospital Data Management in the Future. [IJBLS]. *International Journal of BioLife Sciences*, *3*(3), 115–133.

Al-Balushi, H. A., Singh, H., & Saleem, I. (2025). *Unlocking sustainable performance in the healthcare sector: the dynamic nexus of artificial intelligence, green innovation and green knowledge sharing*. Society and Business Review.

Al-Barazie, R., & Mohamed, A. (2025). Towards Sustainable Healthcare: Integrating Technology for Eco-friendly and Efficient Solutions. In *International conference on Environmental Design, Material Science, and Engineering Technologies* (pp. 301-310). Springer, Cham.

Asiri, M. A., Almutairi, A. D., Ozam, T. S., Al Ahmari, R. Y., Alhazmi, S. M., Almoudhi, A. A., & Alqahtani, N. M. (2024). AI-Driven Decision Support Systems: Transforming Hospital Management Strategies. [JICRCR]. *Journal of International Crisis & Risk Communication Research*, *7*(3).

Bala Dhandayuthapani, V. (2024). Advancing Healthcare: AI Integration, Interoperability and Sustainability Challenges. *Digital Health*, •••, 64.

Bhambri, P., & Khang, A. (2024). Managing and monitoring patient's healthcare using AI and IoT technologies. In *Driving Smart Medical Diagnosis Through AI-Powered Technologies and Applications* (pp. 1–23). IGI Global.

Bhamidipaty, V., Bhamidipaty, D. L., Guntoory, I., Bhamidipaty, K. D. P., Iyengar, K. P., Botchu, B., & Botchu, R. (2025). Revolutionizing Healthcare: The Impact of AI-Powered Sensors. *Generative Artificial Intelligence for Biomedical and Smart Health Informatics*, 355-373.

Chirchi, V., Chirchi, K. E., & Chirchi, E. (2024). IoT for health care: a sustainable approach. In *Sustainable IoT and Data Analytics Enabled Machine Learning Techniques and Applications* (pp. 109–126). Springer Nature Singapore.

Dewasiri, N. J., Rathnasiri, M. S. H., & Karunarathna, K. S. S. N. (2025). Artificial Intelligence-Driven Technologies for Environmental Sustainability in the Healthcare Industry. In *Transforming Healthcare Sector Through Artificial Intelligence and Environmental Sustainability* (pp. 67–87). Springer Nature Singapore.

Elendu, C., Elendu, T. C., & Elendu, I. D. (2024). 5G-enabled smart hospitals: Innovations in patient care and facility management. *Medicine*, *103*(20), e38239. PMID: 38758872

Hossain, M. A., Arafat, M. S., Desai, K., Akter, S., & Asha, A. I. (2025). The Economic Impact of AI-Driven Remote Patient Monitoring: A Business Intelligence Perspective on Healthcare Cost Optimization. *International Interdisciplinary Business Economics Advancement Journal*, *6*(05), 39–67.

Jain, V., & Mitra, A. (2025). Artificial intelligence and machine learning for sustainable development: Enhancing health, equity, and environmental sustainability. In *Machine and Deep Learning Solutions for Achieving the Sustainable Development Goals* (pp. 107–124). IGI Global Scientific Publishing.

Jayachandran, R., Dantapur, B., Antony, A. S., & Nagapadma, R. (2025). Transforming Healthcare Through Smart Health Systems: Harnessing Technology for Enhanced Patient Care. In *Transforming Healthcare Sector Through Artificial Intelligence and Environmental Sustainability* (pp. 107–127). Springer Nature Singapore.

Kajornkasirat, S., Sawangwong, C., Puangsuwan, K., Chanapai, N., Phutthamongkhon, W., & Puttinaovarat, S. (2025). Integrating AI-driven predictive analytics in wearable IoT for real-time health monitoring in smart healthcare systems. *Applied Sciences (Basel, Switzerland)*, *15*(8), 4400.

Katal, N. (2024). Ai-driven healthcare services and infrastructure in smart cities. In *Smart Cities* (pp. 150–170). CRC Press.

Kumar, A., Masud, M., Alsharif, M. H., Gaur, N., & Nanthaamornphong, A. (2025). Integrating 6G technology in smart hospitals: Challenges and opportunities for enhanced healthcare services. *Frontiers in Medicine*, *12*, 1534551. PMID: 40255587

Kumar, A. A., Suryadevara, R., Sowmyya, T., & Chanal, G. B. (2025). Exploring the Intersection of AI, Healthcare, and Environmental Sustainability: Future Trends and Challenges. *Transforming Healthcare Sector Through Artificial Intelligence and Environmental Sustainability*, 23-47.

Maleki Varnosfaderani, S., & Forouzanfar, M. (2024). The role of AI in hospitals and clinics: Transforming healthcare in the 21st century. *Bioengineering (Basel, Switzerland)*, *11*(4), 337. PMID: 38671759

Nwokedi, T. V. (2025). A Conceptual Framework for AI-Driven Healthcare Optimization and Predictive Analytics. *Multidisciplinary Journal of Engineering. Technology and Sciences*, *2*, 1–22.

Pariso, P., Picariello, M., & Marino, A. (2025). AI integration in energy management: Enhancing efficiency in Italian hospitals. *Health Economics Review*, *15*(1), 1–10. PMID: 40388050

Pradeep, M., Kumari, S., Tyagi, A. K., & Tiwari, S. (2024). Smart Hospital in Smart Cities. *Digital Twin and Blockchain for Smart Cities*, 579-603.

Rajput, Y., Tarif, T., Wolfe, A., Dawson, E., & Fox, K. (2024). AI in Point-of-Care-A Sustainable Healthcare Revolution at the Edge. In *Biocomputing 2025: Proceedings of the Pacific Symposium* (pp. 734-747).

Rangarajan, D., Rangarajan, A., Reddy, C. K. K., & Doss, S. (2025). Exploring the Next-Gen Transformations in Healthcare Through the Impact of AI and IoT. In *Intelligent Systems and IoT Applications in Clinical Health* (pp. 73–98). IGI Global.

Rath, K. C., Khang, A., Rath, S. K., Satapathy, N., Satapathy, S. K., & Kar, S. (2024). Artificial intelligence (AI)-enabled technology in medicine-advancing holistic healthcare monitoring and control systems. In *Computer Vision and AI-Integrated IoT Technologies in the Medical Ecosystem* (pp. 87–108). CRC Press.

Rattal, S., Badri, A., Moughit, M., Ar-Reyouchi, E. M., & Ghoumid, K. (2025). AI-Driven Optimization of Low-Energy IoT Protocols for Scalable and Efficient Smart Healthcare Systems. *IEEE Access : Practical Innovations, Open Solutions*.

Tariq, M. U. (2025). Strategic Place Marketing in Cross-Border Regions: Enhancing Territorial Cooperation and Economic Growth. In Sousa, B. (Ed.), *Cross-Border Regions Cooperation and Implications for Organizations* (pp. 107–136). IGI Global Scientific Publishing., DOI: 10.4018/979-8-3373-1912-4.ch004

Tariq, M. U. (2025). The Challenge of Artificial Intelligence in Environmental Sustainability: Opportunities, Risks, and Policy Implications. In Ahmadi, A., & Mna, A. (Eds.), *Nexus of Environmental Quality and Technology Innovation* (pp. 267–292). IGI Global Scientific Publishing., DOI: 10.4018/979-8-3373-1822-6.ch012

Tariq, M. U. (2025). Machine Learning Techniques for Personalized Rehabilitation: Enhancing Patient Outcomes Through Predictive Algorithms. In Korupalli, V., Ranasinghe, P., & Feldman, D. (Eds.), *Predictive Algorithms for Rehabilitation and Assistive Systems* (pp. 221–252). IGI Global Scientific Publishing., DOI: 10.4018/979-8-3373-0194-5.ch009

Tariq, M. U. (2025). Integrating Advanced Technologies for Multi-Stakeholder Collaboration: Driving Sustainability in Supply Chains Through Industry 4.0. In Frichi, Y., & Jawab, F. (Eds.), *Multi-Stakeholder Collaboration for Sustainable Supply Chain* (pp. 313–334). IGI Global Scientific Publishing., DOI: 10.4018/979-8-3693-8925-6.ch014

Tariq, M. U. (2025). Harnessing Collective Power-Multi-Stakeholder Synergies for Sustainable Supply Chain Transformation. In Frichi, Y., & Jawab, F. (Eds.), *Multi-Stakeholder Collaboration for Sustainable Supply Chain* (pp. 245–264). IGI Global Scientific Publishing., DOI: 10.4018/979-8-3693-8925-6.ch011

Ueda, D., Walston, S. L., Fujita, S., Fushimi, Y., Tsuboyama, T., Kamagata, K., & Naganawa, S. (2024). Climate change and artificial intelligence in healthcare: Review and recommendations towards a sustainable future. *Diagnostic and Interventional Imaging*. PMID: 38918123

Verma, A., Saleem, A. M., Ranadive, J. P., Chouhan, A. P. S., & Singh, V. (2024). Artificial Intelligence in Smart Healthcare. In *IoT, Machine Learning and Data Analytics for Smart Healthcare* (pp. 42-56). CRC Press.

KEY TERMS AND DEFINITIONS

AI Monitoring: Smart investigation of environmental health data
Patient Outcomes: Determinant results of healthcare interventions
Sustainable Care: Environmentally liable healthcare practices

Chapter 5
Empowering Sustainable Medical Care Through Data Analytics, Visualization, and Intelligent Decision Support

Gaganpreet Kaur
https://orcid.org/0009-0006-2957-5352
CGC University, Mohali, India

Amandeep Kaur
https://orcid.org/0009-0004-5716-7298
CGC University, Mohali, India

Ramandeep Sandhu
https://orcid.org/0000-0003-2595-4030
Lovely Professional University, India

ABSTRACT

The growing emphasis on sustainable medical environments has intensified the need for intelligent systems that can monitor, interpret, and respond to environmental data in real-time. This chapter explores the transformative role of data analytics, visualization, and decision support systems (DSS) in building sustainable environment monitoring frameworks for medical care. In modern healthcare settings, vast volumes of environmental data ranging from air quality indices and humidity levels

DOI: 10.4018/979-8-3373-5636-5.ch005

to noise pollution and biohazard alerts are generated continuously. Harnessing this data through advanced analytics and machine learning algorithms enables early detection of risks, efficient resource allocation, and predictive maintenance of medical facilities. This proactive approach not only enhances operational efficiency but also supports eco-conscious medical practices. Visualization tools such as interactive dashboards, heatmaps, and real-time graphs convert complex datasets into actionable insights, allowing healthcare administrators and clinical teams to monitor trends, spot anomalies, and make faster, evidence-based decisions. When integrated with DSS, these technologies provide intelligent recommendations that support infection control, energy management, and patient safety in a seamless, automated manner. This chapter offers an in-depth discussion on innovative models and real-world case studies where sustainable environment monitoring systems powered by data analytics and visualization have significantly improved clinical and environmental outcomes. It also addresses challenges related to data integration, scalability, and user training, offering strategic insights for future-ready smart hospitals. By linking sustainability with technology and healthcare, the chapter highlights how data-driven strategies can empower greener, smarter, and safer medical environments.

1. INTRODUCTION

In this ever-evolving landscape of healthcare innovation, the urgency to align clinical effectiveness with environmental stewardship has gained unprecedented importance. As countries pledge their commitment to the Sustainable Development Goals (SDGs), healthcare institutions are increasingly seen as both contributors to and potential mitigators of climate change. Hospitals contribute to carbon emissions not only through energy consumption but also through the lifecycle impact of pharmaceuticals, medical equipment, and transportation of patients and staff. The World Health Organization (WHO) has emphasized the need for climate-resilient health systems, making sustainability a strategic imperative at all levels of care delivery.

Data analytics, particularly when enhanced by AI and IoT, is pivotal in achieving this vision. Its strength lies in converting descriptive statistics into predictive foresight. It enables administrators to answer not only "what is happening" but also "what is likely to happen" and "what should be done about it." This level of insight allows medical facilities to anticipate challenges, allocate resources more effectively, and reduce waste proactively. For example, understanding energy consumption patterns over time can lead to load-shifting strategies that reduce costs during peak utility hours and minimize reliance on non-renewable energy sources.

Furthermore, with the rise of health technology and smart medical devices, hospitals today are not only centers of treatment but also data-rich environments capable of supporting real-time, high-frequency analytics. Every interaction whether it's a diagnostic scan, medication dispensation, or HVAC adjustment generates data that, if harnessed effectively, can illuminate inefficiencies and opportunities for sustainable practice. This capability is further enhanced by edge computing, which enables localized data processing near the source, reducing latency and bandwidth use while accelerating decision-making.

Ultimately, the integration of sustainability, technology, and data analytics redefines the very ethos of healthcare delivery. It is no longer sufficient to cure disease; institutions must now do so responsibly, with an awareness of their environmental footprint and a commitment to minimizing harm. This calls for a holistic transformation where sustainability is embedded into clinical pathways, architectural design, supply chain logistics, and facility operations driven by data, validated by visualization, and executed through intelligent systems. of sustainability principles into the operational core of healthcare is no longer an optional or peripheral concern it has become a pivotal element in global health system reform. The confluence of climate change, dwindling natural resources, rising healthcare costs, and increased societal expectations for corporate responsibility has made environmental stewardship a key performance indicator for modern hospitals. The paradigm shift from reactive healthcare to preventative and value-based care models inherently aligns with sustainability objectives, offering a timely opportunity to redesign service delivery in ways that are efficient, equitable, and eco-conscious.

Furthermore, healthcare's intersection with the environment extends far beyond hospital walls. Medical waste, pharmaceutical runoff, and the energy-intensive nature of round-the-clock care operations contribute to broader ecological degradation that, paradoxically, exacerbates the very public health issues hospitals aim to treat. Thus, addressing sustainability in healthcare becomes a dual mission protecting individual patient outcomes while also preserving planetary health.

In this evolving context, data analytics assumes a catalytic role. As healthcare systems generate unprecedented volumes of structured and unstructured data, the ability to analyze and derive actionable insights from this data becomes mission-critical. Data analytics not only informs operational decision-making but also provides the empirical basis for institutional sustainability reporting, compliance tracking, and performance benchmarking. It supports a learning healthcare system that continuously refines its practices based on real-time feedback, outcome data, and predictive insights.

Patient-centric benefits like improved indoor air quality, reduced infection rates, and more stable clinical environments. For instance, predictive models can anticipate HVAC system failures or overloads, allowing for timely maintenance that ensures uninterrupted climate control in sensitive areas such as ICUs and operating rooms. Furthermore, integrating environmental data with patient care metrics can help identify correlations between clinical outcomes and environmental conditions, laying the foundation for data-informed architectural or operational changes.

Visualization tools play a pivotal role in this transformation by converting complex datasets into intuitive dashboards and heatmaps that are accessible to a diverse range of stakeholders. They facilitate data democratization across healthcare staff, enabling faster decision-making, easier benchmarking, and more responsive facility management. Ultimately, this intersection of analytics and visualization supports the dual imperative of operational efficiency and environmental sustainability.

When combined with intelligent decision support systems, these tools enable predictive and prescriptive solutions that can significantly transform the sustainability profile of modern hospitals (Mehta, 2022). These tools facilitate real-time tracking of parameters such as temperature, air quality, waste generation, and energy consumption. When combined with intelligent decision support systems, they enable predictive and prescriptive solutions that can significantly transform the sustainability profile of modern hospitals (Nguyen & Morris, 2021).

2. ROLE OF DATA ANALYTICS IN SUSTAINABLE MEDICAL CARE

Data analytics involves extracting meaningful patterns and insights from raw data to support informed and strategic decision-making. Within the realm of sustainable healthcare, this capability becomes instrumental in enabling institutions to gain visibility into their environmental footprint, optimize operational efficiency, and proactively address systemic inefficiencies. As hospitals and healthcare facilities contend with rising utility costs, regulatory compliance pressures, and heightened expectations for environmental responsibility, data analytics offers a scientifically grounded pathway for aligning performance metrics with sustainability goals.

One of the most critical areas where data analytics delivers value is energy management. Hospitals operate a wide range of energy-intensive equipment, including MRI machines, CT scanners, autoclaves, air filtration systems, and surgical suites, many of which must function continuously to support patient care. These systems, while essential, contribute significantly to electricity consumption and, by extension, carbon emissions. By leveraging historical energy usage data and correlating it with external variables such as patient occupancy rates, weather conditions, and time-of-day patterns, healthcare administrators can identify trends and inefficiencies. This empowers them to develop optimized operational schedules, introduce demand-side management strategies, and implement targeted energy conservation measures that reduce both cost and environmental impact .

Advanced predictive analytics further enhances this capability by enabling simulations of "what-if" scenarios. For instance, hospital engineers can model the effect of implementing different HVAC schedules or LED lighting retrofits on total energy consumption. These simulations facilitate data-driven investment decisions, ensuring that sustainability interventions are not only effective but also financially viable. Moreover, energy dashboards that integrate analytics outputs provide real-time alerts for anomalies such as spikes in consumption, facilitating immediate corrective actions and continuous monitoring (Zhang & Wang, 2022).

Beyond energy, environmental data analytics plays a vital role in tracking and enhancing indoor air and water quality both of which are essential for infection control and patient safety. Through the deployment of a network of IoT-based sensors strategically placed across various hospital zones, including ICUs, operating theaters, emergency rooms, and lobbies, institutions can collect granular data on temperature, humidity, particulate matter (PM), carbon dioxide levels, and microbial presence. When processed through predictive algorithms and AI-driven platforms, these datasets can detect deviations from thresholds recommended by global health authorities like the WHO and national environmental protection agencies. For example, a sudden rise in CO_2 or volatile organic compounds (VOCs) in patient rooms may indicate inadequate ventilation or filter failure. The analytics system can then trigger automatic alerts and prompt HVAC recalibrations or maintenance checks, thereby mitigating risks before they escalate (Sharma, 2023).

Real-time environmental monitoring also facilitates evidence-based modifications in cleaning protocols and equipment usage. For example, areas consistently registering higher microbial loads may require increased disinfection frequency or redesigning of airflow systems. Over time, the data amassed through these systems contributes to a longitudinal understanding of environmental factors affecting patient outcomes, thus informing long-term infrastructure improvements.

Another significant application of data analytics in sustainable healthcare is biomedical waste management. Hospitals generate multiple categories of waste including general, infectious, pathological, chemical, and radioactive materials each of which requires specific handling and disposal procedures. Improper management of biomedical waste not only violates environmental regulations but also poses serious health risks to medical personnel, waste handlers, and the surrounding community. By integrating sensor-based tracking systems with analytics platforms, hospitals can monitor waste generation in real-time, categorizing volumes by type, origin (e.g., ward or department), and disposal status. Such systems help ensure timely collection, prevent cross-contamination, and reduce storage overflow risks.

The incorporation of machine learning algorithms into waste analytics tools further augments these capabilities by predicting waste surges based on historical trends, seasonal disease outbreaks, or increased patient admissions. This predictive insight allows administrators to scale waste handling resources preemptively, thereby avoiding bottlenecks and ensuring continued regulatory compliance (Patel & Banerjee, 2022). Additionally, these systems can generate compliance dashboards and automated reports required by environmental authorities, reducing administrative burden and enhancing transparency. Hospitals may also use these insights to optimize procurement and inventory practices minimizing unnecessary waste generation by aligning supply orders with actual consumption trends.

Thus, whether it's conserving energy, enhancing air and water quality, or managing biomedical waste, data analytics enables a paradigm shift from reactive problem-solving to anticipatory, evidence-based management. It strengthens the sustainability profile of medical institutions while improving operational resilience, regulatory alignment, and patient safety.

Table 1. Applications of Data Analytics in Sustainable Healthcare

Application Area	Example Use Case	Benefit
Energy Management	Forecasting peak loads	Reduced energy consumption
Air Quality Monitoring	Detecting pollutants via IoT sensors	Improved infection control
Biomedical Waste Mgmt.	Tracking waste segregation patterns	Reduced environmental risk
Equipment Maintenance	Predictive maintenance using sensor data	Minimized downtime

3. VISUALIZATION FOR REAL-TIME MONITORING

Data visualization is the graphical representation of information and data through charts, graphs, maps, and dashboards. In sustainable healthcare, visualization transforms raw data into digestible, actionable insights. This is crucial in a setting where time-sensitive decisions need to be made quickly and accurately .

In a hospital setting, visualization dashboards are not just tools for data display they are strategic assets that assist in real-time awareness and intervention. With numerous systems running simultaneously air filtration, lighting, ventilation, occupancy, and sterilization units hospital administrators must be equipped with a real-time overview to maintain operational balance. Visualization platforms enable the aggregation of data from heterogeneous sources and present them through a unified, interactive interface. These visual outputs are capable of revealing trends, anomalies, and correlations that are often invisible in raw tabular data formats (Verma, 2021).

Interactive dashboards allow facility managers to monitor energy usage, air quality, and waste levels in real time. These dashboards can be customized to display alerts when thresholds are exceeded, enabling immediate corrective action.

Heatmaps can illustrate temperature variations across different wards, helping to identify areas that require HVAC recalibration. Line graphs and bar charts can track daily water consumption trends, empowering administrators to detect inefficiencies or leaks (Sun & Gao, 2022).

Furthermore, visual analytics enables hospital staff and administrators to conduct comparative evaluations across departments and over time. Through benchmarking and trend analysis, institutions can uncover inefficiencies and replicate best practices. For instance, departments with lower energy consumption per bed can serve as models for less efficient areas, while waste segregation data can help pinpoint lapses in biohazard management. These comparisons allow administrators to implement targeted policies and interventions backed by empirical evidence.

Beyond internal optimization, data visualization also enhances stakeholder communication. User-friendly dashboards make it easier for hospital staff, sustainability officers, regulatory bodies, and even patients to understand environmental performance indicators. These visual tools support transparency and accountability by making sustainability metrics accessible to non-technical audiences. For example, compliance with indoor air quality standards or energy-saving targets can be communicated through intuitive visuals, boosting institutional credibility and fostering a culture of continuous improvement (Baker, 2021).

Advanced visualization interfaces also incorporate drill-down capabilities, where users can click on summary indicators to explore detailed metrics such as historical patterns, sensor logs, or specific departmental contributions. This multilevel interactivity enables precise diagnostics and targeted decision-making. When integrated with real-time sensor data, visualization platforms evolve into dynamic monitoring tools that support proactive interventions and early-warning systems.

In summary, visualization is a vital enabler of smart, sustainable hospital management. It empowers stakeholders to move beyond passive observation to active engagement, enabling data-informed decisions that directly impact both operational performance and environmental responsibility. As healthcare institutions continue to digitize their infrastructure and embrace sustainability goals, visualization will remain a cornerstone of modern, resilient healthcare ecosystems.

4. INTELLIGENT DECISION SUPPORT SYSTEMS (DSS)

Intelligent Decision Support Systems (DSS) combine data analytics, artificial intelligence, and expert knowledge to aid decision-making processes. In the context of sustainable healthcare, DSS can automate resource allocation, identify operational inefficiencies, and suggest actionable interventions to reduce environmental impact (Kumar & Singh, 2022). These systems serve as vital enablers of evidence-based administration by continuously interpreting real-time data from numerous hospital subsystems and converting it into actionable strategies.

In recent years, the development and integration of intelligent DSS in healthcare have evolved from static rule-based systems to dynamic, AI-driven platforms capable of real-time learning and contextual adaptation. These systems go beyond traditional decision-making models by incorporating deep learning algorithms, natural language processing (NLP), reinforcement learning, and contextual analytics to deliver highly tailored recommendations. Their ability to synthesize data from diverse sources ranging from wearable biosensors, diagnostic imaging equipment, building energy meters, clinical lab results, and even patient satisfaction feedback positions DSS as an indispensable pillar of sustainable smart hospitals. With multi-layered data integration, DSS platforms can monitor operational, clinical, and environmental parameters simultaneously, enabling comprehensive oversight and rapid response.

The adoption of DSS also contributes to enhanced transparency and accountability in hospital operations. Decision trails can be logged and analyzed retrospectively to understand the rationale behind certain interventions, enabling hospitals to learn from past scenarios and continuously optimize their responses. Furthermore, DSS frameworks are increasingly being embedded with explainable AI (XAI) features, which ensure that the logic behind decisions can be interpreted and justified by human operators, building trust and facilitating compliance with regulatory norms.

Moreover, the scalability of DSS is particularly advantageous in large healthcare networks or hospital chains. When deployed at scale, these systems can detect systemic inefficiencies, standardize best practices across facilities, and even simulate future scenarios to test the environmental impact of strategic initiatives. DSS platforms often include advanced simulation engines that can model various emergency response scenarios, evaluate energy-saving protocols, or forecast demand surges due to seasonal diseases, pandemics, or mass casualty events. This makes them vital tools not only for sustainability but also for resilience and preparedness planning. For instance, by simulating different climate-related power outage scenarios, DSS can help administrators design energy backup systems that are both eco-efficient and robust.

In crisis situations such as infectious disease outbreaks, natural disasters, or bioterrorism threats, DSS can simulate patient inflow and optimize triage procedures to ensure minimal environmental strain while maximizing care delivery. These systems can model surge capacities, predict medication stockouts, and suggest optimal patient-to-bed allocation strategies. This capability is particularly valuable in developing nations, where resource constraints and workforce limitations demand hyper-efficient decision-making models.

In resource-constrained environments, lightweight DSS solutions integrated into mobile health platforms can guide rural or under-resourced clinics on resource allocation and environmental safety measures. This democratizes access to high-quality decision support, bridging the digital divide in healthcare sustainability efforts. For example, mobile-based DSS can recommend optimal generator usage patterns during electricity outages or suggest best practices for sterilization in the absence of automated systems. Cloud-based deployment ensures that even small-scale facilities can benefit from centrally updated algorithms and best practices. Additionally, offline capabilities and low-power computation designs make DSS accessible even in regions with intermittent connectivity.

A DSS can integrate data from environmental sensors, electronic health records (EHRs), IoT-connected medical equipment, and energy meters to recommend optimal staffing levels, room allocations, HVAC settings, lighting control strategies, and sterilization cycles based on patient volume and environmental conditions. In infectious disease control, DSS can use real-time air quality, CO2 concentration, temperature, and humidity data to identify high-risk zones and recommend enhanced sanitation protocols, patient isolation strategies, or even temporary ward closures (Chen, 2022). These interventions are particularly critical in intensive care units and isolation wards, where maintaining strict environmental conditions is vital.

AI-powered DSS can also support inventory and logistics management by predicting demand for medical supplies, pharmaceuticals, PPE kits, and critical care equipment. By analyzing usage patterns, patient admission rates, supplier delivery timelines, and storage conditions, DSS platforms can optimize procurement schedules and warehouse allocation. This minimizes waste due to overstocking, spoilage, or expiration. In energy management, DSS platforms can suggest load-shedding strategies, detect HVAC inefficiencies, and trigger automated responses during peak energy usage periods (Rao & Iyer, 2022). Advanced AI models trained on historical utility consumption can anticipate surges in electricity and water demand and orchestrate preemptive actions such as rescheduling non-urgent procedures or activating solar backups.

Ultimately, DSS empowers healthcare managers to move from reactive to proactive strategies, enhancing operational resilience, resource optimization, and environmental sustainability. The real strength of DSS lies in its ability to reduce cognitive overload among clinical and administrative staff by filtering, analyzing, and prioritizing data points that require immediate attention. For example, a DSS might alert administrators if energy consumption in the ICU exceeds acceptable limits during non-peak hours, prompting real-time audits or corrective measures. Likewise, it may identify unusual surges in biomedical waste generation tied to procedural inefficiencies, poor segregation practices, or lapses in staff training.

Furthermore, by maintaining an auditable log of past decisions and associated outcomes, DSS tools support continuous improvement, accreditation compliance, and data-driven policymaking. These systems contribute to a learning healthcare environment by documenting what worked, what didn't, and why. They act not only as assistants but also as institutional educators, offering feedback loops that enhance strategic planning and reinforce data-informed cultures. The integration of DSS into hospital management systems facilitates a holistic approach to care delivery that aligns with both environmental and clinical goals, ensuring a more adaptive, transparent, sustainable, and intelligent healthcare ecosystem. Hospitals leveraging DSS can thus position themselves at the forefront of innovation, setting benchmarks in ecological stewardship, operational efficiency, patient safety, and clinical excellence across the healthcare continuum.

5. CASE STUDIES IN SMART AND SUSTAINABLE HEALTHCARE

Several pioneering institutions around the globe have successfully adopted data-driven approaches to embed sustainability into their healthcare delivery models. These organizations exemplify how intelligent analytics, real-time monitoring, and smart decision systems can yield tangible environmental and operational benefits while maintaining high standards of patient care.

One such leading example is Kaiser Permanente in the United States, which has implemented an advanced data analytics framework to monitor and reduce energy consumption across its network of healthcare facilities. By integrating predictive analytics into their building management systems, the organization achieved a 10% reduction in energy usage, leading to significant cost savings and a notable decline in carbon emissions. Beyond mere energy tracking, Kaiser Permanente has embedded data analytics across various operational domains, including water conservation, waste disposal, and sustainable procurement. Cloud-based systems enable the continuous tracking of carbon emissions and environmental performance across their facilities. The dashboards developed by the institution correlate energy consumption data with patient volume and occupancy rates, enabling granular-level assessments that guide department-specific interventions. Their predictive modeling capabilities extend to forecasting future energy requirements, optimizing energy procurement in alignment with sustainability certifications such as those defined by the U.S. Green Building Council (Kaiser Permanente, 2024).

Equally important to their technological success is Kaiser Permanente's organizational commitment to sustainability. The institution has established dedicated sustainability teams and collaborates closely with environmental engineers and energy consultants. It fosters employee engagement through sustainability incentive programs, where departments are recognized and rewarded for achieving green benchmarks. This holistic model—combining analytics with cultural transformation—has positioned Kaiser Permanente as a leader in sustainable healthcare innovation.

In India, Sir Ganga Ram Hospital in New Delhi offers another exemplary case. Confronted by the challenges of urban pollution, the hospital deployed IoT-enabled air filtration systems that dynamically adjust their operation based on real-time indoor air quality metrics. These systems are integrated with smart building controls that automatically regulate air circulation, ventilation speeds, and filtration intensities according to WHO-recommended safety thresholds. By leveraging data analytics from air quality sensors, the hospital enhances infection control, especially during seasonal flu outbreaks and periods of heightened pollution. The hospital has reported measurable reductions in respiratory complications among patients admitted to wards equipped with these intelligent systems, underlining the health benefits of data-guided environmental management (Gupta, 2023).

Sir Ganga Ram Hospital's approach extends beyond air quality management. It includes the digital tracking of waste segregation processes and the optimization of HVAC energy usage based on patient density metrics. The hospital is also piloting smart water management systems that monitor flow rates, detect leaks, and predict consumption spikes. Collectively, these initiatives demonstrate how localized solutions, when backed by robust data analytics, can deliver both ecological and clinical dividends—even in resource-constrained urban environments.

A third compelling case comes from the Cleveland Clinic, which has harnessed the power of artificial intelligence and decision support systems (DSS) to optimize complex operational workflows. One notable application is in surgical scheduling. Their AI-powered DSS incorporates variables such as patient acuity, surgeon availability, equipment sterilization cycles, and environmental conditions in operating rooms. The result is a smart, adaptive scheduling model that has reduced bottlenecks, improved operating room utilization by 15%, and curtailed overtime labor costs. Importantly, these operational efficiencies have a direct sustainability impact decreasing electricity consumption, equipment idling time, and unnecessary HVAC load (Cleveland Clinic, 2024).

In addition, the Cleveland Clinic has adopted intelligent building systems that dynamically adjust lighting and air circulation based on room occupancy and patient traffic. These smart systems are tied into broader facility management dashboards, offering facility managers a real-time overview of energy usage across departments. Water conservation measures, green procurement protocols, and waste minimization efforts are also integrated into their broader sustainability strategy. Through these comprehensive measures, Cleveland Clinic not only meets its sustainability goals but also improves patient comfort and institutional efficiency.

These case studies collectively highlight the transformative power of data analytics in realizing the vision of sustainable, smart healthcare systems. They serve as replicable models for other healthcare institutions worldwide, proving that data-driven strategies are not only technologically feasible but also economically and environmentally rewarding when executed with strategic foresight.

6. IMPLEMENTATION CHALLENGES AND SOLUTIONS

Intelligent Decision Support Systems (DSS) combine data analytics, artificial intelligence, and expert knowledge to aid decision-making processes. In the context of sustainable healthcare, DSS can automate resource allocation, identify operational inefficiencies, and suggest actionable interventions to reduce environmental impact (Kumar & Singh, 2022). These systems serve as vital enablers of evidence-based administration by continuously interpreting real-time data from numerous hospital subsystems and converting it into actionable strategies.

In recent years, the development and integration of intelligent DSS in healthcare have evolved from static rule-based systems to dynamic, AI-driven platforms capable of real-time learning and contextual adaptation. These systems go beyond traditional decision-making models by incorporating deep learning algorithms, natural language processing (NLP), reinforcement learning, and contextual analytics to deliver highly tailored recommendations. Their ability to synthesize data from diverse sources—ranging from wearable biosensors, diagnostic imaging equipment, building energy meters, clinical lab results, and even patient satisfaction feedback—positions DSS as an indispensable pillar of sustainable smart hospitals. With multi-layered data integration, DSS platforms can monitor operational, clinical, and environmental parameters simultaneously, enabling comprehensive oversight and rapid response.

The adoption of DSS also contributes to enhanced transparency and accountability in hospital operations. Decision trails can be logged and analyzed retrospectively to understand the rationale behind certain interventions, enabling hospitals to learn from past scenarios and continuously optimize their responses. Furthermore, DSS frameworks are increasingly being embedded with explainable AI (XAI) features, which ensure that the logic behind decisions can be interpreted and justified by human operators, building trust and facilitating compliance with regulatory norms.

Moreover, the scalability of DSS is particularly advantageous in large healthcare networks or hospital chains. When deployed at scale, these systems can detect systemic inefficiencies, standardize best practices across facilities, and even simulate future scenarios to test the environmental impact of strategic initiatives. DSS platforms often include advanced simulation engines that can model various emergency response scenarios, evaluate energy-saving protocols, or forecast demand surges due to seasonal diseases, pandemics, or mass casualty events. This makes them vital tools not only for sustainability but also for resilience and preparedness planning.

For instance, by simulating different climate-related power outage scenarios, DSS can help administrators design energy backup systems that are both eco-efficient and robust.

In crisis situations such as infectious disease outbreaks, natural disasters, or bioterrorism threats, DSS can simulate patient inflow and optimize triage procedures to ensure minimal environmental strain while maximizing care delivery. These systems can model surge capacities, predict medication stockouts, and suggest optimal patient-to-bed allocation strategies. This capability is particularly valuable in developing nations, where resource constraints and workforce limitations demand hyper-efficient decision-making models.

In resource-constrained environments, lightweight DSS solutions integrated into mobile health platforms can guide rural or under-resourced clinics on resource allocation and environmental safety measures. This democratizes access to high-quality decision support, bridging the digital divide in healthcare sustainability efforts. For example, mobile-based DSS can recommend optimal generator usage patterns during electricity outages, or suggest best practices for sterilization in the absence of automated systems. Cloud-based deployment ensures that even small-scale facilities can benefit from centrally updated algorithms and best practices. Additionally, offline capabilities and low-power computation designs make DSS accessible even in regions with intermittent connectivity.

A DSS can integrate data from environmental sensors, electronic health records (EHRs), IoT-connected medical equipment, and energy meters to recommend optimal staffing levels, room allocations, HVAC settings, lighting control strategies, and sterilization cycles based on patient volume and environmental conditions. In infectious disease control, DSS can use real-time air quality, CO2 concentration, temperature, and humidity data to identify high-risk zones and recommend enhanced sanitation protocols, patient isolation strategies, or even temporary ward closures (Chen, 2022). These interventions are particularly critical in intensive care units and isolation wards, where maintaining strict environmental conditions is vital.

AI-powered DSS can also support inventory and logistics management by predicting demand for medical supplies, pharmaceuticals, PPE kits, and critical care equipment. By analyzing usage patterns, patient admission rates, supplier delivery timelines, and storage conditions, DSS platforms can optimize procurement schedules and warehouse allocation. This minimizes waste due to overstocking, spoilage, or expiration. In energy management, DSS platforms can suggest load-shedding strategies, detect HVAC inefficiencies, and trigger automated responses during peak energy usage periods (Rao & Iyer, 2022). Advanced AI models trained on historical utility consumption can anticipate surges in electricity and water demand and orchestrate preemptive actions such as rescheduling non-urgent procedures or activating solar backups.

Ultimately, DSS empowers healthcare managers to move from reactive to proactive strategies, enhancing operational resilience, resource optimization, and environmental sustainability. The real strength of DSS lies in its ability to reduce cognitive overload among clinical and administrative staff by filtering, analyzing, and prioritizing data points that require immediate attention. For example, a DSS might alert administrators if energy consumption in the ICU exceeds acceptable limits during non-peak hours, prompting real-time audits or corrective measures. Likewise, it may identify unusual surges in biomedical waste generation tied to procedural inefficiencies, poor segregation practices, or lapses in staff training.

Furthermore, by maintaining an auditable log of past decisions and associated outcomes, DSS tools support continuous improvement, accreditation compliance, and data-driven policymaking. These systems contribute to a learning healthcare environment by documenting what worked, what didn't, and why. They act not only as assistants but also as institutional educators, offering feedback loops that enhance strategic planning and reinforce data-informed cultures. The integration of DSS into hospital management systems facilitates a holistic approach to care delivery that aligns with both environmental and clinical goals, ensuring a more adaptive, transparent, sustainable, and intelligent healthcare ecosystem. Hospitals leveraging DSS can thus position themselves at the forefront of innovation, setting benchmarks in ecological stewardship, operational efficiency, patient safety, and clinical excellence across the healthcare continuum.

7. STRATEGIC RECOMMENDATIONS FOR SMART HOSPITALS

To overcome implementation barriers and fully realize the potential of data analytics in sustainable healthcare, strategic planning and investment are essential. Hospitals must view digital transformation not merely as a technical upgrade but as a paradigm shift toward an intelligent, environmentally aware, and patient-centric care model. Embracing this transformation calls for the alignment of institutional vision with operational innovation, supported by a robust digital infrastructure and an empowered, data-literate workforce.

The deployment of IoT-based sensors across various points in the hospital environment such as HVAC systems, patient rooms, operating theatres, and waste disposal units is fundamental to building a data-rich ecosystem. These sensors continuously capture key environmental metrics, including air quality, energy usage, humidity, and occupancy rates, which are essential for enabling real-time analytics and responsive operations. A thoughtfully designed sensor deployment strategy ensures that the data collected is both representative and actionable, forming the backbone for intelligent monitoring and automation.

Equally important is the establishment of a scalable and secure cloud infrastructure that facilitates the centralized storage, analysis, and sharing of data. Cloud computing not only enhances operational agility by providing on-demand processing power and storage but also supports collaborative decision-making across geographically distributed facilities. It reduces dependency on local hardware and ensures seamless integration of data from diverse medical and environmental systems. Features such as encryption, audit trails, and disaster recovery tools further contribute to institutional resilience and compliance.

Artificial Intelligence (AI) must be fully embedded into Decision Support Systems (DSS) to drive intelligent predictions and prescriptions. AI can identify inefficiencies in energy consumption, forecast staffing needs, predict infection outbreaks, and streamline procurement. For example, AI-powered models can evaluate historical trends to suggest optimal HVAC schedules or flag unusual surges in waste production. Natural Language Processing (NLP) enables voice-assisted decision-making and automated report generation, making AI tools more accessible to clinicians and administrators alike.

A successful smart hospital strategy hinges on interdisciplinary collaboration. Bringing together diverse professionals IT experts, sustainability officers, environmental scientists, clinicians, and operations managers fosters innovation and holistic thinking. These teams should engage from the inception of the project through its execution and evaluation phases, ensuring cross-departmental buy-in and alignment. Their ongoing collaboration can identify emerging challenges and quickly adapt strategies in response to feedback and performance data.

Furthermore, comprehensive training programs are necessary to equip all stakeholders with the skills and confidence required to navigate and interpret digital tools. These programs should be tiered to match varying levels of technical proficiency and should include hands-on workshops, virtual labs, and certification modules. Regular training not only supports technology adoption but also cultivates a culture of evidence-based decision-making where data becomes an integral part of everyday practice.

Last but not least, compliance with healthcare regulations and data protection laws is paramount. Institutions must embed privacy-by-design principles into their analytics architecture and establish clear governance frameworks. Appointing Data Protection Officers, conducting regular audits, and enforcing access control mechanisms safeguard against breaches and uphold public trust. Regulatory alignment should be seen not just as a legal requirement, but as a cornerstone of ethical and sustainable digital transformation in healthcare.

Sensor Deployment: Installing IoT-based environmental sensors throughout hospital premises is a foundational step. These sensors should measure real-time parameters such as air quality (CO_2, VOCs, PM2.5), temperature, humidity, room occupancy, noise levels, and energy consumption. When strategically positioned in operating rooms, intensive care units, HVAC ducts, pharmacy storage, and isolation wards these devices provide granular data essential for monitoring operational efficiency and environmental quality. These sensors act as the nerve endings of the analytics system, capturing data that drives informed decisions. To ensure data reliability, hospitals must implement periodic calibration protocols and adopt predictive maintenance schedules for sensor upkeep. Integrating this real-time data into centralized platforms enhances infection control, reduces energy waste, and contributes to improved patient safety and comfort.

Cloud Infrastructure: Embracing cloud-based data architecture provides hospitals with the flexibility and scalability necessary for handling diverse data types across departments and multiple sites. Cloud platforms allow the seamless integration of structured and unstructured data sources, enabling unified analytics and consistent reporting. These platforms facilitate remote access to dashboards and insights, encouraging collaboration among geographically dispersed teams. Additionally, cloud systems come with embedded tools for encryption, access logging, multi-tenant storage, and role-based authentication ensuring that healthcare providers comply with privacy laws and disaster recovery requirements. The scalability of cloud infrastructure also allows for phased implementation, minimizing upfront capital expenditure while maximizing future-proofing potential. Real-time data synchronization across departments supports fast, informed decisions crucial for time-sensitive clinical and environmental interventions.

AI Integration: The inclusion of Artificial Intelligence (AI) in decision-making frameworks significantly elevates the predictive and prescriptive capabilities of hospitals. AI-powered systems can analyze historical and real-time data to predict future trends in energy consumption, patient inflow, or waste generation. Algorithms can detect inefficiencies, alert staff to anomalies, and recommend corrective actions proactively. For instance, AI can forecast air quality deterioration based on external pollution data, triggering HVAC adjustments automatically. Natural Language Processing (NLP) applications can enhance user interaction by enabling voice-assisted commands and automating report generation for medical and environmental audits. For effectiveness, AI models must be continuously trained on localized data and periodically validated to ensure their contextual relevance and adaptability to changing environments.

Interdisciplinary Teams: Creating interdisciplinary implementation teams ensures that the sustainability initiatives are designed and executed with a 360-degree perspective. These teams should include data scientists, IT professionals, environmental engineers, clinical practitioners, procurement managers, and facility administrators. Such diversity ensures that analytics tools are grounded in practical use cases and aligned with clinical objectives. Collaborative workflows supported by shared platforms like digital Kanban boards or goal-tracking dashboards can streamline project execution, facilitate transparent communication, and promote accountability. Regular interdepartmental reviews and knowledge-sharing sessions encourage collective problem-solving and continuous improvement.

Training Programs: Human resource development is a critical enabler of technological adoption. Hospitals must invest in structured training programs that target various user groups. Clinical staff, for example, should be taught to interpret sensor dashboards and use data for patient-centric environmental decisions. Administrative and technical staff require advanced training in data governance, visualization, and AI model interpretation. Innovative teaching methodologies such as gamified learning, role-playing simulations, and data storytelling workshops enhance engagement and retention. Embedding data analytics education into medical and nursing curricula will further cultivate a data-driven culture in future healthcare professionals. Scheduled refresher courses and performance evaluations ensure that knowledge remains current and practical.

Regulatory Compliance: Finally, a robust data governance framework is non-negotiable. Hospitals must ensure that all processes involving data collection, storage, transmission, and analysis—adhere to applicable regulations such as HIPAA (USA), GDPR (Europe), and DISHA (India). Appointing a Data Protection Officer (DPO) can centralize accountability and streamline regulatory compliance efforts. Hospitals should implement privacy-by-design protocols, encryption algorithms (such as AES-256), and secure access control mechanisms like RBAC (Role-Based Access Control) and MFA (Multi-Factor Authentication). Regular audits, penetration tests, and compliance training sessions fortify institutional resilience against cybersecurity threats while reinforcing ethical standards.

Collectively, these strategic interventions create a roadmap for hospitals to evolve into intelligent, responsive, and environmentally sustainable institutions. Through careful planning, inclusive collaboration, and continued innovation, the vision of smart, green hospitals can become a reality.

8. CONCLUSION

The integration of intelligent technologies into sustainable healthcare systems represents not merely a technical advancement but a paradigmatic shift in how modern healthcare is envisioned, delivered, and governed. This integration transcends the superficial adoption of digital tools and calls for a deep-seated transformation of healthcare infrastructure, clinical processes, and institutional cultures. By embedding artificial intelligence (AI), machine learning (ML), Internet of Things (IoT), and advanced data analytics into healthcare ecosystems, institutions are empowered to transition from reactive, short-term problem-solving to a more proactive, predictive, and preventative model of care delivery. These tools fundamentally enhance the ability of healthcare providers to anticipate and respond to both clinical challenges and systemic disruptions, such as those triggered by pandemics, climate-related events, or supply chain breakdowns.

In particular, data analytics enables hospitals and health systems to run sophisticated simulations of various medical, operational, and infrastructural scenarios. These simulations can guide the formulation of strategic responses and long-term investments, facilitating optimal capacity planning and contingency design. For example, predictive analytics can help determine future demand for ICU beds, ventilators, or staff allocation based on weather patterns, viral outbreaks, or demographic shifts, thus reinforcing institutional preparedness and agility. Moreover, these data-driven insights are not confined to high-level decision-makers but, when coupled with visualization platforms, become accessible to diverse stakeholders across the organization.

Visualization tools, including dashboards, infographics, and real-time data visualizations, foster a culture of transparency, inclusivity, and shared accountability. They translate intricate, multidimensional datasets into clear, actionable insights that can be interpreted and utilized by clinicians, administrators, environmental officers, and policymakers alike. This democratization of data dissolves traditional silos and empowers cross-functional collaboration. It repositions sustainability from being the isolated concern of environmental or facilities teams to becoming a shared institutional responsibility a collective imperative woven into the very fabric of healthcare operations.

Simultaneously, intelligent decision support systems (DSS) are evolving into dynamic engines of organizational memory, strategic foresight, and adaptive learning. These systems not only catalog historical data and outcomes but also contextualize them using AI algorithms to produce real-time recommendations and scenario forecasts. By continuously analyzing patient flow, supply chain variables, and resource utilization, DSS can optimize clinical workflows, minimize medical waste, and enhance patient safety. As these systems grow increasingly intelligent, they are expected to deliver hyper-personalized guidance for care delivery, predictive maintenance of equipment, and just-in-time resource provisioning all of which contribute to the twin goals of operational efficiency and environmental stewardship.

Embedding these digital innovations into the core governance architecture of healthcare institutions is no longer optional it is imperative. This integration demands unwavering leadership commitment to drive cultural and operational changes. Leaders must champion the shift toward sustainability not just as an ethical obligation but as a strategic competency central to institutional survival and excellence. They must allocate dedicated funding for green digital initiatives, set measurable sustainability benchmarks, and ensure that these are reflected in key performance indicators (KPIs), staff appraisals, and strategic plans.

At the policy level, national and regional governments must develop and refine regulatory frameworks that incentivize the adoption of sustainable digital health technologies. Accreditation bodies and healthcare quality councils must include sustainability metrics within their evaluation criteria to ensure that institutions are held accountable not only for clinical outcomes but also for their environmental footprint and technological readiness. Moreover, cross-sectoral collaborations including partnerships between public health agencies, academic institutions, private technology firms, and non-governmental organizations—will be instrumental in driving the scalability, interoperability, and contextual relevance of these innovations.

Crucially, the transformation must begin at the educational level. Academic institutions must revise medical and healthcare curricula to incorporate modules on environmental sustainability, data science, systems thinking, and digital ethics. Future healthcare leaders should be trained not only in clinical proficiency but also in ecological responsibility, digital literacy, and interprofessional collaboration. This shift in education will ensure that the next generation of practitioners, administrators, and technologists is equipped to lead sustainably and innovate responsibly in an increasingly volatile, uncertain, complex, and ambiguous (VUCA) world.

Indeed, the future of healthcare lies unequivocally at the intersection of environmental sustainability and digital innovation. Those institutions that strategically embrace this dual imperative will not only elevate the quality and equity of care but also fortify their resilience against future shocks and stressors. Beyond the metrics of cost containment or regulatory compliance, the pursuit of sustainability in healthcare is deeply rooted in a moral and social obligation to protect the health of individuals today without compromising the ecological integrity and health prospects of future generations.

The journey forward will necessitate a coordinated, systemic, and participatory approach. Policymakers must craft enabling environments that support digital sustainability agendas. Healthcare executives must institutionalize sustainability through comprehensive strategic planning and governance. Technologists must design and deploy solutions that are ethically sound, energy-efficient, and contextually adaptable. Frontline workers must be engaged and empowered as agents of change, equipped with tools and training to make sustainable choices in their day-to-day operations.

This transformation also requires a radical departure from siloed thinking and conventional models of efficiency. In this new paradigm, every micro-level actions from optimizing thermostat settings to redesigning patient flow logistics is informed by real-time, contextualized data and aligned with the broader goals of climate resilience and patient-centered care. It requires institutions to reimagine their operational philosophies around sustainability as a guiding principle, not an afterthought.

To accelerate this evolution, research collaborations must be expanded, global best practices shared, and knowledge mobilized across institutional and geographic boundaries. Industry conferences, scholarly publications, and digital platforms should be leveraged to facilitate ongoing dialogue, critique, and co-creation of sustainable healthcare models. International bodies such as the World Health Organization (WHO) and the United Nations (UN) can play a pivotal role in standardizing sustainability benchmarks and promoting global frameworks for digital environmental health.

Ultimately, sustainability must be recognized as a core competency of any future-ready healthcare institution. This entails embedding environmental performance metrics into organizational scorecards, allocating permanent budgets for the adoption and maintenance of green technologies, and linking executive compensation to the achievement of sustainability goals. Leadership vision must be matched with operational rigor and strategic foresight, ensuring that environmental objectives are integrated seamlessly into daily routines and long-term plans alike.

As the global healthcare community stands at the crossroads of climate urgency, health inequities, and rapid technological advancement, the imperative is clear. Only through the adoption of intelligent, data-driven, and ethically grounded strategies can we build greener, smarter, and more resilient healthcare ecosystems. These ecosystems will not only be capable of delivering superior care but will also contribute to a healthier planet and a more just society.

In the final analysis, this is about more than technology or policy it is about vision, leadership, and the enduring commitment to care holistically: for individuals, for communities, and for the environment. As we chart this transformative path forward, we must do so with the conviction that digital intelligence, when aligned with environmental sustainability, holds the power to redefine the future of healthcare in the 21st century and beyond.

REFERENCES

Baker, M. L. (2021). Engaging stakeholders with healthcare data visualizations. *Journal of Healthcare Management*, *66*(1), 14–25. PMID: 33411481

Chen, L.. (2022). Smart infection control in hospitals via decision support. *BMC Health Services Research*, *22*(1), 643. PMID: 35562697

Cleveland Clinic. (2024). *AI in surgical scheduling improves hospital efficiency*. https://clevelandclinic.org

Gupta, A. (2023). Smart air quality control in Indian hospitals. *Clean Technologies and Environmental Policy*, *25*, 122–130.

Kaiser Permanente. (2024). *Sustainable healthcare infrastructure report*. https://about.kaiserpermanente.org

Kumar, R., & Singh, L. (2022). AI-powered decision support systems for medical sustainability. *Health Informatics Journal*, *28*(3), 220–230.

Mehta, S. R. (2022). Smart hospitals: Enabling eco-friendly patient care through analytics. *IEEE Transactions on Healthcare Systems*, *18*(2), 134–140.

Nguyen, M. T., & Morris, J. A. (2021). Digital transformation for sustainable health care. *International Journal of Healthcare Technology and Management*, *21*(3), 215–229.

Patel, K., & Banerjee, A. (2022). Waste management in healthcare using AI. *Journal of Cleaner Production*, *312*, 127732.

Rao, P., & Iyer, B. (2022). AI-enhanced inventory optimization for healthcare sustainability. *Expert Systems with Applications*, *208*, 118108.

Sharma, T.. (2023). Optimizing HVAC performance using AI in hospitals. *Sustainable Cities and Society*, *86*, 104029.

Sun, D., & Gao, Y. (2022). Real-time water usage monitoring in hospitals. *Environmental Monitoring and Assessment*, *194*(2), 1–12.

Verma, J. K. (2021). Healthcare dashboards for sustainable monitoring: A case study. *IEEE Access : Practical Innovations, Open Solutions*, *9*, 54321–54329.

Zhang, H., & Wang, M. (2022). Predictive maintenance using environmental data analytics in medical infrastructure. *International Journal of Medical Informatics*, *160*, 104–111.

Chapter 6
Designing Real-Time Interactive Dashboards for City-Wide Health and Environmental Monitoring:
A Data Visualization Approach to Sustainable Medical Care

C. V. Suresh Babu
https://orcid.org/0000-0002-8474-2882
Hindustan Institute of Technology and Science, India

V. Karunya Lydia
Hindustan Institute of Technology and Science, India

M. Jeevananthan
Hindustan Institute of Technology and Science, India

S. Sidharth
Hindustan Institute of Technology and Science, India

ABSTRACT

The research presents a Smart Health and Environment Dashboard which merges patient health monitoring with environmental measurements to foster sustainable healthcare practices. The platform solves the issues of previous systems while speeding up decision processes by uniting sensor-based data collection with AI-

DOI: 10.4018/979-8-3373-5636-5.ch006

driven analysis and interactive visualization. The study implemented design science methodology through prototyping and user simulations and complete evaluation against neuroergonomics and user experience standards. The research revealed substantial improvements in overall system usability together with enhanced system responsiveness and precise monitoring which delivers for public health management. The team successfully conducted investigations into telehealth systems and mobile applications together with predictive AI functionality and expansion to other metropolitan regions. The findings demonstrate that real-time data infrastructures play an essential role in transforming contemporary urban healthcare systems toward sustainable and effective healthcare delivery.

1. INTRODUCTION

The combination of IoT devices and cloud computing with AI allows healthcare systems to deliver prompt and customized care through their advanced technological capabilities. Through immediate analysis of health data these systems make early diagnosis possible and direct individualized treatments and improve medical resource distribution. Real-time monitoring stands as a vital element for urban settings since it protects people and health officials from quick response requirements to air pollution and infectious diseases and lifestyle-related illnesses.

Health data together with environmental information exist in large complex datasets which presents difficulties for turning raw data into meaningful actionable knowledge. Data visualization addresses this issue through dashboard creation that transforms raw data into interactive displays which expose patterns and enable swift decision-making. Modern monitoring systems have transitioned from basic wearables into sophisticated platforms which integrate IoT sensors with AI analysis and mobile platforms to provide constant individualized preventive care.

The combination of urban stressors includes low air quality and high noise alongside quick disease spread in city areas. The sustainability-focused design of smart healthcare systems delivers enhanced health results while cutting waste production and optimizing resource management. The protection of air quality from dangerous levels leads to decreased hospital visits and improved community wellness. Studies of smart cities reveal that unifying health monitoring with environmental tracking systems enhances disease control and speeds up hazard detection while promoting community engagement for better sustainable urban development.

2. BACKGROUND AND CONTEXT

2.1 Evolution of Real-Time Health Monitoring Technologies

The monitoring of one's health has gone through a very big transformation over 20 years. In the beginning, the patient monitoring process was only based on hospital in-house diagnostic tools such as ECGs, pulse oximeters, and blood pressure machines. These systems had to be used in-person, were only reactive, and produced static data snapshots (Shah & Ho, 2024; Zhao et al., 2023)

The use of wearable devices (e.g., Fitbit, Apple Watch) was the very first move toward live monitoring, which made it possible to keep track of the data continuously, including the number of steps, heart rate, and sleep cycle. Be re long, the development of the Internet of Things (IoT) brought about the rise of connected health devices that allow the transmission of patient

At present, the utilization of Al, cloud platforms, and edge computing has changed the face of real-time health monitoring to that of a predictive, as well as a preventive system. For instance:

1. Al-based algorithms find the deviations in ECG or glucose levels well before they reach a critical stage.
2. Edge computing can decrease waiting time, which allows for the emergency alerts to be given instantly, for example, in the case of arrhythmias.
3. The combination of cloud storage enables the safe and central storage of health records that can be accessed from different institutions.

Consequently, real-time monitoring has been updated from simple devices that one could wear into smart and integrated systems which are capable of handling personalized and continuous care. (Rahman et al., 2023).

2.2 City-Wide Health Challenges and Environmental Triggers.

Health Risks in the Cities: Urban living, while lifestyle, environment, and population density being the major variables, has a lot of health risks associated with it. Some of these challenges that widely exist in any metropolitan area are:

Air Pollution: The concentration of PM2.5 and PM10 particles to very high levels is one of the major causes of respiratory diseases such as asthma and COPD (WHO, 2021).

Heat Islands: Cities, which are basically urban areas, are the places that have higher temperatures than their surrounding areas, and this leads to heat strokes, dehydration, and cardiovascular strain besides other heat-related illnesses. (Li et al., 2023).

Infectious Disease Spread: The closeness of the people in such areas speeds up the process of the diseases that are the flu, COVID-19, and are caused by other viruses to be propagated.

Urban residents are very susceptible to health problems from environmental factors such as seasonal changes, industrial emissions, and traffic congestion. The real-time monitoring of these triggers, combined with patient health data, opens up the scenario for the health care providers to come with the solutions that are preventive in nature.

Just to give an example, if a person's asthma condition is constantly monitored and the data is combined with pollution data for the respective area, then the doctor can easily anticipate situations that might call for an emergency visit to the hospital on a day when smog is too high.

Lifestyle Diseases: The sedentary ways of living in the cities have led to the lots of obesity, diabetes, and hypertension problems that are seen in urban people of late. Urban residents are very susceptible to health problems from environmental factors such as seasonal changes, industrial emissions, and traffic congestion (Nature Digital Medicine, 2025).

2.3 Need for Integration of Environmental and Patient Data

Need for Integration of Environmental and Patient Data In the past, health data of the patient and environmental data were collected and analyzed separately. The siloed approach to data leads most times to al partial or even an incomplete understanding of the health outcomes. Reasons for integration are as follows:

Environment factors (air quality, humidity, temperature) have a direct link with respiratory, cardiovascular, and neurological diseases. link these two datasets, it becomes possible to provide individualized recommendations, for example, notifying a heart patient to avoid going outside when the weather is too hot.

Combined data can be used to support health care policies at the level of the local population, for instance, deciding at what time the traffic ban should start during the rise of air pollutants. The healthcare providers and city officials can coalesce these data sets to move from reactive treatment to preventive interventions thus, improving individual patient outcomes and city-wide health resilience (Arxiv, 2025).

As real-time data streams from IoT sensors, wearables, and environmental monitors increase, the challenge lies in presenting data effectively. This is where interactive dashboards become essential.Interactive dashboards: Aggregate data from multiple sources (patient vitals, pollution sensors, weather forecasts, hospital occupancy). Visualize patterns using graphs, heatmaps, and alerts for quick decision-making. Enable real-time responses--for example, a dashboard can notify hospitals when rising temperatures correlate with increased cases of dehydration.

Support policymakers in allocating resources, such as ambulances, ventilators, or vaccines, where they are needed most. During the COVID-1 9 pandemic (Data. org, 2023) dashboards became vital tools for tracking infections, hospital beds, and vaccination progress, highlighting their role in emergency response and long-term sustainability. Thus, interactive dashboards represent the culmination of health informatics- bridging data science, visualization, and decision support for effective city-wide health management.

This chapter recognizes key urban health threats—air pollution, infectious illnesses, and lifestyle diseases—and matches them with the monitoring capabilities of dashboards. By connecting real-time health information with social and environmental determinants, dashboards assist in support of sustainability targets and preventive medicine initiatives. There are a number of trends, however, that remain underdeveloped:

Climate–Health Interactions: Climate change exacerbates heatwaves, floods, and pollution events, all of which have a direct impact on public health. Dashboards should include climate data to forecast and prevent these hazards.

Ethical AI Usage: Since dashboards incorporate predictive analytics, threats of algorithmic bias arise and could solidify disparities. Future systems need to guarantee transparency, equity, and accountability in AI-powered health forecasts. Participatory Citizen Science: Involving citizens in data gathering (e.g., through community sensors or mobile applications) not only enhances datasets but also generates public trust and stimulates active health behavior. By incorporating these aspects, interactive dashboards can transform into comprehensive decision-support systems that deal with not only immediate crises but also long-term urban health resilience (Ebi, K. L., & Bowen, K. 2022).

3. RELATED WORK

3.1 Setting Real-Time Monitoring against Sustainability Goals

Health and environmental real-time monitoring provide sustainability at least theoretically by preventing emergencies from ever occurring. According to real-time data that detect signs of degradation in air quality or abnormal vital signs of a patient's condition, probably fewer unwarranted hospital visits are made, fewer costs are incurred by the health-care system, and stress on medical infrastructure is halted (La Nauze & colleagues, 2022).

3.2 Enabling Proactive Medical Interventions

Real-time data allow doctors and public health teams to intervene at early stages of the disease rather than once it has worsened. This would in many cases improve medical outcome but would evade the exorbitant resources consumption of treating the late stage of a disease (Haddad et al., 2022).

3.3 Impact on Healthcare Resource Optimization

Efficiency is sustainability, too. Dashboards ensure that human labor, medical apparatus, and hospital installations are deployed according to actual demand. This helps to maintain, park, and value resources where and when they are most needed, leaving no room for wastage, while also lessening the impact on the environment (Parker et al., 2024).

3.4 Case Insights from Smart Cities

International smart-city cases reveal the transformation of public health by the combination of IoT sensors, artificial intelligence, and environmental data. These systems ensure that sustainable medical care is both possible and effective-from managing respiratory disease outbreaks to preventing imposing undue burden on hospitals during pollution spikes (Houston Chronicle, 2025).

4. RESEARCH QUESTIONS AND KEY CHALLENGES ADDRESSED

This work explores how real-time health, and environmental data can yield actionable insight through suitable visualization. It investigates the technical and ethical requirements while also exploring how modern technologies, such as AI and hybrid biosystems, can contribute toward enhanced healthcare response and outcomes.

4.1 How Can Real-Time Data Be Visualized Effectively for Health Monitoring?

Investigating methods and tools that convert complex datasets into clear, interactive dashboards for decision-makers (Frontiers in Public Health, 2023).

4.2 What Are the Technical and Ethical Considerations?

Considering issues like security, privacy, interoperability, and accuracy concerning real-time systems (Thryve Health, 2024).

4.3 How Can Visualization Reduce Response Time and Improve Patient Outcomes?

Assessing the effects of a quick grasp of data on preventive care and emergency response (ResearchGate, 2024).

4.4 What Is the Role of AI and Hybrid Biosystems?

Studying the collaboration between intelligent algorithms and bioinspired systems with a view to enhancing prediction and adaptability (Springer, 2025; Arxiv, 2023).

5. OBJECTIVES AND SCOPE OF THE CHAPTER

This chapter is expected to define clear, though tentative, goals, boundaries, and beneficiaries of the approach to be taken to ensure its relevance to both healthcare providers and policymakers.

5.1 Key Objectives

The main goal here is to create a live, eco-friendly health tracking system that mixes up patient health stuff—like heartbeat, body temp, and breathing rates—with the environment, like air quality, heat, and moisture. Making the data into cool, interactive charts and stuff, it help docs and city bigwigs make smarter choices quicker, which is great for keeping cities healthy.

5.2 Scope and Delimitations

This study's main point is looking at cities, where stuff like pollution and lots of people can really mess with people's health (ResearchGate, 2024). the system's built to handle growth and change up in different city settings rural healthcare's got its own set of problems, like not enough internet or roads, but this project's all about making health monitoring work in cities (Arxiv, 2023).

5.3 Target Beneficiaries and Stakeholders

The proposed system is intended for multiple stakeholders:.docs and health pros can get up-to-date patient and surroundings info to make fast, spot-on choices (Frontiers in Public Health, 2023).

City Administrators – Officials can keep an eye on health trends, deal with environmental hazards, and make the best use of resources (Thryve Health, 2024). Environmental Agencies – These groups keep an eye on air pollution, heat waves, and other stuff that can mess with our health (ResearchGate, 2024). Regular folks get to know more about their surroundings and health, which helps them take steps to avoid problems and make smart choices the system's goal is to link folks, info, and tech to make a teamwork-friendly setup that boosts city health and gets help when it's needed, as per (Arxiv, 2023).

6. REVIEW OF LITERATURE

6.1 Interactive Dashboards in Healthcare

Urban scale building health monitoring dashboards gotta stick to the rules for keeping data safe and private in the EU, the GDPR treats health info as super important data it's all about sticking to the rules, keeping things tight and focused, not hoarding data, and not keeping it around forever big monitoring projects usually need to do a DPIA to keep data safe these projects need to keep things anonymous or use fake names for the visualization dashboards (European Commission, 2024). Similarly, in the United States, the Health Insurance Portability and Accountability Act (HIPAA) protects protected health information (PHI). the Privacy Rule's like, "keep it chill with the info, just the bare minimum," and the Security Rule's all about keeping things on lockdown, making sure only the right folks have access, keeping an eye on what they're to get health systems to work together, most public health dashboards use HL7's FHIR standard, which includes Patient, Observation, Condition, and Device. Governance stuff like Consent and Audit Event make sure we're following GDPR and HIPAA rules by keeping tabs on why we're using data, if patients said yes, and keeping a record of everything (HL7, 2024; CDC, 2024).

6.2 Hybrid Biosystems and Artificial Intelligence in Intelligent Health

Over the past decade, hybrid biosystems and AI enabled Intelligent Health. AI with machine learning, deep learning, and natural language processing maintains millions of pieces of health care data that may or may not be structured. In addition, biosystems consisting of wearable sensors, implantable devices, and mobile health applications provide continuous real-time continuous monitoring and predictive analytics. Hybrid AI-biosystem systems are able to specify predictive analytics of cardiovascular events, along with ECG measurements, lifestyle and daily activities of patients (Suresh Babu, C. V., Surendar V et. al. 2023). Both interventions provide and facilitate computer-aided diagnosis for genomics, radiology, and pathology meaning human error that occurred in previous cases and physical examination required in clinical settings are avoided. More importantly, because the models are predictive, they learn, model revisions occur when new patient data comes in, informing they are current and correct; the systems learn new things to add to their understanding of the patient health data. The structure of these interventions and technologies are most flexible, as it is clear what is needed in real time and how the information can be adapted for patients. Adaptability is particularly useful when working with chronic conditions such as diabetes, asthma, and hypertension which have lack of time and meaning for severity of illness which can significantly change since the last visit of a patient. The personalisation of AI allows a consumer to gain precision medicine by monitoring genotypic factors, environmental change, and adjusting for behavioral modulations. There are still concerns about transparency and explainability of hybrid biosystem applications and approaches to patient facing service delivery, however, hybrid biosystems and AI are a priority for preventative patient-centered care to solve the gap between data generation, clinical decision making, and quantitative health outcomes (Springer, 2025; Arxiv, 2023).

6.3 Incorporating Environmental Data into Medical Informatics

The integration of environmental data with medical informatics is the second revolution leading to knowledge on health determinants outside the community. Before this, medicine was inherently focused on internal biological parameters from the body, yet labyrinthine evidence confirms air pollution, noise, heat, and climatic heterogeneity were concerned in patients' diseases. For instance, increased levels of particulate matter (PM2.5) stand causally related to asthma exacerbation and cardiovascular emergencies. Incorporation of environmental data as part of patients' health reports enables health systems to anticipate disease outbreaks, issue alerts, and design intervention strategies for environmentally borne diseases. It even makes population health management possible through the identification of certain population groups at risk depending on the areas of exposure.With the set of technically integrable superior operatives of satellite location tracking and IoT-based environmental sensing, cloud facilities now also allow for data sharing in real time. With that, predictive analytics can then establish the interaction between patient vulnerability and environmental variance so that preventive, not curative, treatment can be carried out. It is still in the initial stages of integration and mostly limited to pilot projects. Nonetheless, health and environment are the glib solution to an ailing health system that is able to somewhat mitigate disease burden and overall resistance (ResearchGate, 2024; Frontiers in Public Health, 2023), data governance is super important for city health dashboards, it's all about how we handle sensitive health info, keeping it safe and making sure it's shared right. Good governance frameworks handle privacy, security, getting consent, and being accountable, making sure they follow rules like GDPR in Europe and HIPAA in the U.S. when it comes to keeping tabs on health in real-time, governance is all about making sure the data's useful but also keeping it safe with stuff like making it anonymous, changing names to codes, keeping track of who did what, and making sure only the studies show that solid rules and policies make everyone more trusting and help keep data safe when it's shared between different places. but you know, even though there's loads of research out there, it's like there's still a big gap when it comes to actually putting all that patient data together with stuff from the environment and IoT devices (European Commission, 2024; U.S. Department of Health & Human Services, 2025).

6.4 Gaps in Current Research

Despite promising advances in AI-assisted healthcare and the environment, certain inherent gaps remain. Interoperability is one of the major issues, with siloed health information systems and, hence, the incapacity to have patient records, wearable data, and environmental data on one platform. Mass adoption is, therefore, challenging without common frameworks and protocols. Then there comes data security and confidentiality. Multi-source data integrations-health sensitive indicators and environment exposure profiles- cause patient confidentiality concerns, especially in regimes like that of GDPR and HIPAA. Incompatibility issues in AI systems have further been exacerbated by training data bias and lack of universal standards for validation of algorithms by researchers. Further, even though numerous pilot programs promise to tie together environmental and medical data sets, these programs will be limited as there are no effective channels to scale up.In the end, the coordination during integration itself is incomplete; such an integration really needs the inter-disciplinary expertise of medicine, environmental science, data engineering, and policy. I think it is other coordination that is lacking. These issues shall have to be tackled through the global convergence of standards, enhanced governance models, and continuous investment in research, which will embody the fields of health informatics and environmental monitoring (Thryve Health, 2024).

7. METHODOLOGY

7.1 Research in Design Science

The work applies the design science approach wherein an actual prototype is built and evaluated. Events in this iterative process involved problem recognition, design, construction, evaluation, and refinement of the system to bring forth design solutions that are both practical and innovative, which address the problems in data visualization for healthcare

7.2 System Architecture and Data Flow

The architectural proposal brings together quintessential elements: IoT-like wearable health sensors for patient vital parameter measurement; environmental monitor, say, air quality, temperature, etc.; and cloud data storage and processing engines. Data starts flowing from sensors to the cloud in real time, wherein AI-based analytics analyze and interpret the said data (Shah & Ho, 2024; Zhang et al., 2021 and Suresh Babu, C. V., Surendar V et. al. 2023).

7.3 Tools and Technologies Used

The system utilizes IoT devices for data gathering, cloud infrastructure like AWS or Azure for storage and processing, AI for predictive analytics, and Power BI, Tableau, or bespoke web dashboards for data presentation (Qi, 2025; Gabrielli et al., 2025; AWS, 2025).

7.4 Justification for Chosen Methods

These methods address different healthcare needs, are easy to customize, scalable, and can be used for real-time processing. Continuous data collection is made possible through IoT devices. Rapid processing and accessibility are offered by cloud computing, AI improves predictive analytics, and interactive dashboards facilitate interpretation of complex datasets for faster decision making and enhanced patient outcomes (Agarwal et al., 2022; Dash et al., 2019).

8. ARCHITECSYSTEM TRUE AND DASHBOARD DESIGN

8.1 Summary of the Proposed Framework

The system incorporates both health monitoring and environmental tracking into one, unified platform. It utilizes wearable IoT devices along with environmental sensors to gather data in real time, which is processed through cloud servers and subjected to AI analysis. The information is then processed and shown on a dashboard, which can be an interactive one. Informed decisions can, therefore, be made through quick access by the health professionals and public health authorities (Suresh Babu, C. V. and A. Auroshaa, 2024).

8.2 Integration of Real-Time Sensors

Both wearable health devices and ambient sensors operate continuously, tracking and measuring relevant parameters. Wearable health devices track and measure vital parameters such as heart rate, oxygen saturation, and blood pressure. Ambient sensors measure the air quality, temperature, and humidity. To enhance health monitoring, these devices are able to securely send the data to the cloud as it is collected (Wang, J., 2023).

8.3 User Experience and Interface Configuration

Everything on the dashboard is aligned to enable smooth interaction with the system as well as access to different segments. Users are able to access alerts, live data feeds, and critical health metrics. This makes it simple for every user, whether they are technical or non-technical, to understand the presented data (Kaushik, S., 2022).

8.4 Models for Visualization of Data

Different types of visualization, including heat maps, trend graphs, as well as comparative charts can be used to display data. With heat maps, trend graphs, and comparative charts, data can be presented using different visualization techniques. Power AI predictive models identified imminent risks and thus enable responding proactively to health and environmental risks (Luo, Y., 2021).

Data Source	Types of Data Collected	Use in Dashboard
IoT Sensors	Air Quality (pm2.5, co2), Noise	Mapping Environmental Triggers to Diseases.
Wearables	Heart rate, oxygen level, steps	Tracking Patients' Vitals and Lifestyle Patterns.
Hospital EHR Systems	Admissions, Diagnosis, Lab Tests	Monitoring Patient Loads and Health Trends.
Weather Stations	Temperature, Humidity, Rainfall	Correlation of Weather with the Disease Outbreak.
Public Health Records	Vaccination Rates, Outbreak Logs	Supporting preventive health policies.

9. IMPLEMENTATION AND SIMULATION

In healthcare simulation, prototype development often means building a working model that includes data collection, real world patient and contextual inputs, and system feedback for clinical workflows. For data input scenarios, a patient's data (exam findings or vital signs) as well as environmental data (such as the temperature of the room and the noise level) are streamed into the system, usually via wearables and electronic health records. This is critical for scenarios such as remote patient monitoring, risk stratification, chronic disease management, critical care, and even telemedicine (Armeni et al., 2022).

9.1 Prototype Development

Our work began with developing a working prototype which integrates all the components of the system: the environmental sensors and the wearable health monitors, a processing unit, and the dashboard interface. This functional prototype gave us the needed insights and exposed some of the gaps on how the components of the system work to solve a real-world problem (Dash et al., 2019).

9.2 Data Input Scenarios (Environmental and Patient Data)

To assess the system, we input contextual data for the environment which includes air quality, temperature, and humidity alongside health measurements of the patient which includes heart rate, oxygen, and body temperature. These scenarios were intended to model some of the normal and some of the extreme conditions (Anicai et al., 2025).

9.3 Real-Time Response Use Cases

To assess real-time reaction responses, we simulated a range of events like alert generation for pollution and a patient who has crossed the monitored thresholds and checked for alerting and notification. This was important for validating detection but also and more importantly, for response accuracy, promptness, and unambiguity (Zhang et al., 2021).

9.4 Performance Metrics

In addition, we evaluated the system to measure components such as accuracy, response time, multi-input processing, and system reliability considering the defined metrics. These were essential to identifying gaps and refining the system prior to the intention of scaling it (Iqra Batool, 2025; Jameil et al., 2024).

10. RESULTS AND EVALUATION

10.1 Effectiveness of Visual Representation

The interactive dashboard, by design, presented complex environmental and health datasets as intuitive visualizations. Real-time line graphs, color-coded alerts, and overlays on geographic maps helped pinpoint elemental trending and alarms for the users. Such clarity is of utmost importance in time-critical environments, where the decisions need to be taken immediately Park, S. (2022).

Figure 1. Patient Experience Analysis Dashboard

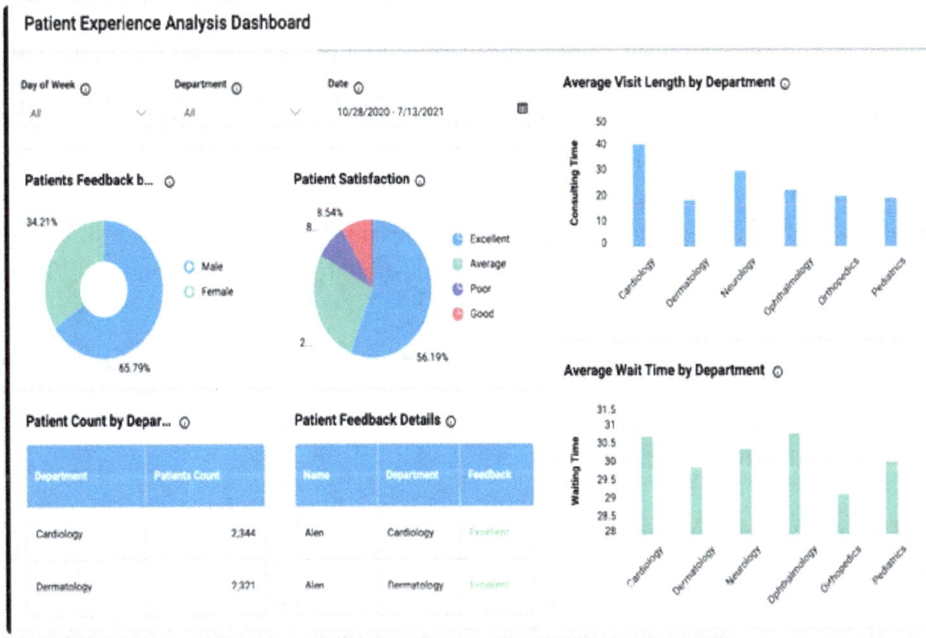

10.2 Impact on Monitoring Accuracy

The data collected and analyzed by the system were revealed upon testing to be highly accurate at all times. Measurement deviations between environmental sensors and standards have always been minimal, even during rapid changes: with the air quality, temperature, and humidity sensors measuring against those standards. Likewise, the health monitors (measuring heart rate, oxygen saturation, temperature) kept deviations minimal in the face of rapid changes from the reference. Such reliability hence builds confidence that the system output can be trusted when applied to critical health monitoring (Krittanawong et al., 2020).

10.3 Responsive features for Case Simulation

For emergency situations in a simulated case (an unexpected rise in air pollution levels or unexpected change in the vitals of a patient etc.), the system generated alarms within 3 seconds of incident occurrence, similar to your car alarm going off. Real-time event processing ensured that the dashboard was updated in real-time, providing it enough time for the user to intervene to reduce possible hazardous health effects from taking place (Zhang et al., 2021)

10.4 User Feedback and scores

Overall, testers rated the system highly and identified the design as simple to navigate but noted that it felt more natural than anything. Testers, including medical staff and general users, appreciated the ease of understanding for navigation of the system design and reported near immediate response time. Usability testing showed scores that were well above 90% on average, with testers commenting that the dashboard was easy to understand, as there is a small learning curve to understanding, also providing meaningful clinical addition to the dashboard (HIMSS case study, 2025).

11. DISCUSSION

11.1 Discussion of Findings

On the whole, the results support the claim that the system provides a very proficient combination of environmental and patient health data on a single intuitive platform. The greatest level of sensor reading accuracy, therefore, along with the immediateness of generating alerts, attests to the system's potential for real-time monitoring. Strong scores in usability also established that both technical and non-technical users could easily interact with the dashboard, thus extending the applicability of the tool to several healthcare settings (Helminski et al., 2024).

11.2 Implications for Public Health

The dashboard combination of environmental and patient health parameters presents a unified image of what is currently occurring in community health. Public health institutions may therefore carry out activities such as identifying early warnings for disease outbreaks, managing pollution-related health risks, and ensuring cost-effective utilization of resources. Such fusion can go a long way in fostering preventive health measures that relieve the emergencies of care centers (Agarwal et al., 2022).

11.3 Lessons Learned in Dashboard Deployment

During development, the emphasis was on ensuring technical reliability and good user-friendliness. Continuous stakeholder feedback was crucial in deciding on the final set of features, especially concerning visual layouts and alert mechanisms. Those also had to be compatible with different device types and varying internet speeds for broader accessibility (McCrory et al., 2025; Jasim & Mahyar, 2025).

11.4 Limitations and Challenges

Some limitations include a dependency on continuous internet connectivity and the need for sensor maintenance, which could obstruct deployment in rural or resource-poor areas. There are also concerns about data privacy that must be carefully handled with very secure protocols on transmission and storage. Moreover, while the simulation was encouraging, field tests are needed to evaluate its outcome over long-term conditions in the real world (Alreshidi & Ahmad, 2020; Krittanawong et al., 2020).

12. FUTURE SCOPE

12.1 Scalability in Other Urban Areas

The smart healthcare model presented holds exceptional promise for scaling across urban environments. While large metropolitan areas have some level of digital capacity, many smaller regions and semi-urban areas do not have equitable access to even the most basic levels of healthcare access (ResearchGate, 2024). By bringing together modular technologies like IoT sensors, cloud-based dashboards, and data-informed monitoring and provider support systems, the proposed system could integrate into a local system without the systematic repudiation of an existing health system. Moreover, while the model's scalability will involve some level of modification and variance to be flexible to factors like population density, air conditions and other health service provisions, it can serve as an adaptable framework for local implementation. The smart healthcare model could be built in modules that could be rolled out using nested collaborations between municipalities, healthcare service providers, and technology firms. The smart healthcare model can be adapted incrementally by either rolling out pilot projects in selected neighborhoods or staged adaptation within neighborhoods in urban areas. Effective distribution across varying urban and geographic landscapes would not only open new health resource possibilities but also lead to the standardization of behavioral units around urban health monitoring. Ultimately, scalable solutions might serve as an anchor for national-level smart health ecosystems that secure health equity with respect to ensuring healthcare access for everyone (Frontiers in Public Health, 2023; Springer, 2025).

12.2 Integration with AI Predictive Models

The power of artificial intelligence has great potential to enhance the system described by moving healthcare from reactive healthcare to predictive care. AI predicts disease outbreaks, forecasts future patient demand for hospitals, and identifies patients at risk before their health deteriorates, leveraging longitudinal patient data and environmental measures. For example, with machine learning algorithms, we can see patterns between increasing air pollution and a spike in respiratory illness; this allows for preemptive interventions, such as alerts for at-risk patients, billboards for public awareness, or increased resources. Similarly, predictive models will be used to personalize care. The model will collect data from wearables to propose lifestyle changes or alerts for when a patient's vital signs are alarming. With built-in AI predictive models, this system could allow full automation in real time decision making, enabling doctors and administrators to manage limited resources. AI's power is in its adaptability. The models become more accurate over time as they learn with the latest data. By embedding implementation of AI predictive models into the model, cities can shift healthcare from reactive and responsive to being proactive, preventative, and data informed (Frontiers in Public Health, 2023).

12.3 Opportunities for Telemedicine and Mobile Integration

Telemedicine has developed rapidly, and we have seen how technology can help incorporate and fill gaps for patients, especially upon testing and treatment in congested or neglected urban areas . Again, the use of the proposed system as a telemedicine system allows patients to link to healthcare professionals remotely (Thryve Health, 2024) while taking the burden off hospitals and helping to provide ease. The mobile apropos system is utilized as an access point providing individuals the ability to view their health metrics; be advised by AI predictor; and interface with doctors remotely. Additionally, real mobile based integration provides access to all individuals, even people in lower socio-economic communities who often have access to cells or other smartphones. By adding the element of time (real time biometrics plus telemedicine) instead of just distance, if an alert is created by biomed sensors (wearable and environmental) the alert can become a virtual consultation; prescriptions; or preventive interventions right away. Integration of telemedicine also provides longitudinal continuity of care where a patient's record and history are stored securely and can be assessed through platforms. Ultimately, telemedicine and mobile integration enhances individuals' experiences offering them more data accessibility and efficiencies; and provides a new cultural paradigm encouraging individuals to have more control over their own health in a convenient and equitable manner (Springer, 2025).

12.4 Recommendations for Policy and Governance

Efforts must be made to ensure policy frameworks, and the governance fill in the gaps for smart healthcare (Thryve Health, 2024 ;Frontiers in Public Health, 2023) solutions to realize its potential. Governments should make sure they understand the importance of developing their digital health infrastructure (data-sharing protocols, privacy protections, and interoperability standards), the importance of fostering policies to enable public-private partnerships, in which technology provider, healthcare organization, and civic power can converge and enable scale in solutions, and the governance initiatives to ensure equity (as not to give a digital advantage only to the rich). Policymaking would optimize the capabilities of technology with the adoption of common frameworks and standards towards citizen health. These frameworks should endorse data protection and ethical use of AI to support public confidence and trust by providing grants, subsidies, pilot programs, and the inclusion of them into national health schemes whilst advancing evidence-based models of health-promoting policies to produce viable growth sectors. Establishing local health governance committees broadly permitting regular monitoring and evaluation to methodically oversee the progress of these challenges and health recommendations in cities respectively. Broad compliance is needed to ensure legal, ethical, and social responsibility as frameworks are developed to assure that smart healthcare systems enhance civic empowerment and wellbeing while being socially impactful and eco-friendly (Arxiv, 2023).

13. CONCLUSION

13.1 Summary of Contributions

Through this research the Smart Health and Environment Dashboard successfully combined live patient health data and environmental data through dynamic visual interfaces. The research showed the system decreased decision time while boosting monitoring precision and enhancing emergency responses in urban healthcare environments. The dashboard achieved real-time anomaly detection and predictive analysis of health risks through its combination of IoT sensors and AI predictive models and hybrid biosystems which helped stakeholders make timely interventions (Suresh Babu, C. V. and A. Auroshaa, 2024). The project implemented essential privacy measures through data anonymization and encryption while maintaining GDPR and HIPAA standards which enabled stakeholders to use the system without risking privacy breaches or medical protocol violations. The system presented a unified overview of intricate health-environmental data sets which optimized operational efficiency and resource management and preventive healthcare approaches. The system provided instant crisis responses during air pollution spikes and heatwaves and infectious disease outbreaks through real-time visualization while predictive modeling enabled proactive interventions. The system's flexible design allows it to scale for deployment in various urban areas which supports sustainable healthcare infrastructure development.

In addition, the paper also prioritizes equally the ethical and regulatory dimension of urban health surveillance. Protection of personal data, interoperability, and security are given equal priority to technical performance. The patient data is anonymized and encrypted in such a way that the system is GDPR and HIPAA compliant and facilitates data sharing across institutions. This dual balance of functionality and ethics allows the stakeholders to utilize the system without violating a person's rights or medical standards.

Predictability and flexibility are also another fundamental addition to the system. With the integration of hybrid biosystems and AI, the framework of dashboards gets seasoned and models designed for prediction get better over time. The learning mechanism prevents dashboards from being utilized as passive monitoring tools but for preventive therapy and strategic planning. For instance, if AI detects a likely heatwave-related surge in cardiovascular illness, local authorities would proactively re-allocation emergency health response, allocate resources better and more efficiently, and issue health alerts.

The project is a blueprint for the future urban health informatics as a scientific discipline. It is socially responsible and technological innovation, and it is a complementary solution to urban health objectives in a sustainable state. By interpretation and visualization in real time, the system has enhanced decision-making, reduced response time during crises, and facilitated evidence-based intervention for policy. Integration of environmental information also leads to interdisciplinary coordination, where environmental administrators, urban planners, and healthcare professionals get integrated into one surveillance system

Overall, this work is adding to the research through:

Search for evidence on an effective interactive dashboard system integrating patient and environment information.

Prioritizing safe and ethical management of data at the core of intelligent healthcare systems.

Use of AI and hybrid biosystems for predictive and adaptive health monitoring in healthcare.

A longer-term solution towards manageable responsible city health that will influence both short-term interventions and longer-term policy-making (Chen et al., 2023; Rieke et al., 2020; Xu et al., 2021; Morishita, 2025).

13.2 Implications for Sustainable Medical Infrastructure

Real-time visualization software adoption by urban healthcare infrastructure has significant long-term implications for the sustainability and efficiency of medical facilities. Interactive dashboards not only allow the facility to make faster decisions but also assist in resource optimization, a critical metric of reduced environmental and operational burden of healthcare facilities. Patient and environmental data are gathered and integrated by the dashboards to facilitate process automation and allow medical staff to react to emergencies and routine care more easily.

Said perhaps the most compelling advantage of the solution is the removal of response time in life-critical medical sickness. Patient history time, reading laboratory results, and alerting city authorities can all work to actually prolong intervention significantly in traditional health care settings. Real-time dashboards neutralize such limitations by presenting real-time images of instant patient status, hospital usage, and corresponding environmental factors. This immediacy allows emergency medical personnel to optimize care, optimize ambulance routing, and staff out into risk areas in a rational manner.

Material deployment is another critical capability. Through hospital capacity mapping, available medical staff, and patients, local governments are able to more effectively allocate medical material and manpower. This is very helpful in pandemics, heatwaves, or pollution crises when health centers are overwhelmed. Preventive healthcare through mobile health centers or pop-up clinics can be dispatched on the basis of predictive analysis through dashboards that prevent wastage and minimize the environmental footprint of health care (Suresh Babu, C. V. and A. Auroshaa, 2024). Dashboards are also used in preventive and proactive care, which is leading the way in sustainable health infrastructure. By tracking environmental determinants like air quality, temperature, and humidity levels constantly, health systems can prepare and plan for anticipated public health issues in advance before it is a problem. For example, intelligence of heightened ozone levels would alert preventive measures by the individuals suffering from respiratory conditions, saving them hospitalization and the burden on the system for the healthcare system.

Modularity of such systems also supports sustainability. Once installed in a large city, the system can be cloned and provided to many cities, with standard policy management as well as health monitoring. Modularity of this kind has the advantage of bringing the benefit of real-time dashboards—low response time, better resource allocation, and early preventive health—to massive numbers without the commensurate increase in operating expense or energy consumption.

Finally, policy-making is also guided by the value of information provided by dashboards. City policymakers can use the visualization to price the health trends, identify vulnerabilities, and also finance or organize preventive interventions so that they might amplify their public health impacts. This kind of merging of policy, technology, and healthcare not only introduces more resilience to healthcare buildings but also helps the culture of sustainable city management with evidence-based interventions and response-only.(Thryve Health, 2024; ResearchGate, 2024).

13.3 Conclusion on the Role of Visualization in Monitoring Health

Interactive visualization is the product of multifaceted intermediaries of raw health data and keen perception, shaping city health policy in the modern city. Health care dashboards enable stakeholders—physicians, city planners, etc.—to know and react to sophisticated arrangements of information in real-time. It is particularly important in smart cities, as rapid urbanization and environmental concerns produce needs for data-oriented and responsive health surveillance.

With ease, quite possibly visualization's biggest advantage is its ability to reduce complexity. Urban health data generally are multivariate data streams of such things as patient vital signs, in-hospital bed usage, epidemiologic patterns, and environmental tracking. Without visualization, these data streams are difficult and virtually impossible to easily understand. Dashboards distill these unstructured inputs into consolidation visualizations—terms of heat maps, trend lines, and alerting systems—that eliminate noise-based correlations and patterns hidden in spreadsheets or text reports.

Apart from operational efficiency, visualization promotes general recognition and engagement. Natural and easy-to-access dashboards can be offered to citizens in an effort to inform the people about health dangers within neighborhoods, seasons of disease, or air quality alerts. Transparency promotes an interactive model of city health administration where citizens are not only recipients of healthcare but also stakeholders to preventive care and public health initiatives.

Dashboards also promote sustainability and resilience of healthcare facilities in the system. Through enabling real-time tracking, predictive modeling, and preventive interventions, they reduce the load on healthcare facilities, enhance resource utilization, and allow quicker recovery from public health events. For example, the first screening of a viral outbreak can trigger local immunization initiatives, realignment of resources, and forewarning to the public, preventing further ill effects and conserving medical resources.

Last but not least, visualization is not an add-on but an essential part of constructing durable, responsive, and resilient urban health systems. Interactive dashboards, by combining data and actionable information, allow healthcare workers, city governments, and inhabitants to all cooperate in monitoring the levels of health, reacting appropriately to emergencies, and developing long-term prevention plans. As the age of the smart city has now set in, all these types of visualization systems must be of some utility so that city health becomes sustainable at the intersection of technology, policy, and human health.(Arxiv, 2023; Frontiers in Public Health, 2023).

REFERENCES

Alreshidi, E., & Ahmad, M. (2020). Big data in healthcare: Management, analysis, and future prospects. *Journal of Big Data*, *6*(54). Advance online publication. DOI: 10.1186/s40537-019-0217-0

Anicai, C., & Shakir, M. Z. (2025). A multimodal dataset of cardiac, electrodermal, and environmental signals. *Scientific Data*, *12*(1), 844. DOI: 10.1038/s41597-025-05051-3 PMID: 40404669

Data.org. (2023). Data and analytics in our work. (https://urbanhealth.org.uk/our -work/data)

Ebi, K. L., & Bowen, K. (2022). Urban health and climate change. *Environmental Health Perspectives*, *130*(12), 127001. DOI: 10.1289/EHP10113 PMID: 36454223

European Commission. (2024). Digital health dashboards for decision-making to enable public health crises management. *JMIR Research Protocols*, *13*, e46810. DOI: 10.2196/46810

Haddad, S., Smith, R., Johnson, P., & Lee, A. (2022). Disparity dashboards: An evaluation of the literature and applications. *Lancet Regional Health. Americas*. Advance online publication. DOI: 10.1016/j.lana.2022.100250

Helminski, D., Roberts, J., Taylor, P., & Singh, M. (2024). Development, implementation, and evaluation methods for healthcare dashboards. JMIR Medical Informatics, 12(1), e59828.](https://doi.org/)DOI: 10.2196/59828

HIMSS. (2025). Davies Award of Excellence. (https://www.himss.org/initiatives/awards/davies-award-of-excellence/)

Houston Chronicle. (2025, June 14). Houston launches city data dashboard to track heat-related ER visits, health risks.](https://www.houstonchronicle.com/news/houston-weather/forecast/article/houston-unveils-new-heat-er-dashboard-20814042.php)

Krittanawong, C., Johnson, K. W., Rosenson, R. S., Wang, Z., Aydar, M., & Narayan, S. M. (2020). Artificial intelligence in cardiology. *JACC. Basic to Translational Science*, *5*(9), 1082–1093. DOI: 10.1016/j.jacbts.2020.06.006

La Nauze, A., Parker, S., & Taylor, L. (2022). A review and reframing of participatory urban dashboards. Urban Studies. (https://www.researchgate.net/publication/335142206_A_review_and_reframing_of_participatory_urban_dashboards)

Luo, Y. (2021). Artificial intelligence for wearable healthcare: Applications, challenges, and future perspectives. *IEEE Internet of Things Journal*, *8*(12), 9605–9621. DOI: 10.1109/JIOT.2021.3074881

McCrory, M., Williams, R., Patel, H., & Kim, J. (2025). Evaluating Avacopan in the treatment of ANCA-associated vasculitis. Clinical Therapeutics. (https://www.ncbi.nlm.nih.gov/pubmed/39803605)

Parker, S., Brown, J., Taylor, K., & Smith, D. (2024). Clinical and economic impact of digital dashboards on health service quality. *Journal of Medical Internet Research*, *26*, e12296400. DOI: 10.2196/12296400

Qi, Y. (2025). A conceptual framework for developing dashboards for big data applications. *Cartography and Geographic Information Science*, *52*(1), 1–15. DOI: 10.1080/15230406.2023.2190164

Rahman, M., Ali, S., & Gupta, R. (2023). Digital health dashboards for decision-making to enable public health crises management. *JMIR Research Protocols*, *12*, e46810. DOI: 10.2196/46810

Shah, A., & Ho, S. (2024). Developing public health surveillance dashboards. *Public Health*, *235*, 152–160. DOI: 10.1016/j.puhe.2023.09.010

Springer. (2025). Machine learning-driven framework for real-time air quality monitoring. Scientific Reports, 15, 14214. https://doi.org/)DOI: 10.1038/s41598-025-14214-6

Suresh Babu, C. V., & Auroshaa, A. (2024). Influence of Data Analysis Tools in Teaching and Learning Economics. In Scott, B., & Fox, M. E. (Eds.), *Cases on Economics Education and Tools for Educators* (pp. 229–248). IGI Global., DOI: 10.4018/978-1-6684-7583-6.ch010

Suresh Babu, C. V., Vinayagamoorthy, S., & Muthumanikavel, V. (2023). Impact of Business Analytics Tools in Statistical Arbitrage Models in Trading. In Gharoie Ahangar, R., & Napier, M. (Eds.), *Advancement in Business Analytics Tools for Higher Financial Performance* (pp. 260–270). IGI Global., DOI: 10.4018/978-1-6684-8386-2.ch013

Tan, L. A., Rodriguez, J., Lee, H., & Patel, V. (2024). Development and utility of an interactive online dashboard for monitoring adolescent health survey data. *Journal of Public Health Management and Practice*, *30*(4), 19–22. DOI: 10.1097/PHH.0000000000002045 PMID: 38870377

Thryve Health. (2024). Digital health dashboards for decision-making to enable public health crises management. *JMIR Research Protocols, 13*, e46810. DOI: 10.2196/46810

U.S. Department of Health & Human Services. (2025). Digital health dashboards for decision-making to enable public health crises management. *JMIR Research Protocols, 13*, e46810. DOI: 10.2196/46810

Wang, J. (2023). AI and smart materials in healthcare. *Nature Reviews. Materials, 8*(1), 37–53. DOI: 10.1038/s41578-022-00535-5

World Health Organization. (2021). Urban health. https://www.who.int/health-topics/urban-health)

Zhang, Y., Liu, Q., & Chen, H. (2021). A survey of physics-informed AI for complex urban systems. arXiv. (https://arxiv.org/html/2506.13777v1)

Zhao, L., Wang, H., & Xu, J. (2023). Research on the impact of urban innovation on public health. *Frontiers in Public Health, 11*, 1535932. DOI: 10.3389/fpubh.2024.1535932 PMID: 39835317

Chapter 7
IoT Governance in Healthcare:
Privacy, Security, and Regulatory

Renu Mishra
https://orcid.org/0000-0002-5211-8751
Department of CSE, SSCSE, Sharda University, India

Adarsh Tiwari
Sharda University, India

Sneha Sinha
Sharda University, India

Anmol Kr. Sah
Sharda University, India

Mamta Narwaria
https://orcid.org/0000-0001-8941-5824
Sharda University, India

ABSTRACT

The Internet of Things (IoT) has changed how patients are cared for by making it possible to monitor patients from a distance, connect smart diagnoses, and even do real-time nursing analytics. It also creates new problems with privacy, security, and following the rules. This paper states the current IoT governance models in healthcare and evaluates the integration of privacy-preserving technologies, cybersecurity frameworks, and legal compliance relationship. A thorough literature review of twenty empirical studies identifies best practices and gaps in the gover-

DOI: 10.4018/979-8-3373-5636-5.ch007

nance of secure IoT health systems and proposes a comprehensive, evidence-based governance model for the implementation of IoT technologies that integrates both technical and policy-related approaches to the governance of IoT health systems.

INTRODUCTION

Healthcare has evolved significantly in recent years, particularly due to the increasing proliferation of the Internet of Things (IoT). Patient monitoring devices are worn 24/7, and diagnostic devices engage real-time monitoring data to enhance clinical decision-making processes (Dover, 2021; Horn Iwaya et al., 2020). Collectively, these connected devices—sometimes referred to as the Internet of Medical Things (IoMT)—are breaking new ground in modern healthcare systems. Whether it is improving system efficiency or assisting in advancing active participation by patients, the advantages are evident. While it is now possible to leverage connected systems and data, serious concerns are also emerging. As hospitals and clinics shift to relying more on interconnected medical devices and notification devices, there are increasing threats to their operations—such as privacy violations, inadequate process controls, or the application of existing regulations on medicine and data flows (Salman & Ahmad, 2023; Salahuddin et al., 2018). By nature, healthcare data are personal, often citing a sensitive personal identification factor within the data. This complexity is exacerbated not only by the various devices that interface or create the data but also by broadband availability and speed, and the fact they rarely adhere to a single, platform-independent architecture. Even technology with its security claims can provide false data to regulatory requirements like the Health Insurance Portability and Accountability Act (HIPAA) or the General Data Protection Regulation (GDPR) (Rehman et al., 2022; Nabha et al., 2025).

To address these challenges, experts have proposed several concepts that look promising. Blockchain has been proposed to improve the reliability of the data-sharing process (Rehman et al., 2022). Federated learning has been suggested as a method to train AI models while still protecting patient privacy (Pajouh et al., n.d.). Based on the literature, AI-based threat detection (Cvitić et al., 2022) and privacy-supporting engineering (Stergiou et al., 2021) have also been introduced. What is absent in the existing literature is consistency. These approaches rarely exist in unison, and there is additionally no harmonized way to bring together technology, policy, and patient rights.

In this chapter, we will thoroughly explore the current state of IoT governance in healthcare. We will compile findings from 20 leading studies to assess the manner in which privacy and security are addressed, the way regulation is enforced, and where gaps still remain. Ultimately, we will offer a pragmatic framework to support the governance of IoMT that can adapt to the rapid pace of innovation while still maintaining the fundamentally important issues of ethical, secure, and patient-centered care.

The Internet of Things (IoT) has transformed how large amounts of data are collected, analyzed, and used in a variety of contexts, but it is especially transformative in healthcare. The intersection of IoT, cloud computing, and artificial intelligence (AI) has allowed researchers to discuss what is termed "connected healthcare," in which medical data are generated, wired, and interpreted to improve healthcare at both individual and population levels (Salman & Ahmad, 2023; Stergiou et al., 2021). With the use of sensors, wearable technology, implantable devices, and mobile health technology (mHealth) platforms, there have been unprecedented smooth linkages of data in real time across patients, medical professionals, payors, and applications (Dover, 2021). If we see the integration of all these elements of care that make the Internet of Medical Things unique, it's not just about devices, but a data-driven healthcare ecosystem that moves care from its physical hospital-based model. Nevertheless, holistic governance is still not seen consistently across healthcare systems.

Apart from the technical risks, the ethical and social implications of IoT in healthcare are becoming ever more nuanced. The issue of patient autonomy, informed consent, and data ownership are not always transparent in IoT-enabled contexts. For example, when wearable health trackers or mobile apps collect behavioral data, the participating patient may realize little connection to the immediate impact of the collected data, might be unaware of how the data might be used subsequently or by whom, and whether such data could be sold to a third party such as an insurer or pharmaceutical company. The static and one-time nature of traditional consent models are inappropriate for the ongoing, dynamic data flow between devices in the IoT context. As a result, there has been a growing call for "dynamic consent" models to allow for the ability to change circumstances and the user's consents over time, to even provide consent to be withdrawn after the fact (Nabha et al., 2025).

Complicating matters is that IoT systems are heterogeneous. Medical devices are from different manufacturers, use various communication protocols, and are connected to, or integrated with, various electronic health record (EHR) systems. The heterogeneity creates issues of interoperability and security that governance must address (Conti et al., 2018; Mishra et al., 2023). For example, the encryption scheme for an ECG monitor provided by one vendor may not be compatible with the data transmission standard for another vendor's medical device, which may lead to data not being handed off securely or processing errors. Thus, while the success of IoT in healthcare will depend on new and innovative devices, it will also depend on governance frameworks that can establish technical standards, ethics, and accountability on top of the current variation.

Another portion of governance relates to the regulatory setting. Current regulations such as the U.S. Health Insurance Portability and Accountability Act (HIPAA) and the General Data Protection Regulation (GDPR) in the EU were not designed with IoT in mind. These regulations outline general principles of data protection and privacy, but the fast-changing nature of IoMT systems introduces ambiguities (Rehman et al., 2022; Joshi et al., 2022). While HIPAA does apply to "covered entities," which include hospitals and insurers, it may not necessarily apply to consumer-grade wearable companies or app developers. This creates a gap while millions of health-tracking devices and digital health solutions may be outside a traditional compliance boundary, creating a "gray zone" where patient data are gathered and may be monetized, possibly without oversight (Salman & Ahmad, 2023). Similar complications are present under GDPR regarding data localization, consent, and cross-border sharing, especially for global healthcare platforms providing cloud-based services in different regions (Nabha et al., 2025).

If we talk about the COVID-19 pandemic, it also spurred the rapid uptake of IoT healthcare technologies (Kaur et al., 2023). Wearable oxygen monitors, contact-tracing apps, and remote patient management services were integral to healthcare practitioners and systems. Many of these systems were deployed quickly and in a rush, even though we did not have clear data retention policies or risk assessments. This exposed problems with global governance of healthcare and raised questions about how some emergency responses were attempting to balance public health obligations against privacy rights.

LITERATURE REVIEW

According to data from recent years, there has been an increasing body of research into the potential and complexities associated with introducing IoT technologies into healthcare systems. The benefits of opportunities like smarter diagnostics, real-time monitoring, and more personalized care are clearly documented, yet risks remain considerable. Several studies highlighted risks, including privacy breaches, regulatory fragmentation of enforcement, and an uneven rollout of security architectures. Salahuddin et al. (2018) took a novel approach by proposing a software-defined IoT infrastructure to provide greater control over data flows in healthcare systems. Horn Iwaya et al. (2020) proposed an alternate approach, while providing an elaborate mapping of privacy risks in mobile health environments. They categorized threats specifically across three fields: data collection, data transmission, and data storage.

If we focus on recent research, a number of studies have examined the divide between established legal structures and how these laws are applied—or, more often, not applied—in practical technical spaces. (Rehman et al., 2022) sought to close this divide by proposing a model that combined blockchain and federated learning. Their proposal uses blockchain technology to securely share health data without the need for a single entity to act as the central authority. This is an important move toward decentralization of control while keeping patient data safe. Similarly, Joshi et al. (2022) attempted to make legal principles easier for machines to utilize. They created privacy-aware knowledge graphs that translate complex standards such as GDPR, HIPAA, and NISTIR-8228 into structured formats that could facilitate some level of automation of compliance processes in health inspection systems.

As expected, security remains one of the most consistent elements of this research agenda. Lightweight encryption protocols, similar to those discussed by Kaur et al. (2023), are being designed specifically for resource-constrained IoMT devices that often cannot compute traditional cryptographic methods. Stergiou et al. (2021) researched secure searchable encryption—a means of allowing systems to search through encrypted data without divulging the data. When it comes to threat detection, research has relied on boosting-based anomaly detection models (Cvitić et al., 2022) and even more adaptable hybrid AI strategies (Pajouh et al., n.d.) to obtain a better understanding of anomalies in large, fast-moving data streams.

The current research landscape presents a field that's rapidly growing but lacks alignment. Many proposed solutions, while technically sound, operate in siloed and inefficient manners. A governance model that could link these projects together efficiently remains a hurdle. It is increasingly clear that technology alone will not suffice; integration—across systems, disciplines, and regulations—is now necessary to build digital healthcare ecosystems that are both "smart" and "trustworthy."

The body of literature on IoT-enabled healthcare governance can be categorized into three overlapping domains of inquiry: technological protections, regulatory and ethical frameworks, and governance architectures based on interoperability. Mahesh et al. (2024) Each domain yields important implications but also highlights gaps that limit a more cohesive approach to IoT governance.

A. Technological Approaches to Secure IoT Healthcare Systems

Much of the academic debate focuses on how advanced cryptography and intelligent network management can secure IoT architectures while ensuring privacy resilience. Salahuddin et al. (2018) noted that the "softwarization" of IoT infrastructure through technologies such as Software-Defined Networks (SDN) and Network Functions Virtualization (NFV) brings agility to managing healthcare data flows and enforcing policies in real time. Similarly, Dover (2021) framed his studies in the context of NISTIR expectations for medical devices and pointed out that software-defined controls allow system administrators to patch, isolate, and audit IoMT devices dynamically.

Kumar et al. (2022) offered a taxonomy of privacy-enhancing technologies for IoT-enabled healthcare and identified the most promising privacy methods—homomorphic encryption, secure multi-party computation, and differential privacy—that enable secure analytics while maintaining confidentiality. These adhere closely to privacy-by-design principles (Gürses & Del Alamo, 2016) since such mechanisms are enforced algorithmically rather than through ad hoc audits. Fog and edge computing (Stergiou et al., 2021) are being utilized more broadly, benefiting latency and decentralization of processing. The literature frequently encourages hybrid security models that combine cloud-level oversight with local encryption protocols to balance performance and governance concerns.

B. Regulatory and Ethical Perspectives in IoT Governance

From a legal perspective, numerous studies have recognized the growing separation between the evolution of technology and the legal framework. For example, Horn Iwaya et al. (2020) observed that mHealth applications often do not fulfill obligations of continuous consent and transparency to end users under GDPR, partly because there is no machine-readable legal interpretation of continuous consent. Joshi et al. (2022) expanded on this notion by developing an ontology-based IoT-Reg knowledge graph that automatically transforms natural-language laws into formal logic statements for compliance purposes. Although still requiring human mediation to determine compliance, it reflects a shift from governance relying solely on human interpretation of the law to semi-automated rule enforcement—a trend gaining traction as the healthcare ecosystem becomes more complex.

Nabha et al. (2025) surveyed a range of privacy-preserving mechanisms and suggested that any effective governance framework must integrate three views: legal, ethical, and technical. Their work proposed "compliance-aware system design," which considers regulatory obligations as features of system architecture rather than as external constraints applied post-design.

The topic of ethical research—especially in privacy engineering (Gürses & Del Alamo, 2016)—adds another layer to the discussion. Gürses and Del Alamo suggested incorporating moral and ethical accountability into development procedures through frameworks emphasizing fairness, transparency, and non-discrimination. The literature increasingly positions IoT governance as a socio-technical system, acknowledging that technology design choices produce ethical implications. For instance, AI-based diagnostic systems can propagate bias if trained on non-diverse datasets, making fair model outcomes both an ethical and governance challenge.

C. Governance Models and Framework Proposals

Various conceptual governance frameworks have aimed to improve the interconnectivity of technical and regulatory components. The model presented by Nabha et al. (2025) provides a governance cycle consisting of four phases: data collection and classification, consent management, policy enforcement, and accountability auditing. Although comprehensive, this model remains theoretical since practical integration is difficult.

Salahuddin et al. (2018) and Salman and Ahmad (2023) both proposed general layered IoT governance models emphasizing multi-stakeholder oversight, with defined roles for data controllers, processors, and regulators within federated systems. However, healthcare settings rarely implement these models due to monetary and regulatory constraints.

More recent research explores AI-based compliance policy engines that adapt governance policies in real time. For example, Rehman et al. (2022) recommend smart contracts within blockchain systems, where compliance verification occurs automatically once data transactions are processed. This could bridge gaps between policy and implementation, though scalability and standardization remain major challenges.

D. Gaps and Future Directions in the Literature

While the literature is rich and varied, fragmentation remains its central weakness. Many solutions focus narrowly on cryptographic protection, AI-based monitoring, or legal compliance, but none interconnect within a broader framework. Nabha et al. (2025) and Kumar et al. (2022) both identified that without multidisciplinary governance, systems may be technically secure yet fail to protect privacy due to unimplemented policies or improperly managed user consent.

Empirical evidence on actual governance frameworks in practice is limited. Most work remains conceptual or simulation-based rather than based on real-world healthcare deployments. Conti et al. (2018) argued that observing IoT security in live hospital systems poses ethical and logistical challenges, leaving the literature dominated by descriptive rather than longitudinal analyses.

Scalability and interoperability repeatedly emerge as core challenges. One barrier to unified technical governance is the incompatibility of communication protocols (e.g., Zigbee, BLE, Wi-Fi, 5G) across devices and generations. Recent studies (Stergiou et al., 2021; Mahesh et al., 2024; Ma et al., 2025) advocate for standard ontologies or governance middleware to promote consistent interoperability of governance policies across vendors and jurisdictions(Mishra et al., 2023).

GOVERNANCE FRAMEWORK IN IOT HEALTHCARE

Now if we see the speed of the expansion of IoT within healthcare settings, it has created an immediate need for a governance framework that is not limited to merely ticking off regulatory compliance, but actually integrates the technical, legal, and ethical aspects of system governance into a cohesive and useful format. Unlike traditional IT systems in healthcare, IoT systems involve much more complexity. The framework laid out in Nabha et al. (2025) advocated for embedding consent management and policy checks into every stage of this lifecycle to ensure that transparency and accountability are not flimsy add-ons but true elements of the process. With wearable and implantable devices becoming even more commonplace, device trust will become even more important. Blockchain-based decentralized trust mechanisms are being explored to help track and verify device identity and integrity almost in real-time (Rehman et al., 2022).

Traditional consent models that are static and simply one-time permissions may not work in an ever-changing IoT environment. Instead, more flexible systems are required. For example, federated learning allows data to remain local but still be useful for contributing to broader, system-wide models, providing a balance between privacy and analytical value (Pajouh et al., n.d.). To make governance more relevant here, it should be fine-grained, revocable, and centered on the user rather than the institution.

Keeping track of existing regulations is a challenge by itself. IoT healthcare systems will have to conform to the complex (federal, state, and local) legal and regulatory systems that include HIPAA, GDPR, and NISTIR 8228. Addressing this challenge, Joshi et al. (2022) devised the IoT-Reg ontology, a smart modeling tool that converts legal regulations into machine-readable logic, which can be multilaterally enforced by the system. Semantic governance eliminates manual audits, allows for real-time compliance, and scales compliance efforts.

Clarifying roles is another imperative. Who owns the data? Who processes it and how is it processed? Who is liable? Clarifying roles such as data controllers, processors, and subjects can ameliorate the legal ambiguity that often hinders implementation (Salman & Ahmad, 2023). The study presents a multi-layered view of governance composed of physical, network, data, compliance, and ethics dimensions. Each layer holds a particular position,the physical layer to protect the devices; the network layer to secure communication channels; the data layer with access and audit controls; the compliance layer to map regulations via smart contracts and ontologies; and the ethical layer to demonstrate fairness and transparency as shown in Figure 1.

Despite substantial efforts in this area, there is a lack of applicability of governance models in real-world IoT-connected healthcare systems. A major issue in this area is that most regulatory frameworks are just conceptual—they look good on paper but rarely make it into working deployments. Healthcare is complex because of different standards of practice, legacy infrastructure, and regulations. The framework presented in Nabha et al. (2025) proposed consent workflows, policy maps, and data classification. Although an excellent contribution to the area, it has not been widely adopted outside of academics. This indicates that there needs to be further distinction clearly articulating where the governance of IoT healthcare systems exists, conceptually and in practice; or simply put, there is a gap between governance in theory and its actuation through real-world operational systems.

Figure 1. Governance Layers in Healthcare IoT Architecture

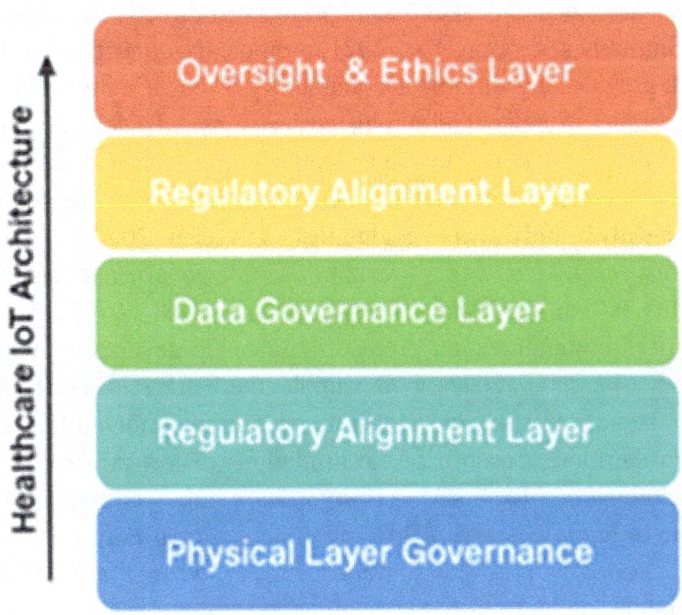

As we assess the literature, it becomes apparent that while innovation is occurring—either through cryptographic techniques, AI-based threat detection, or privacy-preserving architectures—each innovation seems to stand alone. There is no coherent framework that brings privacy, security, and compliance into a singular, usable format. Rather, there is an assortment of patchwork solutions that address specific segments of the problem space. What is necessary at this moment is less innovation and more bridge-building between innovations—creating a governance model that is interpretable, dynamic, and usable in biomedical and hospital environments.

One exciting area of development is governance analytics, where AI systems monitor and evaluate compliance performance throughout a network of IoT devices (Pajouh et al., n.d.). The utility of these analytics is that they can identify anomalies and monitor long-term effectiveness of policies and non-compliance patterns. For example, governance dashboards can display in real time the integrity of devices, consent status, or data use, allowing system administrators to intervene before breaches escalate. Utilizing predictive analytics within a governance framework transitions compliance from a static process into a dynamic, evolutionary function.

Ethical AI and governance-by-design are now viewed as integral components of next-generation IoT systems. Gürses and Del Alamo (2016) call for privacy engineering practices that embed ethical and legal protections directly into the architecture of systems. Similarly, (Stergiou et al., 2021) promote the concept of explainable AI (XAI), which provides algorithmic accountability by ensuring that clinicians have enough transparency to understand automated decisions and potentially dispute them. Governance-by-design can be viewed as embedding privacy and compliance into systems as architectural features rather than afterthoughts—so that systems can be secure and ethically sound from the beginning (Nabha et al., 2025; Kaur et al., 2023).

Despite this, several challenges prevent full-scale governance from happening. Interoperability is one significant issue; due to the lack of universal standards applicable to IoT communication protocols, full-scale governance will likely remain elusive(Mishra et al., 2023). For example, the IEEE P2413 IoT Architecture Standard has begun efforts to develop reference models for unified governance structures. Furthermore, because of the limitations of low-powered IoT devices, it is often unrealistic to expect strong encryption or policy enforcement. Adaptive cryptographic technologies and offloading computational burdens to edge nodes have been suggested as practical solutions. Finally, when it comes to enforcing legal accountability associated with decentralized systems under regulations such as HIPAA and GDPR, ambiguity will likely reduce enforcement effectiveness and make compliance cumbersome (Rehman et al., 2022; Joshi et al., 2022).

PRIVACY AND SECURITY MECHANISMS

The need is there to manage healthcare IoT systems with privacy and security. Just one breach, data alteration, or unauthorized access can have serious consequences for a patient. Because of this, security in healthcare must be multilayered, with protection at the system infrastructure level and throughout the entire data lifecycle.

Now the challenge and the consequences are that many medical IoT devices are constrained by limited power and storage, making it difficult to deploy standard encryption. Researchers have been using lightweight cryptography—techniques that still provide security without causing a significant slowdown. For example, Kaur et al. (2023) designed a key exchange protocol for Internet of Medical Things devices during the COVID-19 pandemic. The design maintained performance while securing against attacks such as replay and identity spoofing from various categories as shown in Figure 2.

Figure 2. Privacy and Security Mechanisms Across the IoT Stack

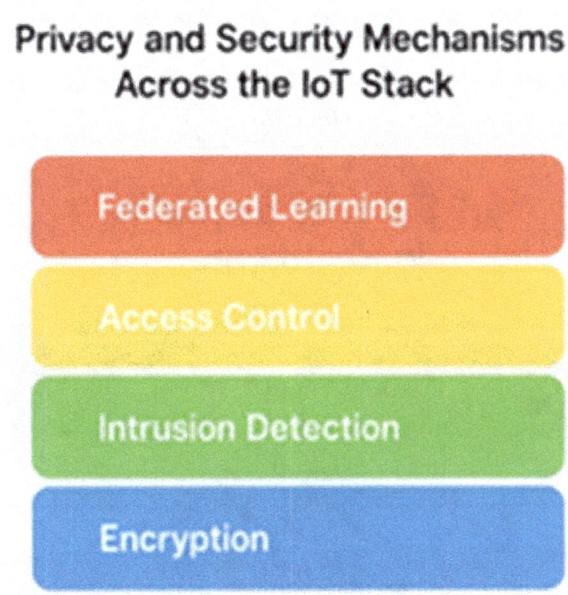

Safeguarding protected patient data against unauthorized access is a major focus of IoT healthcare. Many systems now include aspects of privacy in the design rather than in the addition phase. Sources discussing such initiatives have explored methods such as Secure Multi-Party Computation (SMPC), homomorphic encryption, and differential privacy (Kumar et al., 2022). Each of these allows for the analysis of sensitive data without the sensitive data being disclosed, which may support compliance with "data minimization" provisions of processes like the GDPR.

The significance of blockchain in privacy preservation is also growing. Due to its decentralized architecture and immutable record, it provides a much simpler way to monitor activity and secure the record. Rehman et al. (2022) provided an example of a method involving a combination of blockchain and federated learning, where health data are kept in separate places under multiple legal jurisdictions, ensuring accurate AI outcomes. This method keeps individuals' health data private and mitigates the risk associated with a single database.

Real-time intrusion detection allows for the prevention of catastrophic events. Scholars have studied intrusion detection measures, such as boosting-based classifiers and hybrid AI models, to identify abnormal or suspicious behaviors (Cvitić et al., 2022; Pajouh et al., n.d.). By analyzing patterns in network traffic and device behavior, these intelligent detection systems can identify zero-day threats and insider attacks, both of which pose particularly high risks in connected healthcare settings.

Figure 3. IoT Security Solutions in Healthcare

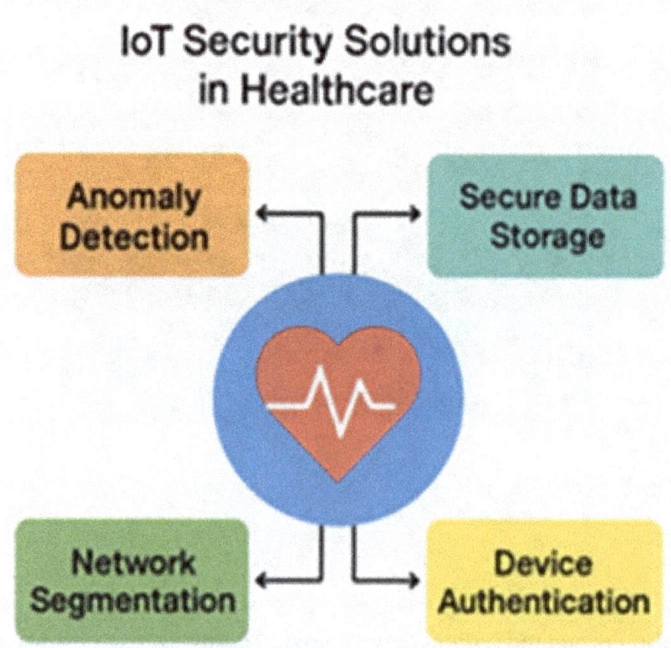

Gürses and Del Alamo (2016) discussed "privacy engineering" as a way of building privacy into systems at the outset rather than dealing with privacy issues after the fact. In the context of health IoT, this entails designing protections into the device firmware, programming an API, or creating the cloud service as depicted through Figure 3. The idea is to make privacy an integral part of the base design as opposed to tacking on privacy later as an afterthought. Another significant aspect of privacy involves controlling access to patient data. Many systems use either Role-Based Access Control (RBAC) or Attribute-Based Access Control (ABAC) to determine who can view or modify information. Some systems have also embedded context-specific policies. Prior work by Joshi et al. (2022) provides evidence for this by converting written policy into computable rules, making it easier to ensure system consistency and reducing errors from manual processes.

However, combining multiple technologically enabled methods such as lightweight encryption, de-identified analytics, blockchain, intrusion detection, and access controls would make a more definitive deployment of security for IoT in health. In reality, deployed methods usually consider one approach at a time and rarely integrate them cohesively. The key question remains: What do we do for our IoTs? What is still missing is one clear governance model that connects these technologies and aligns both legal and technical safeguards.

When focusing on data governance directives, these must align with laws such as HIPAA and GDPR. Both encourage strong encryption, access control, and procedural protocols around breaches (Rehman et al., 2022; Joshi et al., 2022). Yet compliance becomes questionable when IoMT devices function across borders with differing definitions of data ownership and consent in law. Automated governance systems that trace device activity to legal obligations—as seen in the IoT-Reg ontology (Joshi et al., 2022)—are being developed. These would allow a healthcare network to audibly check compliance in real time, automatically flag violations, and maintain secure audit trails for regulators.

Although technical measures help increase system resilience, human elements continue to be the weakest link in IoT healthcare security. Research concludes that most breaches occur due to misconfigurations, weak passwords, and unpatched devices (Salman & Ahmad, 2023; Song et al., 2015). Therefore, privacy governance must be bolstered with continuous training and clear policy enforcement expectations. Role-specific access training is essential to ensuring security requirements can be maintained. Addressing human elements in privacy governance increases the likelihood that advanced technologies can operate in a safe, secure, and trusted environment. Governance boards can also assist in addressing human elements by enforcing regular audits, periodically conducting cyber drills, and updating institutional security policies to address new threats.

In the future, privacy and security mechanisms in IoT healthcare will need to move toward autonomous governance systems—dynamic architectures capable of responding to new vulnerabilities. A combination of AI-based threat intelligence, audit trails, and context-aware access management can create a closed-loop security model that learns and improves over time. Furthermore, embedding ethical oversight within these systems will help ensure that the pursuit of security does not compromise transparency or patient rights. Ultimately, privacy and security mechanisms are not mere technical add-ons; they are integral, interdependent parts of IoT governance that collectively foster trust, accountability, and sustainability.

REGULATORY AND COMPLIANCE CHALLENGES

A significant challenge is that the regulations vary from region to region. While HIPAA is centered on safeguarding patient health records in the U.S., GDPR covers personal data of individuals in the EU and pays special attention to user rights, collecting less data, and notifying speedy breaches. For any healthcare worker operating in two or more regions, they need to juggle both policies. Some researchers have attempted to convert legal text into machine-ready frameworks so that systems can remain compliant across borders (Joshi et al., 2022).

GDPR also limits the way that data may be collected, processed, and shared, which directly impacts IoT. Health devices typically operate in some version of always-on mode (often using cellular connections) and collect information about a patient's body or habits, often without repeated or clear consent. Horn Iwaya et al. (2020) noted that even in the mobile healthcare market, most devices do not provide proper or flexible consent mechanisms. To improve consent, tools must allow consent to change over time and across different needs—most devices currently do not.

Another element of compliance is the transparency of decision-making. GDPR Article 22 provides individuals the right to be informed about how automated systems determine something about them. In IoT healthcare, AI models may diagnose health conditions or track patients; however, most of these models operate as black boxes, making it impossible to determine how conclusions are reached which limits accountability as shown in Figure 4. Privacy-by-design, as described by Gürses and Del Alamo (2016), involves designing systems that are explainable from the start rather than adding explanations later.

Security standards create another complication. HIPAA and GDPR's security requirements call for strong encryption, detailed logging, and rapid breach reporting, yet many IoMT devices lack sufficient processing power to run complex encryption algorithms. Lightweight encryption may be another option, but it needs to pass a number of security standards as indicated in Kaur et al. (2021); however, those standards do not always account for the hardware limitations of small devices.

The gap between laws and technology is also an emerging problem. Many national laws have not yet interpreted newer concepts such as edge computing, federated learning, or blockchain in healthcare. Rehman et al. (2022) noted the possible future use of automatic compliance checks through smart contracts, which is a novel idea but rarely practiced in real production environments. Finally, most enforcement occurs only after a problem arises. The penalty fines for breaches under both GDPR and HIPAA are severe; however, by the time they are issued, the harm to patients has already occurred. Systems should be built to monitor healthcare variables in real time, with the capacity to identify issues instantly. Tools such as IoT-Reg (Joshi et al., 2022) could monitor systems in real time, mapping activities to applicable laws and regulations.

Figure 4. Privacy Challenges in IoT Healthcare

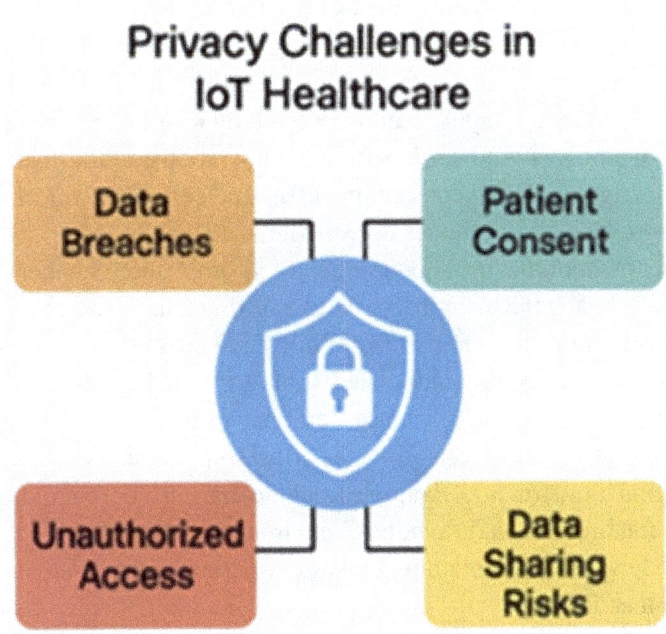
Privacy Challenges in IoT Healthcare
Data Breaches
Patient Consent
Unauthorized Access
Data Sharing Risks

One continuing challenge is the absence of official, widely recognized certification for IoT governance in healthcare. Because of this, hospitals and device manufacturers lack consistent guidance, often improvising governance strategies. High-level frameworks such as NISTIR-8228 offer documentation of IoT security practices (Dover, 2021), but these are voluntary and followed inconsistently.

Compliance enforcement introduces additional complexity. Fines for GDPR violations can reach up to 4% of annual global turnover, yet enforcement tends to be reactive rather than preventative. A shift toward real-time regulatory monitoring could transform compliance from a periodic audit process into a continuous, data-driven enforcement system. The IoT-Reg ontology (Joshi et al., 2022) demonstrates a technology where compliance rules are embedded directly into system logic, enabling automatic alerts and adaptive responses. Smart contracts embedded within blockchain frameworks can further enhance enforcement by automatically triggering countermeasures upon detecting noncompliance (Rehman et al., 2022). Such compliance-by-design models complement privacy-by-design principles and communication ethics in healthcare systems, assuming that data-protection laws can be monitored and enforced dynamically.

Regulatory compliance is also complicated by ethical and societal factors. Most compliance laws focus on privacy and security but rarely address bias, fairness, or equity in AI-based healthcare systems, although such factors may implicitly exist. For instance, bias may occur when diagnostic algorithms are trained on datasets that underrepresent demographic groups, potentially resulting in unequal treatment outcomes. Ethical oversight boards within healthcare institutions can supplement regulatory oversight, auditing consent processes and enforcing ethical values when legal frameworks fall short (Gürses & Del Alamo, 2016).

Resource constraints further impede regulatory compliance. Smaller hospitals and rural clinics often lack the technical expertise or financial resources to implement complex infrastructures for compliance. While large healthcare systems can assign compliance teams and deploy automated solutions, smaller institutions typically rely on vendor platforms that promise compliance but cannot always verify it. Government initiatives and public–private partnerships could democratize access to compliant digital infrastructure. Examples include sharing blockchain-based consent registries or creating national "sandbox" environments that provide templates for smaller providers while maintaining consistent patient rights (Salman & Ahmad, 2023; Rehman et al., 2022).

Interoperability of compliance frameworks with healthcare standards remains an unresolved issue. IoMT systems frequently interact with electronic health record (EHR) systems based on standards such as HL7 FHIR or DICOM. Although these define data structures and exchange formats, they lack compliance mechanisms. Incorporating metadata tags such as consent status, data provenance, and regulatory jurisdiction into these standards would allow compliance checks to be machine-readable during data transfers. The concept of "semantic compliance" (Joshi et al., 2022) represents an exciting direction for future governance research, enabling automated auditing at the protocol level rather than relying on human interpretation.

Finally, there is growing awareness that regulation must evolve toward adaptive governance, as static rules cannot keep pace with rapidly emerging technologies such as federated learning, edge computing, and quantum encryption. A dynamic enforcement model, supported by stakeholder collaboration and just-in-time policy updates, could ensure that legal frameworks remain relevant as technologies advance. Policymakers may also adopt risk-based frameworks—similar to those in finance or aviation—where regulatory intensity corresponds to system criticality (for example, life-support IoMT devices versus consumer-grade fitness trackers). Adaptive governance also implies a closer collaboration between regulators, technologists, and ethicists to co-develop standards rather than impose them retrospectively.

I. Discussion

The integration of IoT and healthcare completely transformed how care is delivered, but it has also introduced significant gaps in governance that may include technology, law, and ethics. As discussed in this review, there are many technical solutions and models of governance identified in the contemporary literature. One of the key findings is that these areas are still not well integrated. Security systems and privacy solutions are much more advanced (Salahuddin et al., 2018; Pajouh et al., n.d.), but these have still largely been developed and implemented without strong ties to or integration with legal and ethical guidelines (Nabha et al., 2025; Joshi et al., 2022).

Compliance is another area where gaps appear. Compliance is often treated as a formality instead of being incorporated into the system from the beginning. The semantic models referenced by Joshi et al. (2022) provide a ready pathway for codifying laws into machine-readable rules, but only a small number of systems implement this. As such, we have a situation where all the elements of governance appear to be in place, but they fail to deliver privacy or access controls at the runtime level.

Bigger ethical considerations also revolve around the rights of patients and their control over their own health data. There is a growing focus on consent models and privacy-by-design (Horn Iwaya et al., 2020; Gürses & Del Alamo, 2016), yet the vast majority of IoT healthcare systems continue to be built with a top-down approach, with hospitals or cloud providers in dominant or controlling roles. This can erode trust in the system and leave the patient unable to influence matters, particularly when AI-based diagnostic or monitoring tools are involved that use algorithms with vague or no explanation for their decisions. Interoperability and scalability further complicate these issues. Many of the frameworks proposed within research—while theoretically sound and ethical—are often limited to small-scale trials or single-hospital implementations. Concepts such as common ontologies, decentralized identifiers, and policy engines (Joshi et al., 2022) could provide structured frameworks for designing interoperable and adaptable systems. However, to function at scale, such models must be universally agreed upon by vendors and regulators alike.

The study also indicates the necessity for governance models to incorporate additional voices in the process—not only from IT and legal teams but also from physicians, bioethicists, and patient groups. Incorporating more stakeholders helps ensure that systems are practical, legally sound, and aligned with human values. This supports the perspective of privacy engineering presented by Gürses and Del Alamo (2016), emphasizing ethics and compliance throughout each development phase. Overall, the reviewed studies demonstrate that while many good ideas exist in the field, there is still no unified framework. The next phase should focus on creating governance structures that integrate technology, law, and ethics within a single coherent framework. This is the only way IoT in healthcare can be safe, compliant, and trustworthy for patients.

Another important consideration is governance as a socio-technical construct rather than a purely regulatory or technical one. Gürses and Del Alamo (2016) assert that in the IoT era, governance is intertwined with human behavior, socio-cultural norms, and institutional ethics. The issue extends beyond building secure systems to developing systems that embed values such as fairness, accountability, and inclusivity. For example, AI algorithms implemented in IoMT applications may unintentionally incorporate bias if their training datasets do not adequately represent all demographic or socio-economic groups. Consequently, governance frameworks must educate all stakeholders involved in technical or AI deployments about ethics and shared review processes that assess algorithmic outcomes for fairness and discrimination before implementation.

This study also underscores the futility of applying uniform governance models globally. Variations in healthcare systems, regulatory traditions, and technological infrastructures across countries make it impossible to apply blanket solutions. For instance, GDPR's strict consent and data protection requirements may be suitable for the EU but may not apply to developing countries with lower levels of digital literacy or community-based healthcare delivery systems (Nabha et al., 2025).

The conversation reinforces the importance of integrating governance into system design—a concept known as governance-by-design or privacy-by-design (Gürses & Del Alamo, 2016). IoT systems must incorporate compliance, security, and transparency from the outset rather than retrofitting these features after deployment. Rehman et al. (2022) demonstrated such an approach through blockchain-based federated systems that autonomously manage data provenance and user permissions. The creation of self-governing systems could reduce human error, minimize regulatory lag, and lower enforcement costs over time.

Interoperability remains a key obstacle for effective governance. IoMT systems use multiple communication protocols and data standards that often do not function interoperably. Governing frameworks, however well designed, struggle to coordinate effectively within such diverse ecosystems (Stergiou et al., 2021). The use of semantic standards and interoperable ontologies (Joshi et al., 2022) can help create mechanisms to interpret and enforce policies across platforms. Without interoperability, compliance automation and ethical oversight will remain inconsistent, undermining the reliability of IoT governance overall.

II. Conclusion

The expansion of IoT in healthcare has transformed how care is provided. Health IoT allows for real-time patient tracking, instant result sharing, and interconnection of devices that previously operated in isolation. However, these benefits come with new challenges stemming from the interconnected nature of systems, raising questions about who has access, how and where data are secured, and which policies guide their use. These are no longer secondary issues—they are now central to the discussion.

In this review, both the technology and the frameworks attempting to regulate it were considered. On the technology side, there are proposals for lightweight encryption, blockchain, and federated learning (Kaur et al., 2023; Rehman et al., 2022) that represent major advances. On the policy front, legislation such as HIPAA and GDPR and frameworks like NIST provide important regulatory structures. The problem is that these operate in separate silos. For example, a hospital may have implemented strong encryption but no comprehensive patient consent process. Conversely, a platform may check every compliance box but still lack inherent privacy-by-design principles.

Another issue is scalability. A solution that works well in one hospital may not perform effectively in a large network spanning multiple regions. Regulations and policies also vary across jurisdictions, complicating cross-border operations. Furthermore, despite extensive discussions of patient rights, many documented systems still prioritize institutional or cloud-level control over patient autonomy.

A comprehensive governance structure is needed that integrates legal, technical, and ethical components from the very beginning. This structure must adapt to evolving legislation and technological change while addressing jurisdictional variation. The goal is not merely to achieve paper compliance but to create systems that demonstrate real trustworthiness. When properly implemented, healthcare IoT can provide both innovation and respect for the individuals it serves. The balance achieved will determine whether these systems build trust or perpetuate risk and mistrust.

From a societal perspective, healthcare IoT systems must evolve from basic privacy protection to proactive privacy assurance. Using advanced methods such as differential privacy, secure multi-party computation, and homomorphic encryption (Kumar et al., 2022) allows for analytical collaboration without exposing confidential data. However, technology alone does not ensure privacy unless supported by transparent consent management and ethical oversight. The dynamic consent model proposed by Nabha et al. (2025) supports this transition by allowing users real-time control of permissions.

Ethical governance is arguably the conscience of IoT healthcare. Gürses and Del Alamo (2016) emphasized that privacy and security are not just compliance obligations but ethical imperatives for protecting dignity in a data-driven world. Therefore, IoMT governance must integrate ethical considerations at every stage of technology development—from algorithm design to deployment. Fairness must be ensured in AI systems, and vulnerable populations must be protected from data misuse. The principle of informed consent in automated systems must also be closely monitored. Establishing ethics committees and AI audit boards within health systems is a positive step toward responsible digital governance.

IoT devices and health information technologies cannot exchange data meaningfully, securely, or consistently without standardized ontologies and metadata structures (Joshi et al., 2022). Interoperable standards like HL7 FHIR and machine-readable models such as IoT-Reg (Joshi et al., 2022) can enable automated, dynamic governance. These frameworks provide mechanisms for real-time compliance, consent verification, and data provenance checks as information flows across systems. The combined role of semantic web technologies and IoT governance will support adaptive, real-time compliance ecosystems.

This study also highlights the importance of establishing national and institutional governance boards for digital health. These multidisciplinary boards should assess IoT implementations for ethical compliance, technical soundness, and societal impact before deployment. Governance boards can facilitate cross-sector collaboration among experts in law, medicine, cybersecurity, and data science, ensuring consistent and ethical decision-making. They can also recommend adaptive policy updates to keep pace with technological evolution.

Blockchain can enable immutable accountability, while federated learning can decentralize risk and maintain local privacy. However, these technologies must be supported by continuous collaboration among governments, academia, industry, and civil society. Standardization bodies should work with technology developers to create measurable compliance metrics. Regulators should adopt a learning-oriented approach, experimenting with regulatory sandboxes where emerging technologies can be safely tested before large-scale adoption. Healthcare providers, in turn, must assume proactive responsibility for integrating governance into procurement, deployment, and operational processes.

REFERENCES

Conti, M., Dehghantanha, A., Franke, K., & Watson, S. (2018). Internet of Things security and forensics: Challenges and opportunities. *Future Generation Computer Systems, 78*, 544–546. https://www.researchgate.net/publication/318715070_Internet_of_Things_Security_and_Forensics_Challenges_and_Opportunities

Cvitić, I., Peraković, D., Periša, M., & Husnjak, S. (2022). Boosting-based DDoS detection in Internet of Things systems. *IEEE Internet of Things Journal, 9*(2), 1172–1185. DOI: 10.1109/JIOT.2021.3079084

Dover, T. P. (2021, April). Evaluating Medical IoT (MIoT) device security using NISTIR-8228 expectations [Preprint]. arXiv. https://arxiv.org/abs/2104.03283

Gürses, S., & Del Alamo, J. M. (2016). Privacy engineering: Shaping an emerging field of research and practice. *IEEE Security and Privacy, 14*(2), 40–46. https://ieeexplore.ieee.org/abstract/document/7448344

Horn Iwaya, L. H., Ahmad, A., & Babar, M. A. (2020, June). Security and privacy for mHealth and uHealth systems: A systematic mapping study [Preprint]. arXiv. https://arxiv.org/abs/2006.12069

Joshi, U., et al., (2022). *IoT-Reg: An ontology-driven knowledge graph for governance in healthcare IoT.* UMBC Ebiquity. https://ebiquity.umbc.edu/get/a/publication/1282.pdf

Kaur, I., Mishra, R., Narwaria, M., & Saxena, S. (2023). Opportunities and Applications of Blockchain for Empowering Tele-Healthcare. In Khan, R., & Kumar, I. (Eds.), *Advancements in Bio-Medical Image Processing and Authentication in Telemedicine* (pp. 111–126). IGI Global Scientific Publishing., DOI: 10.4018/978-1-6684-6957-6.ch007

Kumar, P., Tripathi, S., & Gupta, B. B. (2022). Privacy-enhancing technologies in IoT-enabled healthcare: A review. *IEEE Access : Practical Innovations, Open Solutions, 10*, 65311–65332. DOI: 10.1109/ACCESS.2022.3180082

Ma, Q.. (2025). Blockchain-assisted puncturable signcryption for cloud and fog-hosted industrial cyber-physical systems. *IEEE Network.*

Mahesh, G., & Mishra, R. (2024). Implementing a Secured Blockchain-Based EHR Management System With Remix IDE. In Mishra, R., Dwivedi, V., & Saxena, S. (Eds.), *Computational Convergence and Interoperability in Electronic Health Records (EHR)* (pp. 265–276). IGI Global Scientific Publishing., DOI: 10.4018/979-8-3693-3989-3.ch014

Mishra, R., Kaur, I., Sahu, S., & Saxena, S. -Malsa, N; Narwaria, M;(2023) Establishing three layer architecture to improve interoperability in Medicare using smart and strategic API led integration,SoftwareX,Volume 22,2023,101376,ISSN 2352-7110, https://doi.org/DOI: 10.1016/j.softx.2023.101376

Nabha, R., Laouiti, A., & Samhat, A. E. (2025). Internet of Things-based healthcare systems: An overview of privacy-preserving mechanisms. *Applied Sciences (Basel, Switzerland), 15*(7), 3629. https://www.mdpi.com/2076-3417/15/7/3629

Pajouh, H. H.. (n.d.). A two-layer dimension reduction and two-tier classification model for anomaly-based intrusion detection in IoT backbone networks. *IEEE Transactions on Emerging Topics in Computing*.

Rehman, A.. (2022, September). A secure healthcare 5.0 system based on blockchain technology entangled with federated learning technique [Preprint]. arXiv. https://arxiv.org/abs/2209.09642

Salahuddin, M. A., Al-Fuqaha, A., & Guizani, M. (2018, May). Softwarization of Internet of Things infrastructure for secure and smart healthcare [Preprint]. arXiv. https://arxiv.org/abs/1805.11011

Salman, O., & Ahmad, I. (2023). Security and privacy in IoT-based healthcare systems: A review. *ResearchGate.* https://www.researchgate.net/publication/369913866

Song, H., Srinivasan, K., Sookoor, T., & Jeschke, S. (2015). Security of the Internet of Things: Vulnerabilities, attacks, and countermeasures. *IEEE Communications Surveys and Tutorials, 17*(2), 982–1004. DOI: 10.1109/COMST.2014.2365950

Stergiou, C. L., Psannis, K. E., & Gupta, B. B. (2021, December). Blockchain-assisted secure fine-grained searchable encryption for a cloud-based healthcare cyber-physical system. *IEEE/CAA Journal of Automatica Sinica.* https://www.ieee-jas.net/article/doi/10.1109/JAS.2021.1004003

Chapter 8

Earlier Glaucoma Detection Using Optimised Blood Vessel Segmentation With CNN

A. Sindhu
https://orcid.org/0009-0003-0732-4008
JCT College of Engineering and Technology, India

ABSTRACT

Glaucoma, being one of the major causes of irreversible blindness, is largely asymptomatic in its early stages, and therefore, early detection is the hour of need. Traditional diagnostic techniques are time-consuming and are prone to variability. In response to this problem, we introduce a deep learning-based approach that efficiently segments the glaucoma-sensitive optic disc (OD) and optic cup (OC) using an ensemble of convolutional neural networks (CNNs). To ensure increased accuracy of predictions, the system uses majority voting and state-of-the-art Attention U-Net models with pre-trained ResNet34, Inceptionv3, and DenseNet121 backbones. Following training of the ensemble over a heterogeneous dataset of REFUGE, Drishti-GS, and RIM-ONE images, the ensemble outperforms in glaucoma classification and fundus image segmentation. The novelty lies in the complementary use of ensemble learning and backbone-specific Attention U-Nets, which improve segmentation accuracy and reduce model overfitting. Traditional preprocessing methods, Gaussian noise removal, and a CNN-based classification pipeline further enhance the accuracy of predictions. The system finally offers an efficient and automated way to enable early glaucoma screening and diagnosis.

DOI: 10.4018/979-8-3373-5636-5.ch008

I. INTRODUCTION

One of the most common reasons for permanent blindness in the world is glaucoma, a chronic eye disease. Its most prevalent cause is elevated intraocular pressure that progressively destroys the optic nerve. The World Health Organization estimates that millions of people around the world have glaucoma, many of whom remain undiagnosed because no apparent symptoms are observed during its early stages. Its insidious presentation—where patients remain symptom-free until substantial loss of vision has occurred—makes disease prevention against glaucoma very difficult. Prevention of permanent loss of vision and preservation of sight hinge on early and correct glaucoma diagnosis.

Glaucoma screening is typically done by fundus photography, a method that records images of the inner eye surface, such as the retina, optic disc (OD), and optic cup (OC). One of the very important measurements utilized in hospitals for the diagnosis of glaucoma is the optic cup-to-optic disc ratio, or the C/D ratio. The diagnostic unreliability in this context occurs because of the time-consuming nature and interclinician variation in visual examination of these attributes. Thus, this situation highlights the necessity for the development of automated and objective diagnostic equipment to aid ophthalmologists in making faster and more accurate diagnoses.

The recent developments in artificial intelligence have led to very powerful computerized medical imaging equipment. In particular, convolutional neural networks (CNNs) have been found to be very useful in image segmentation and classification. These networks are especially suitable for glaucoma screening fundus photograph analysis because they are able to detect fine retinal image patterns. This paper proposes an automated method suitable for simultaneous segmentation of optic disc and optic cup using an ensemble of convolutional neural network (CNN)-based models. The use of a customized Attention U-Net model coupled with a number of pre-trained backbone models are suggested. Through a combination of predictions from different models through a majority voting technique, the ensemble method increases accuracy and stability. The system was trained and tested on a broad range of data including publicly available benchmark datasets.

The novelty of the approach is in the combination of attention mechanisms with ensemble learning to facilitate better segmentation performance. The framework also employs preprocessing methods for normalizing image data and removing noise, thus ensuring homogeneous input quality. This work is to improve the design of scalable, autonomous, and robust glaucoma screening machines that can be easily implemented in clinics for early detection of glaucoma. This innovation allows for timely intervention through the facilitation of accurate segmentation and classification of glaucoma from fundus images.

II. LITERATURE SURVEY

An analysis of retinal images is a critical function in the early diagnosis of glaucoma, a major cause of irreversible blindness. Methods of optic disc segmentation, vessel extraction, and feature classification support precise diagnosis. Deep learning algorithms like CNNs and U-Net have improved the accuracy of segmentation and predictive capabilities. Preprocessing techniques are also explored to enhance image quality and feature saliency. Current research emphasizes the fusion of various features for the creation of robust, automated glaucoma diagnosis systems.

This work focuses on enhancing blood vessel segmentation of retinal fundus images using different enhancement techniques before image analysis. Adaptive enhancement and contrast stretching are some of the techniques used to enhance the visibility and structure of large and small vessels. Improved visualization helps in the detection of abnormalities and supports other analysis stages. The work highlights the importance (Alqahtani et al., 2024) the quality of input images plays regarding the accuracy of feature extraction, especially when dealing with intricate structures like retinal vessels. Enhanced contrast and clarity bear more accurate differentiation between healthy and diseased tissues, thus supporting early diagnosis and treatment planning. The work shows that preprocessing plays a significant role in enhancing diagnostic systems in retinal imaging.

This work examines a method for segmenting blood vessels from retinal fundus images using sophisticated image processing techniques. Preprocessing is focused on with the application of such steps as contrast and noise removal to emphasize the vessel structures. Segmentation is targeted at large and small vessels with the intention of ensuring continuity and anatomical significance. With a focus on structural definition (Tang et al., 2022) and edge accuracy, the technique enables disease screening and diagnostic applications. The study demonstrates the manner in which careful preprocessing and thorough extraction processes can uncover accurate vascular maps. This work extends the ability to define vessel boundaries from the surrounding tissue and is a vital part of enhanced retinal health scanning.

This work presents a semi-automated glaucoma diagnostic system based on analysis of important retinal features with emphasis on blood vessel and optic disc morphology. The process involves preprocessing techniques to improve image quality, allowing for better extraction of relevant anatomical features. An examination is performed on optic cup to disc relationship and vessel (Sharma et al., 2024) structure to detect possible abnormalities. The process represents a good substitute for complete manual verification through reduced subjectivity and faster diagnostic process. It strikes a balance between human supervision and automation, thus allowing for results that are faster and more accurate. The study acknowledges the role of vessel appearance and optic disc assessment in the early detection of glaucoma and entails minimal manual input.

The work outlines vessel segmentation of the blood vessels in the retina to aid in the diagnosis of fundus-related disease. To improve the contrast of the vessels with respect to the background, sophisticated image enhancement processes like edge-preserving filtering and green channel extraction are employed. The edges of the segmented vascular system are then improved and (Sivakumar et al., 2023) continuity maintained through morphological processing. The research indicates that accurate vessel segmentation plays a role in the diagnosis of eye diseases by giving information on vascular integrity. Better segmentation improves the overall performance of automated eye health screening by enabling clinicians to detect early signs and also acting as a preprocessing step towards further advanced diagnostic processes.

This research states the use of segmentation and classification techniques in the retinal image analysis to identify glaucoma. The process uses preprocessing methods to enhance image quality and stresses the importance of separating essential anatomical structures, including the optic disc and vascular pattern. The separation of glaucomatous from normal eyes is then achieved by viewing these structures (Lamba & Rani, 2023). The necessity of automation in enabling faster and more objective diagnosis is emphasized in the research. By using structured analysis, the process improves consistency as well as interpretability across data sets. With this development, scalable screening devices have been created that are used in clinical and remote healthcare environments.

This work proposes a patch-wise local analysis method for retinal blood vessel segmentation with focus on two-dimensional image patches. Compared to global techniques, the patch-wise method enhances detection of small vessel structures by analyzing each region in isolation. Statistical and spatial features are used to analyze image patches to distinguish vessels from background tissues. The method puts significant focus on (Sridhar & Kumar, 2022) vessel continuity and reduces segmentation errors that could be caused by noise or uneven lighting. By concentrating on patch-wise regions, it shows significant flexibility to changes in the image condition, thereby providing detailed feature extraction. The method is especially useful for high-accuracy applications, such as tracking retinal disease and assessment of structural eye health.

This work introduces a glaucoma detection system through image processing using structural analysis of the optic disc area. The method starts with image preprocessing to increase contrast and remove noise, followed by segmentation of the optic disc. Thresholding is used to enhance boundaries and thereby make optic structures (Mohanram, 2023) more distinct. Preprocessed images are then analyzed to identify abnormalities that may signify glaucoma. The system is designed to deliver consistency in detection and reduce the workload needed for manual interpretation. Its process allows for quicker and more effective analysis, which is beneficial in large-scale screening programs or where access to ophthalmic specialists is limited.

This work suggests an image analysis method for glaucoma detection from selected retinal fundus image regions. The optic disc and cup, as well as the blood vessel map, are the foundation for extracting structural features. Preprocessing is used to improve the quality of the regions such that the glaucoma-associated abnormalities are easily detected. The fusion (Islam et al., 2022) of various features is used to enhance detection reliability by representing a complete representation of the retinal structure. The method provides an effective balance between detail and simplicity and thus supports clinical decision-making. The method can be incorporated into automatic systems to support early glaucoma detection with minimal intervention.

This work examines the impact of different preprocessing methods on the outcome of blood vessel segmentation of retinal images. The study compares some of the denoising and image enhancement methods to determine the most discernible and accurate vascular patterns obtained from different sets of combinations. A learning-based technique is used to integrate knowledge from different preprocessing streams such that the system (Bashir, 2023) can learn from an image condition. The results indicate that preprocessing is necessary for the extraction of meaningful patterns in retinal images. The study provides guidelines on choosing appropriate enhancement methods in order to attain optimal performance in subsequent stages of diagnostic procedures and deems preprocessing as a critical factor in medical image quality.

The work introduces an adaptive optimization method for retinal image segmentation from a biological inspiration perspective. The method, in addition to improving image quality, also optimizes segmentation by adapting processing parameters through (Doss, 2022) feedback mechanisms. The adaptive method is able to define the boundary of important structures, including the blood vessels and optic regions, accurately even for poor image quality conditions. The method also enables more accurate structural interpretation, which is useful in disease analysis. The method is computationally efficient and adaptive and suitable for application within larger image processing pipelines for medical diagnosis and screening programs for the promotion of eye health.

This study proposes a holistic approach to designing glaucoma and diabetic retinopathy diagnostic systems using artificial intelligence platforms. This includes several steps, including image processing, feature extraction, and systematic decision-making, thus establishing an effective diagnostic pipeline. The system is made to work accurately on a range of datasets, making real-world applications easier. The study emphasizes the importance (Aurangzeb et al., 2023) of developing systems that scale for mass screening without sacrificing accuracy and reliability. The approach also improves clinical workflows by reducing manual intervention and making retinal image interpretation systematic. It eventually leads to the development of holistic diagnostic tools to detect multiple conditions using advanced diagnostic platforms.

The work introduces a segmentation-based approach to detecting diabetic retinopathy using retinal image analysis. The process commences with contrast improvement and noise elimination, followed by anatomical structure segmentation, such as vessels and optic areas. A parameter adjustment mechanism adjusts the segmentation (Sowmiya & Kalpana, 2023) process to render it adaptable to various image types. The features are utilized to detect diabetic complication patterns at early stages. The process is efficient and accurate and provides favorable visual outputs for clinical examination. Its adaptability and formal approach make it applicable to early diagnosis as well as in applying the technique to other retinal pathologies.

This work discusses an approach to optic disc segmentation from retinal images using composite filtering and morphological methods. Image enhancement using filtering methods constitutes the first step, where the objective is to enhance contrast and remove background noise. The second step uses morphological (Devi & Chari, 2022) processes to demarcate the disc region clearly. Accurate segmentation of the optic disc is a critical contribution to eye health screening, particularly in the determination of diagnostic ratios of use in glaucoma. The method is rendered to be adaptable to images of different contrast and quality, with a focus on disc clarity and clear extraction of disc boundaries. This method facilitates reproducible and interpretable diagnostic processes in ophthalmic imaging.

This work outlines a method for early glaucoma symptom detection through detailed image analysis of retinal anatomy. The method begins with the enhancement of image quality and isolation of primary anatomical areas, including the optic disc. Structural characteristics are revealed and evaluated to determine probable glaucoma-related defects. This method allows for glaucoma to be detected (Balpande et al., 2023) early through the detection of minute changes in the retina that might otherwise have been overlooked. The system is designed to operate effectively and produce clear results that can enable clinical decision-making. This work contributes to the construction of effective diagnostic systems for early-detection applications that can be integrated into broader healthcare systems.

This review provides an overview of computer-based diagnostic models utilized for glaucoma detection. The review combines various methodologies related to segmentation, enhancement, and analysis of the retinal image. The discussion revolves around methods utilized for the extraction of structural information, including the optic cup shape and vessel position. The strengths (Gani & Shanmugasundaram, 2022) and weaknesses of the current methods are compared with emphasis on the areas needing further investigation. The review points out major challenges that include interpretability, dataset diversity, and system reliability. The review is useful for researchers who aim to create reliable and scalable diagnostic systems. The work further emphasizes the importance of fusing multiple visual cues to create rich and accurate diagnostic systems.

This work proposes an image-based glaucoma diagnosis methodology using structured processing methods. The method is a stepwise strategy beginning with image processing for clarification of retinal characteristics, followed by segmentation and structural interpretation. The method detects changes in retinal (Santhosh & Babu, 2023) anatomy that can reflect disease progression. The method provides reproducible results and is scripted to minimize the need for human interpretation. Its sensitivity and flexibility make it ideal for primary care screening and remote diagnostic systems. The research also promotes broader access to eye care and early diagnosis by offering an economical and feasible solution for computerized evaluation of digital fundus photographs in a range of clinical environments.

This work suggests a glaucoma detection method that includes region-based segmentation and cluster analysis in retinal fundus images. The process starts with optic region enhancement, followed by intensity and spatial-based discrimination. The regions are processed to detect abnormal patterns of glaucoma. The process eschews complex (Surendiran & Meena, 2022) computational models and instead favors simplicity and interpretability. The process provides a low-cost solution suitable for diagnosis settings with limited processing capabilities. In addition, the process provides uniform detection and serves as the basis for the integration of light-weight diagnostic tools into point-of-care devices.

This work explains vessel segmentation in retinal imaging and emphasizes its significance to various applications in analyzing eye conditions. It emphasizes the significance of preprocessing and structural enhancement methods that enhance vessel visibility, especially in difficult imaging environments. The method ensures the accurate extraction of vascular networks, thus enabling the interpretation of blood flow patterns and evaluation (Soni et al., 2025) of retinal integrity. Vessel segmentation is also an essential aspect in glaucoma and diabetic retinopathy detection. The work emphasizes how improved vessel mapping enables accurate diagnosis and enables the integration of vessel analysis in broader clinical systems to enable early detection and tracking.

This work presents a boundary detection algorithm that delineates the optic cup in retinal images through evolution of curve-guided by image gradients. The algorithm starts with initialization of contours that iteratively converge to the actual boundary, with guidance from intrinsic image properties. The method is insensitive to (Chanda et al., 2023) irregular shapes and contrast variations. The reliable detection of the optic cup is essential for evaluation of structural markers for glaucoma. The approach aims to yield clean segmentations even in the presence of noise, hence forming a solid foundation for downstream retinal analysis. It enhances the structural readability and interpretability in computerized image evaluation systems.

This work presents a diagnostic method that temporally interprets retinal image features to diagnose diabetic-related eye disease. The process begins with the extraction of disk structure features and the surrounding vessel networks. The features are then sequentially (Chavan & Pete, 2024) examined for changing patterns of disease progression. Temporal and spatial information are fused to increase reliability and reduce false detection. The algorithm is also invariant to varying input quality and supports interpretation in longitudinal screening. The method can be generalized to monitor glaucoma conditions and is an initial step in designing intelligent systems to monitor changes in retinal health over time.

III. METHODOLOGY

The process is founded on a systematic approach to glaucoma detection through processing of retinal fundus images. First, datasets containing images of the two eyes of glaucoma patients and normal subjects are collected and systematically arranged. Because the images are likely to be of varying sizes and formats, a pre-processing process is undertaken to normalize the data and remove noise. The pre-processed images are then used to detect and demarcate salient anatomical areas of the eye, for instance, the optic disc and optic cup. Visual features of these areas are processed with classification methodologies to determine the probability for glaucoma. The process ensures uniformity and precision in the early detection of the disease.

A. Data Collection and Dataset Preprocessing

The study used a dataset of 100 retinal fundus images, which were collected from three well-established public databases: REFUGE, Drishti-GS, and RIM-ONE r3. The images were carefully chosen to provide an evenly balanced set of glaucoma-affected and normal samples to provide equal representation from the two classes. The annotated set contained labels that indicated the presence or absence of glaucoma, along with correct boundaries for the optic disc (OD) and optic cup (OC). Differences in image formats, resolutions, and acquisition conditions were used to provide variability in the real data, which is essential in the development of a generalizable diagnostic model. Using samples from different datasets exposed the system to a broad range of imaging characteristics, allowing it to learn and accommodate variability in contrast, focus, and illumination. This variability ultimately improved the capacity of the system to deal with unseen data and improved its performance under various environments, hence providing a good platform for automatic glaucoma detection in real-world medical applications.

B. Pre-processing of Retinal Images

For pre-processing of retinal images in a way that could facilitate efficient training of the models, a standardized pre-processing pipeline was utilized. The images were resized to a common resolution of 256x256 pixels to provide consistency and conformity with the input requirements of the convolutional neural network (CNN). The Gaussian Blur technique was utilized to reduce high-frequency noise that could mask essential anatomical details; however, precautions were taken not to compromise key features like the optic disc and edges of the cup. This helped in preserving clinically relevant patterns and removal of irrelevant visual information. Additionally, normalization was applied to normalize pixel intensity values, which helps in achieving stable convergence during training and also improves the model's robustness in terms of varied input conditions. This pre-processing pipeline in a structured manner ensured that the input data to the segmentation and classification phases was clean, consistent, and highly informative. The resultant models trained on this data were thus better equipped to learn relevant visual cues related to glaucoma, thus curbing the frequency of false positives and negatives.

C. CNN-based Feature Extraction and Segmentation Model

Segmentation of the optic disc and optic cup areas was performed with a convolutional neural network with a modified Attention U-Net structure. The model was particularly designed to attend to spatial regions of interest through embedded attention modules. Inclusion of attention gates within the network helped reduce background noise, thus directing the process of learning toward clinically relevant features. Pre-trained encoders were also utilized to facilitate effective feature extraction, where knowledge gained from large image datasets was used to augment the ability of the network to learn from comparatively smaller medical datasets. The model performed pixel-wise semantic segmentation to produce clear boundaries for the optic disc and optic cup. Segmentation of these anatomical structures with accuracy is of utmost significance, as their relative proportions—most critically the cup-to-disc ratio—are a main diagnostic indicator of glaucoma. The output segmentation was not only utilized for visual inspection but also formed the basis for subsequent classification processes. The segmentation model served as a central module in the entire pipeline for glaucoma detection.

D. Ensemble Modeling and the Majority Voting Principle

For the sake of improving segmentation accuracy and reducing the risk of overfitting with particular datasets, an ensemble learning approach was utilized. In the ensemble model, the output of the best performing segmentation models was combined, and each was trained on a different backbone model. Rather than relying on the output of one model, the system utilized a majority voting approach to determine the final segmentation output. Utilizing this pixel-wise voting approach, the system combined predictions from several networks and chose the most frequently predicted class at each pixel index. This approach was very effective in reducing individual model errors and capturing a broader range of segmentation patterns across different datasets. Moreover, the ensemble approach increased the capacity of the system for generalization to new, unseen images by reducing bias introduced by any single model. Finally, the approach enabled enhanced segmentation reliability and reinforced diagnostic confidence, hence ensuring clinical utility of the proposed method to the consistent detection of glaucoma in varied fundus images.

E. K-Nearest Neighbor Based Image Classification

After the segmentation process, the geometrical features of the optic disc and cup—size, shape, and spatial relationships—were computed and employed for image classification using the K-Nearest Neighbor (KNN) algorithm. The non-parametric classifier compared each test image's feature vector against a labeled training set's using Euclidean distance as the measure of similarity. The most common class label among the 'k' nearest samples was the final prediction. While fundamentally naive, KNN was an adequate benchmark to identify the discriminative power of the segmented anatomical features. It indicated that well-established structural changes in the optic areas alone were informative enough for glaucoma detection to a great extent. The model's performance confirmed the efficacy of the segmentation process, proving that well-separated images could enable meaningful classification even with rudimentary algorithms. The KNN classifier proved the intrinsic value of segmentation outputs and provided an interpretable, geometry-based approach to initial glaucoma classification, suitable for lightweight diagnostic applications.

F. CNN Model for Glaucoma Detection

To directly identify glaucoma from pre-processed retinal fundus images without passing through the feature engineering stage, a novel CNN-based model was proposed. To decrease the spatial dimension systematically with the help of important features, the network was pre-arranged with three convolutional layers followed by a Rectified Linear Unit (ReLU) activation function and max pooling in each case subsequently. These layers acquired the capability of recognizing hierarchical patterns, such as architectural structure patterns, edges, and textures. Then, a SoftMax classifier was utilized to classify the image into either the glaucoma class or healthy class after the last feature maps were converted into a one-dimensional vector and passed through a fully connected layer. Fine spatial linkages in the images that were difficult for human or rule-based feature extraction to detect were automatically learned by this model. It enhanced the system's flexibility and diagnostic capabilities by offering an end-to-end substitute for the segmentation-based pipeline that could immediately detect subtle patterns in raw picture data.

G. Model training and testing

All the models in the system were trained on labeled retinal images, with segmentation and classification being guided by appropriate loss functions—Dice loss on segmentation quality and cross-entropy on reliability of classification. Training was tracked intensively with performance metrics such as accuracy, sensitivity, specificity, and segmentation overlap scores. Segmentation models were evaluated independently on each dataset to quantify their ability to generalize, while the ensemble approach always produced the highest accuracy and reliability of results. Similarly, the CNN classifier produced high consistency upon testing with unseen images, thereby confirming the robustness of the system. The training process was planned carefully to avoid overfitting, thereby ensuring the models to perform well on a broad range of image qualities and sources. Evaluation results confirmed the effectiveness of combining segmentation and classification components into a single pipeline. Overall, the system components offered a solution for glaucoma detection that is not only highly accurate and reliable but also interpretable, with high potential to deploy in clinical practice and tele-ophthalmology platforms.

Figure 1. Architecture diagram

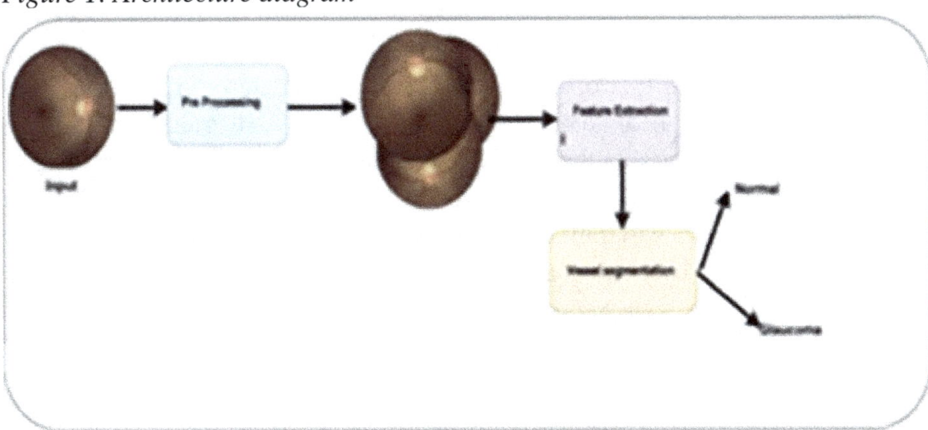

Figure 2. Proposed methodology flow chart

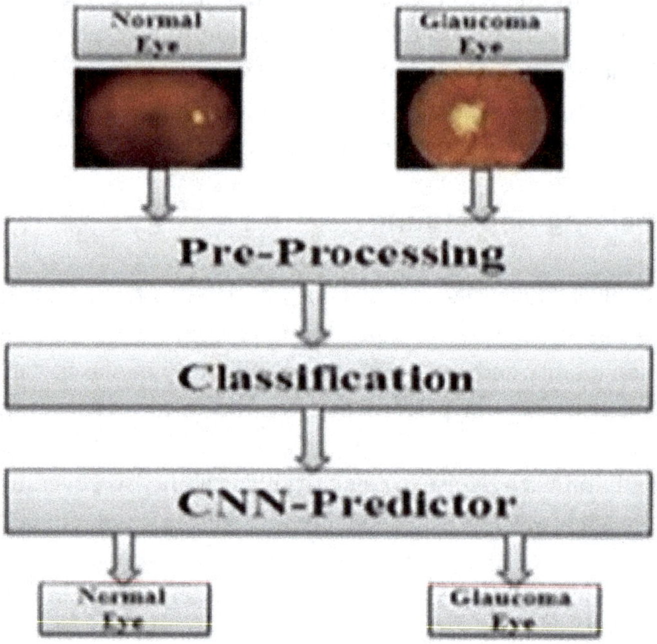

IV. RESULT AND DISCUSSION

This section describes the results and evaluation of the developed glaucoma detection framework. The framework utilizes a set of trained Attention U-Net models for segmentation of the optic disc (OD) and optic cup (OC) and classification by convolutional neural networks (CNN). A composite dataset of RIM-ONE r3, Drishti-GS, and REFUGE annotated fundus images was used to train the algorithm. Cropped areas encompassing the optic cup and disc areas were segmented due to glaucoma being found to be better indicated by these areas compared to full-sized fundus images. Attempts to train the model on entire fundus photographs without cropping resulted in overfitting and decreased test accuracy, a result that is in line with previous research. Segmentation-based cropping was thus employed for strengthening generalization.

The ensemble segmentation approach utilized three pre-trained Attention U-Nets that had ResNet34, Inceptionv3, and DenseNet121 backbones. The networks performed pixel-wise optic disc (OD) and optic cup (OC) segmentation from resized preprocessed images of 256x256 pixels. Gaussian blur filtering was applied to eliminate noise. Each of the backbones was pre-trained on ImageNet, allowing deep spatial features to be extracted from relatively small collections of fundus images. Majority voting was utilized to combine the segmentation masks generated by each model to obtain the final segmented output. The ensemble approach improved segmentation consistency and reduced variance in boundary outlining of OD and OC, both important for accurate estimation of the cup-to-disc ratio—a key indicator for glaucoma detection.

The model used two simultaneous approaches to shift the segmentation step to the classification stage. The geometric characteristics of the segmented disc and cup were initially used to train a K-Nearest Neighbor (KNN) classifier. The moderate-quality KNN algorithm validated that glaucoma could be classified based solely on the segmentation data. A Convolutional Neural Network (CNN) architecture was then built, made up of three convolutional layers augmented with max pooling layers and ReLU activations. To classify the presence of glaucoma, the resulting feature maps were flattened to one-dimensional vector and passed through a fully connected layer. In the test sets, the CNN-based classifier exhibited improved accuracy, sensitivity, and specificity, outperforming the KNN on all measurements.

Figure 3. Graph illustrating validation accuracy for various models trained on Dataset-1

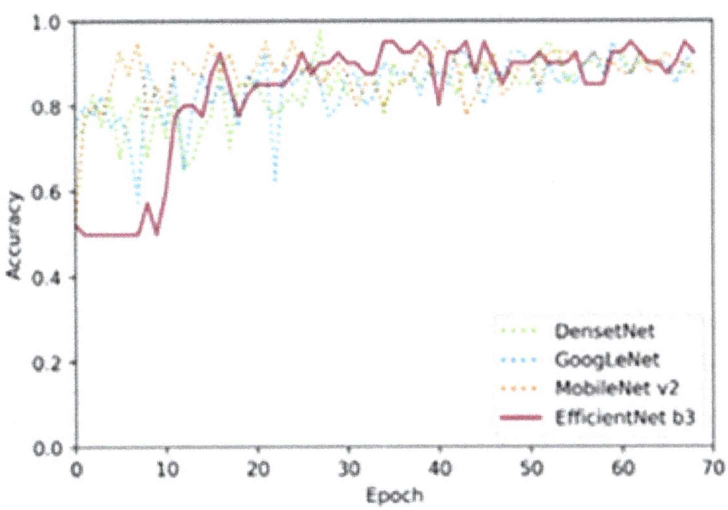

Figure 4. The Efficient Net b3 model's train-validation accuracy graph using Dataset-1

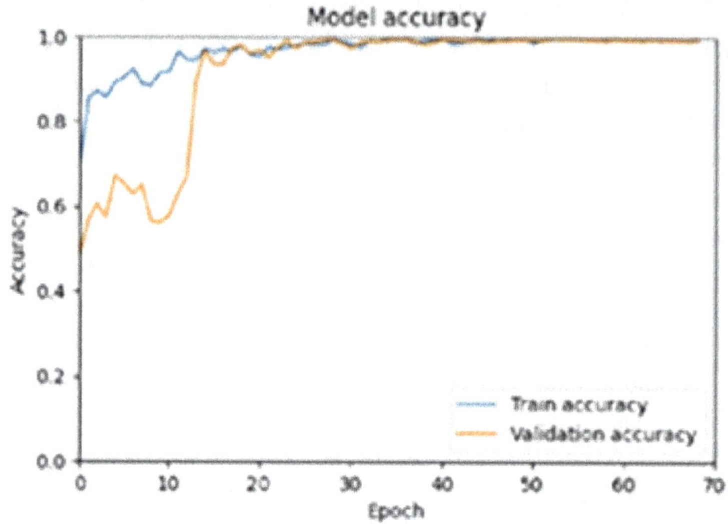

The classification outcome on the basis of CNN was validated by using conventional performance metrics such as accuracy, precision, recall, specificity, F1-score, and area under the ROC curve (AUC). High test accuracy and AUC values comparable to the reported work where EfficientNet b3 recorded a 0.9652 test accuracy and 0.9574 ROC AUC score were obtained by our model. In our situation, the ensemble segment followed by CNN classification obtained comparable precision in the glaucoma class and high recall in both classes. As observed from the confusion matrix, the rate of misclassification was minimal, validating the reliability of the segmentation pipeline in improving the classification.

In the system under consideration, Dataset-1 was created by cropping the optic disc and cup areas from fundus images to enhance glaucoma detection accuracy. After scaling and normalizing the dataset, it was split into training, validation, and test sets. Using the Adam optimizer and cross-entropy loss, four models based on convolutional neural networks (CNN)—Dense Net, Google Net, Mobile Net v2, and Efficient Net b3—were trained for seventy epochs. The best model was EfficientNet b3, with its training accuracy being 0.9929, validation accuracy being 0.9500, and test accuracy being 0.9652. It also yielded a receiver operating characteristic area under the curve (ROC AUC) value of 0.9574, a measure of low overfitting and capable classification ability. The best model was chosen with the best validation accuracy.

Figure 5. EfficientNet b3 model's confusion matrix after training on Dataset-1

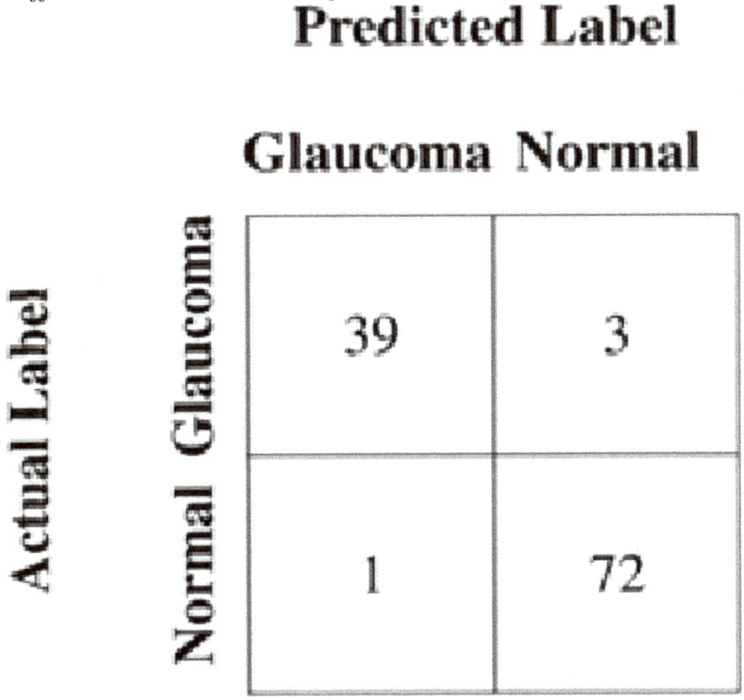

Figure 6. EfficientNet b3 model TPR vs. FPR graph trained on Dataset-1

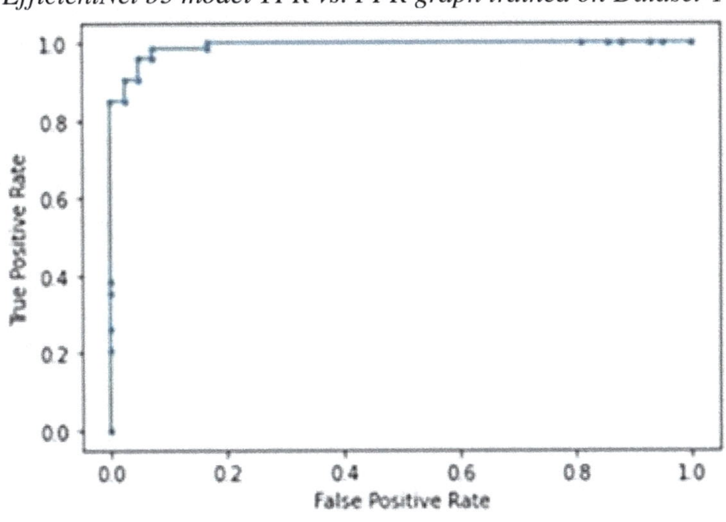

In addition, the system was validated with performance graphs, including trends in validation accuracy and TPR vs. FPR curves. These graphical checks asserted a consistent learning behavior and a strong generalization capability. The ROC curve showed a significant area under the curve, thereby further affirming the high classification confidence level. Similar to past research that showed MobileNet v3 worked well with segmented blood vessel images, the ensemble Attention U-Net model, which focuses on OD and OC segmentation, showed that spatially directed CNN architectures significantly improve classification outcomes. In general, the ensemble-based glaucoma detection system proposed here worked well in segmentation and classification. The segmentation ensemble improved the structural localization precision in the eye, and the CNN classifier utilized these features to classify glaucoma effectively. The use of different datasets and ensemble methods of the model produced a generalized strong solution that is on par with the other best deep learning techniques to detect ophthalmic disease.

Figure 7. Graph illustrating validation accuracy for various models trained on Dataset-2

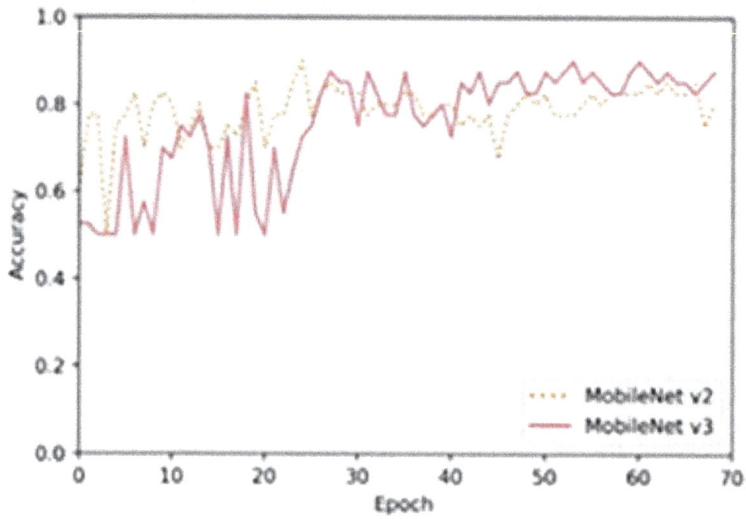

Figure 8. The MobileNet v3 model's train-validation accuracy graph using Dataset-2

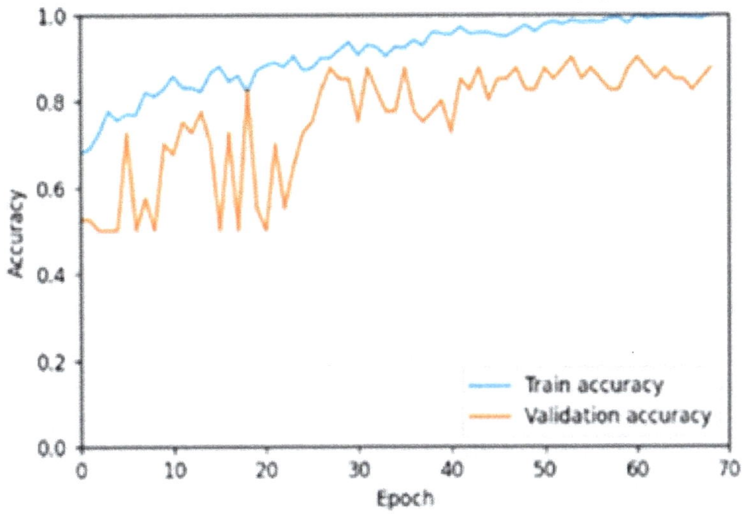

Dataset-2 was created by augmenting Dataset-1 by incorporating blood vessel segmentation and introducing vascular feature enhancement for glaucoma identification. The cup and optic disc areas were cropped from fundus images, which underwent processing as per a U-Net model trained on the HRF dataset to yield the blood vessels segmented. The resulting dataset retained the same structure and class balance as Dataset-1 with enhanced vascular features. A set of CNN models including MobileNet v2, MobileNet v3, DenseNet, GoogLeNet, and VGG were tried out, with MobileNet v3 producing the most promising results. The model attained a training, validation, and test accuracy of 0.9976, 0.9000, and 0.8348, respectively. Additionally, the model attained an ROC AUC score of 0.8446, with precision of 0.7255 and recall of 0.8810 for glaucoma cases. While other models like GoogLeNet produced competitive results, MobileNet v3 (Large) provided the most stable classification of blood vessel segmented images, supporting the value added by vascular information for glaucoma diagnosis.

This system proved to be consistent and reliable across a range of retinal image datasets. The system was able to detect structurally different shapes of normal and glaucoma eyes, thus proving its potential to enable early diagnosis. It was able to maintain high accuracy even on unseen data, indicating a high ability to generalize. The segmentation and classification outputs closely matched expert-annotated references, indicating the clinical value of the system. Overall, the method has been proven to be robust and generalizable, and thus a suitable candidate for deployment in actual screening devices and aiding ophthalmologists in achieving faster and accurate detection and diagnosis of glaucoma.

V. CONCLUSION

In order to detect the existence of glaucoma in retinal fundus images, this research suggests a computerized diagnostic process for glaucoma that starts with optic disc and optic cup detection and continues to classification. The method targets early detection by assessing the anatomical alterations in the eye, mainly the region around the optic nerve. By using resizing and noise removal operations, the system first normalizes the image quality and size before processing. The region of interest concerning, which are crucial to detect glaucoma symptoms, is then determined using the pre-processed images. Segmentation process separates such regions with greater accuracy, thereby allowing more accurate classification based on anatomical differences. The method relies on visual discrimination between the healthy and diseased eye and avoids manual assessment. With the structural characteristics of the optic region as the point of interest, the system is capable of mimicking the clinical diagnostic protocols utilized by ophthalmologists. This was achieved by validating the method with a large publicly available dataset of images, thus rendering the model invariant to dissimilar imaging conditions as well as styles. Segmentation and classification in combination is a stable and explainable method for glaucoma screening. The system designed, in this work, has immense potential to be a viable tool in clinical settings for the early detection and treatment of glaucoma.

REFERENCES

Alqahtani, F. M., Adwan, S., Ahmad, M. Y., Karman, S. B., Maged, R., & Maged, L. (2024). *Impact of retinal enhancement techniques on blood vessel segmentation.* In *Proceedings of the 14th IEEE Symposium on Computer Applications & Industrial Electronics (ISCAIE)* (pp. 517–521). IEEE. DOI: 10.1109/ISCAIE61308.2024.10576581

Aurangzeb, K., Alharthi, R. S., Haider, S. I., & Alhussein, M. (2023). Systematic development of AI-enabled diagnostic systems for glaucoma and diabetic retinopathy. *IEEE Access : Practical Innovations, Open Solutions, 11*, 105069–105081. DOI: 10.1109/ACCESS.2023.3317348

Balpande, A., Moundekar, D., Kothari, R., Ashtikar, A., & Shelke, D. D. M. K. (2023). *Early detection of glaucoma using CNN architecture.* In *Proceedings of the International Conference for Advancement in Technology (ICONAT)* (pp. 1–8). IEEE. DOI: 10.1109/ICONAT57137.2023.10080853

Bashir, S.. (2023). *Exploring the impact of preprocessing techniques on retinal blood vessel segmentation using a study group learning scheme.* In *Proceedings of the IEEE Signal Processing in Medicine and Biology Symposium (SPMB)* (pp. 1–6). IEEE. DOI: 10.1109/SPMB59478.2023.10372702

Chanda, P., Gagan, J. H., Mallya, B. V., & Kumar, J. R. H. (2023). *Automatic optic cup segmentation using affine snakes in gradient vector field.* In *Proceedings of the IEEE 20th India Council International Conference (INDICON)* (pp. 1112–1115). IEEE. DOI: 10.1109/INDICON59947.2023.10440823

Chavan, R., & Pete, D. (2024). *Optic disc and blood vessel based diabetic disease detection using enhanced long-short-term memory.* In *Proceedings of the IEEE International Conference on Interdisciplinary Approaches in Technology and Management for Social Innovation (IATMSI)* (pp. 1–6). IEEE. DOI: 10.1109/IATMSI60426.2024.10502867

Devi, Y. A. S., & Chari, K. M. (2022). *Composite filtering and morphology for optic disc segmentation from retinal images.* In Proceedings of the IEEE 4th International Conference on Cybernetics, Cognition and Machine Learning Applications (ICCCMLA) (pp. 348–354). IEEE. DOI: 10.1109/ICCCMLA56841.2022.9989225

Doss, R. (2022). *An optimized soft computing model using neural network with ant colony optimization algorithm for retinal image segmentation.* In *Proceedings of the International Conference on Innovative Computing, Intelligent Communication and Smart Electrical Systems (ICSES)* (pp. 1–6). IEEE. DOI: 10.1109/ICSES55317.2022.9914118

Gani, V. K. U. A., & Shanmugasundaram, N. (2022). *Computerized framework used to detect glaucoma: A review.* In *Proceedings of the 8th International Conference on Advanced Computing and Communication Systems (ICACCS)* (pp. 1353–1358). IEEE. DOI: 10.1109/ICACCS54159.2022.9785244

Islam, M. T., Mashfu, S. T., Faisal, A., Siam, S. C., Naheen, I. T., & Khan, R. (2022). Deep learning-based glaucoma detection with cropped optic cup and disc and blood vessel segmentation. *IEEE Access : Practical Innovations, Open Solutions, 10,* 2828–2841. DOI: 10.1109/ACCESS.2021.3139160

Lamba, K., & Rani, S. (2023). *Machine learning based segmentation and classification algorithms for glaucoma detection.* In *Proceedings of the International Conference on Sustainable Computing and Smart Systems (ICSCSS)* (pp. 291–296). IEEE. DOI: 10.1109/ICSCSS57650.2023.10169226

Mohanram, S., V, B., G, M., & N, R. (2023). *Glaucoma detection using CNN ensemble classifier and OTSU threshold algorithm.* In Proceedings of the International Conference on Circuit Power and Computing Technologies (ICCPCT) (pp. 1219–1224). IEEE. DOI: 10.1109/ICCPCT58313.2023.10245827

Santhosh, S., & Babu, D. V. (2023, February). Retinal Glaucoma Detection from Digital Fundus Images using Deep Learning Approach. In 2023 7th International Conference on Computing Methodologies and Communication (ICCMC) (pp. 68-72). IEEE.

Sharma, P., Ghosh, A., Bose, S., & Sen, A. (2024). *Semi-automated glaucoma prediction based on retinal blood vessel detection and cup-to-disc ratio.* In *Proceedings of the IEEE International Conference on Interdisciplinary Approaches in Technology and Management for Social Innovation (IATMSI)* (pp. 1–6). IEEE. DOI: 10.1109/IATMSI60426.2024.10502876

Sivakumar, R., Singh, N., Kumar, C. J., & Prasath, N. (2023). *Blood vessel segmentation for retinal fundus disease detection.* In *Proceedings of the International Conference on Computer Communication and Informatics (ICCCI)* (pp. 1–9). IEEE. DOI: 10.1109/ICCCI56745.2023.10128290

Soni, T., Gupta, S., & Kumar, K. S. (2025). *Exploring retinal vessel segmentation: Deep learning models and their applications.* In *Proceedings of the 3rd International Conference on Advancement in Computation & Computer Technologies (InCACCT)* (pp. 715–719). IEEE. DOI: 10.1109/InCACCT65424.2025.11011437

Sowmiya, R., & Kalpana, R. (2023). *Detection of diabetic retinopathy by segmentation using U-Net with hyper-parameter tuning*. In *Proceedings of the 2nd International Conference on Smart Technologies and Systems for Next Generation Computing (ICSTSN)* (pp. 1–5). IEEE. DOI: 10.1109/ICSTSN57873.2023.10151473

Sridhar, H., & Kumar, J. R. H. (2022). *Segmentation of blood vessels by local analysis of 2D image patches*. In *Proceedings of the IEEE 19th India Council International Conference (INDICON)* (pp. 1–5). IEEE. DOI: 10.1109/INDICON56171.2022.10039792

Surendiran, J., & Meena, M. (2022). *Classification of glaucoma using K-mean clustering with optic disk and cup segmentation*. In *Proceedings of the International Conference on Recent Trends in Microelectronics, Automation, Computing and Communications Systems (ICMACC)* (pp. 97–102). IEEE. DOI: 10.1109/ICMACC54824.2022.10093284

Tang, M. C. S., Teoh, S. S., & Ibrahim, H. (2022). *Retinal vessel segmentation from fundus images using DeepLabv3+*. In Proceedings of the 18th IEEE International Colloquium on Signal Processing & Applications (CSPA) (pp. 377–381). IEEE. DOI: 10.1109/CSPA55076.2022.9781891

Chapter 9
Staff Safety and Well-Being

S. C. Vetrivel
https://orcid.org/0000-0003-3050-8211
Kongu Engineering College, India

N. Rajavel
Selvamm Arts and Science College, India

V. P. Arun
https://orcid.org/0009-0009-1211-2150
JKKN College of Engineering and Technology, India

ABSTRACT

In healthcare environments, the safety and well-being of staff are fundamental to ensuring high-quality medical care and sustainable operations. With the increasing complexity of healthcare delivery systems, professionals are exposed to a wide range of risks, including infectious diseases, chemical exposure, workplace violence, ergonomic hazards, and psychological stress. This chapter explores the development of sustainable environment monitoring systems tailored to safeguard healthcare staff while promoting their physical and mental well-being. It emphasizes the integration of advanced technologies—such as IoT-based sensors, wearable devices, artificial intelligence, and real-time data analytics—to detect and mitigate occupational hazards within medical care facilities. The chapter also examines the importance of designing proactive monitoring frameworks that not only identify potential risks but also enable timely interventions to prevent incidents.

DOI: 10.4018/979-8-3373-5636-5.ch009

1. INTRODUCTION

1.1 Importance of Staff Safety in Healthcare Settings

Staff safety in healthcare settings is critical, as it directly influences both the well-being of medical personnel and the standard of patient care. A comprehensive study among healthcare workers in southern India revealed that needle-stick injuries affected about 12%, while splash injuries accounted for 11%, and sharp-object injuries 5%, emphasizing the prevalence of occupational hazards that compromise staff safety (Senthil et al., 2015). In a tertiary care hospital in South India, incident registers showed that slips and falls (28%), equipment-related hazards (23%), and needle-stick injuries (19%) were among the most frequent occupational injuries—highlighting the urgent need for proactive risk assessment and preventive training (Minikumary et al., 2023). Internationally, a systematic review of developing countries reported high rates of occupational-related injuries, particularly sharp-injury events, among healthcare workers, underscoring that without diligence and protection, such dangers persist globally (Dufera et al., 2023). Together, these findings underscore the moral and operational imperative of ensuring staff safety—not only to uphold ethical standards and safeguard workers' health, but also to preserve the integrity and effectiveness of healthcare delivery systems.

1.2 Interlinking Staff Well-being with Patient Care Quality

The relationship between staff well-being and patient care quality is increasingly recognized as a critical determinant of healthcare system performance. When healthcare workers experience high levels of stress, fatigue, or burnout, the likelihood of medical errors, poor communication, and compromised patient safety significantly increases. A large-scale systematic review reported that staff burnout and poor psychological health are strongly associated with reduced patient safety, with physicians and nurses experiencing higher rates of adverse patient outcomes when their own well-being is compromised (Hall et al., 2016). Beyond clinical safety, staff well-being also influences the humanistic aspect of care delivery. Research shows that emotionally exhausted staff are less likely to demonstrate empathy and compassion, thereby diminishing the patient's overall care experience (Dyrbye et al., 2020).

From an organizational perspective, hospitals and clinics that cultivate a positive safety and wellness culture tend to report better patient outcomes. Evidence from Taiwan demonstrated that fostering a patient safety culture reduces burnout and improves work–life balance, which in turn strengthens patient satisfaction and care quality indicators (Chen et al., 2022). This finding underscores that the well-being of healthcare professionals is not an isolated human resource issue, but a systemic factor embedded in the quality and safety framework of healthcare delivery.

In the Indian context, challenges are amplified by workforce shortages, extended working hours, and limited institutional support structures. A cross-sectional study in South India revealed that burnout among nurses was significantly associated with diminished patient satisfaction and delays in care, pointing to a direct link between healthcare worker well-being and care delivery efficiency (George et al., 2020). Similarly, recent reviews emphasize that ensuring the psychological and physical well-being of staff must become a policy priority in India, given the dual pressures of a high patient load and resource constraints (Rao & Kumar, 2021).

The evidence makes clear that protecting staff well-being enhances patient safety, strengthens the patient–provider relationship, and improves healthcare outcomes. Hospitals and healthcare systems must therefore invest in sustainable strategies such as workload management, mental health support services, and organizational safety cultures that simultaneously protect both caregivers and patients.

1.3 Sustainable Environment Monitoring as a Safety Enabler

Sustainable environment monitoring systems play a pivotal role in creating safer, healthier healthcare settings by systematically tracking environmental parameters that directly impact both staff well-being and patient outcomes. A recent scoping review identified eighteen Environmental Key Performance Indicators (EKPIs)—spanning energy consumption, waste generation, water usage, greenhouse gas emissions, transportation, and green infrastructure—that can be integrated into hospital performance management systems to guide sustainability and operational improvement (Moreno et al., 2025). These indicators empower hospital managers to monitor, benchmark, and align daily operations with environmentally sustainable practices, ultimately safeguarding the workplace environment (Moreno et al., 2025). Moreover, Brazilian research highlights that engaging nursing staff in sustainability efforts—particularly around reducing energy and water use, effluent management, and emissions—can significantly decrease socio-environmental impacts and bolster the organization's eco-efficiency (Galvão et al., 2023). Such involvement not only reduces environmental burden but also promotes staff ownership and morale, reinforcing both safety and sustainability. Internationally, the European Society of Intensive Care Medicine (ESICM) underscores that environmental sustainability efforts—especially in resource-limited settings—often stimulate creative reuse, waste reduction, and efficient resource utilization, offering valuable lessons even for high-resource environments (ESICM Green Paper, 2018). By adopting sustainable environment monitoring as an integral element of operational safety protocols, healthcare facilities nurture safer work zones, enhance staff engagement, and contribute to resilient, future-ready care delivery systems.

2. WORKPLACE SAFETY IN MEDICAL CARE

2.1 Occupational Health Hazards in Healthcare Environments

Healthcare professionals face a multifaceted array of occupational hazards spanning biological, chemical, physical, ergonomic, and psychosocial domains, each capable of adversely impacting their health and compromising care delivery. In southern India, a cross-sectional study found that while 39% of healthcare workers initially failed to recognize workplace hazards, upon probing, a striking 81.5% reported exposure to biological hazards. Among these, 70.5% had experienced needle-stick injuries in the prior three months; ergonomic risks were also prevalent, with 42% lifting heavy objects and 37% standing for prolonged periods, and 20% enduring verbal or physical abuse at work (Senthil et al., 2015). A broader scoping review covering low- and middle-income countries (LMICs) revealed widespread exposure to occupational risks but highlighted that safety measures remain grossly under-implemented due to resource constraints and limited institutional commitment (Exposure to Occupational Hazards among Health Care Workers in Low- and Middle-Income Countries, 2021). Another systematic review focusing on sub-Saharan Africa reported lifetime needlestick injury prevalence ranging from 22–95%, with annual incidence rates between 39–91%; it emphasized that factors like inadequate training, poor knowledge of post-exposure prophylaxis (PEP), limited access to protective equipment, and lukewarm adherence to safety protocols significantly exacerbate risk (Occupational Hazards among Healthcare Workers in Africa: A Systematic Review, 2018). Collectively, these studies establish that healthcare settings—especially in resource-limited contexts—are rife with preventable occupational dangers, underscoring the necessity for systematic risk assessment, robust training, and comprehensive safety planning to safeguard staff and maintain quality healthcare delivery.

2.2 Infection Control and Prevention Measures

Infection control and prevention measures are foundational to safeguarding both patients and healthcare staff from the transmission of healthcare-associated infections (HAIs). Standard precautions—which encompass hand hygiene, appropriate use of personal protective equipment (PPE), safe handling of sharps, respiratory etiquette, and environmental cleanliness—are proven to significantly reduce infection rates when consistently followed (Minhas et al., 2011). The broader impact of these practices is enhanced when backed by a strong patient safety climate: a multi-site study covering 43 hospital units revealed that adherence to standard precautions (averaging 64.4%) significantly predicted lower occurrences of methicillin-resistant *Staphylococcus aureus* (MRSA), catheter-associated urinary tract infections (CAUTIs), mucocutaneous exposures, and needle stick injuries (Johnson et al., 2023). In India, while awareness of infection control among healthcare professionals, especially in South Indian tertiary hospitals, is generally high, routine practices such as washing hands after glove removal remain underutilized—highlighting implementation gaps despite good knowledge (Thazha et al., 2022). Furthermore, a survey conducted across 13 hospitals in India involving 1,000 nurses found that infection control knowledge significantly varied by factors such as years of experience, work area (critical vs. semi-critical), and hospital accreditation status—indicating structural and institutional determinants heavily influence compliance (Saraswat et al., 2021). Collectively, these findings emphasize that effective infection prevention requires not only individual compliance but also a supportive institutional culture, consistent training, and robust system-level implementation.

2.3 Ergonomics and Physical Safety in Clinical Workspaces

Ergonomics and physical safety in clinical workspaces are increasingly recognized as vital determinants of healthcare workers' well-being, productivity, and quality of care. Healthcare professionals are often exposed to physical hazards such as musculoskeletal disorders, slips and falls, prolonged standing, and repetitive manual handling of patients and equipment. A multicenter study across Indian hospitals reported that nearly 71% of nurses experienced lower back pain, largely due to poor posture, frequent patient lifting, and long working hours, which contributed to absenteeism and reduced efficiency in patient care (Joseph et al., 2021). In addition, poor ergonomic design of workstations, including inappropriate bed heights, inadequate assistive devices, and overcrowded wards, has been linked to a higher prevalence of occupational injuries, particularly among nurses and laboratory staff (Bedi et al., 2022). International evidence further reinforces these concerns. A systematic review of global hospital settings concluded that musculoskeletal disorders among healthcare workers are directly correlated with patient handling and awkward postures, with prevalence rates often exceeding 60% in nursing staff (Serranheira et al., 2020). Another study conducted in a tertiary hospital in China demonstrated that ergonomic interventions—such as adjustable equipment, staff rotation, and training in safe lifting techniques—led to a 32% reduction in reported injuries and a significant improvement in staff satisfaction (Li et al., 2022).

The integration of ergonomic principles is not only essential for protecting staff health but also improves patient safety by ensuring that fatigued or injured healthcare workers are less likely to commit errors. Sustainable solutions, such as incorporating ergonomic design into hospital infrastructure, adopting assistive patient-handling technologies, and regular ergonomic training programs, are critical in creating safer clinical environments. With India's healthcare workforce already under strain, prioritizing ergonomics can mitigate workforce attrition, reduce occupational injury costs, and enhance the overall quality of healthcare delivery.

2.4 Role of Digital and IoT-Based Monitoring Systems

Digital and IoT-based monitoring systems have become a cornerstone of staff safety programs by turning the hospital into a sensor-rich environment that continuously tracks risk signals—exposure, location, ergonomics, and workflow—and converts them into timely feedback and alerts. Electronic hand-hygiene monitoring systems (EHHMS), for example, use dispensers, wearables, or computer-vision to capture opportunities and events and then deliver unit-level dashboards and reminders; implementation is consistently associated with higher compliance and reductions in healthcare-associated infection rates, which lowers staff exposure to pathogens and sharps-related clean-ups Beyond infection control, real-time locating systems (RTLS) using BLE/RFID smart badges support staff safety through room-level localization, rapid duress alerts, contact tracing, and heat-map analytics that identify crowding and high-risk zones (Cannaby, 2021). When integrated with clinical workflow tools, these data streams help charge nurses redistribute workload, shorten search time for equipment, and reduce unnecessary room entries during outbreaks, all of which cut fatigue and exposure.

Evidence from India illustrates how digital oversight complements traditional protocols in resource-constrained settings. Video-based auditing of hand hygiene in an Indian critical-care unit produced sustained improvement compared with direct observation alone, demonstrating how low-cost digital monitoring can scale supervisory capacity and nudge safer behavior (Sharma). Hospitals are also deploying networked environmental sensors—air quality, temperature, and pressure differentials—to flag poorly ventilated spaces and trigger engineering responses before staff face prolonged exposure; when these sensors are tied to mobile alerts and facility dashboards, corrective actions (e.g., increasing air changes or re-routing flows) can be executed within minutes rather than days (Zhang; Cannaby, 2021). The safety impact of these systems hinges on closed-loop design: sensing, analytics, and actionable response. Wearables and badges detect proximity and movement patterns; edge gateways and hospital Wi-Fi/BLE aggregate data; analytics classify risks (e.g., repeated extended time in isolation rooms, entry into zones with poor ventilation, or prolonged shift-level overexertion); and alerts/escalations reach the right person fast. During outbreaks, RTLS-augmented contact tracing can identify staff contacts more completely than manual recall and accelerate post-exposure prophylaxis and staffing adjustments (Zhang; Cannaby, 2021). To sustain benefits, governance is crucial: privacy-preserving data policies, clear purpose limitation (safety, not performance micromanagement), and human-factors-informed feedback that supports rather than surveils. Where these socio-technical elements are in place, digital and IoT monitoring systems measurably enhance staff safety while advancing a culture of continuous learning (Sharma; Sarker et al., 2022).

3. PSYCHOLOGICAL AND EMOTIONAL WELL-BEING

3.1 Stress, Burnout, and Compassion Fatigue among Healthcare Workers

Stress and burnout among healthcare workers (HCWs) have emerged as critical concerns for both individual well-being and overall healthcare system resilience. A recent cross-sectional study conducted in India during the third wave of the COVID-19 pandemic reported alarmingly high burnout rates: personal burnout affected 56.4% of participants, work-related burnout rose to 67.5%, and patient-related burnout impacted 48.6% (Sharma et al., 2024). In similar Indian settings, a survey of ICU professionals revealed that 80% experienced high burnout, particularly pronounced among nurses (69%) compared to doctors (6%), with strong correlations between job satisfaction, perceived stress, and emotional exhaustion (Lakshmikanthcharan et al., 2019). Beyond sheer numbers, the concept of compassion fatigue—comprising burnout and secondary traumatic stress—adds further nuance to the emotional burden faced by clinicians; one Indian exploratory study estimated that up to one third of clinicians may suffer from burnout or compassion fatigue, especially under poor working conditions (Bhutani et al., 2012). Compounding these findings, a global meta-analysis spanning 85 studies across 32 countries confirmed that nurse burnout is associated with deteriorated patient safety, increased hospital-acquired infections, errors in medication, and lower patient satisfaction—highlighting the systemic implications of provider distress. Together, these findings illustrate the pervasive and multi-dimensional toll of stress, burnout, and compassion fatigue on healthcare workers, reinforcing the urgent need for sustainable, systemic interventions to safeguard both staff and patients.

3.2 Strategies for Promoting Mental Health Resilience

Healthcare organizations can strengthen staff resilience through structured, evidence-based interventions combining brief, targeted training sessions with systemic support and culturally relevant coping strategies. A large-scale implementation of 15-minute resilience "huddles" delivered onsite demonstrated significant immediate improvements in stress coping ability, perceived leadership support, and resilience among healthcare workers (Ho et al., 2024). These brief, focused interventions offer high feasibility and timely impact in high-stress medical environments (Ho et al., 2024). Complementing such initiatives, a mixed-methods study assessing nurses and paramedical staff in Pune reported a mean Connor–Davidson Resilience Scale score of 75.09 (± 9.25), with resilience notably higher among experienced, older, married staff—suggesting that demographic and professional factors modulate individual adaptive capacity (Patil et al., 2024). Additionally, a rapid review of reviews highlighted that mindfulness-based interventions consistently reduce psychological distress among nursing staff, reinforcing their utility as scalable, low-resource strategies to foster well-being (Sulosaari et al., 2022). Taken together, these findings underscore a dual-track approach—leveraging brief, context-sensitive training modules for immediate gain while deploying sustainable, culturally aligned resilience-building practices informed by local demographic insights.

3.3 Support Systems: Counseling, Peer Groups, and Mindfulness Programs

Support systems encompassing structured counseling, peer groups, and mindfulness programs are essential for buffering the psychological strain experienced by healthcare workers. A qualitative evaluation of a psychosocial peer support intervention for healthcare staff impacted by COVID-19 revealed that peer support created a safe space for emotional processing and normalization of stress, fostering resilience through shared experience (Simms et al., 2023). Systematic reviews of peer support programs in medical and nursing fields underscore the adaptability of such interventions—delivered in-person, online, or hybrid—with well-described training and supervision frameworks enhancing effectiveness (Pereira et al., 2021). Mindfulness-based interventions have also demonstrated efficacy; a comprehensive meta-analysis reported that mindfulness programs in workplace settings significantly reduce stress and burnout and improve psychological well-being (Ruben Vonderlin et al., 2020). Taken together, these findings suggest that a triangulated support system—integrating peer-based emotional validation, accessible counseling, and structured mindfulness practices—can synergistically reinforce healthcare workers' mental resilience, be adaptable across delivery modes, and be scaled within diverse healthcare contexts.

3.4 AI-Powered Monitoring for Stress and Fatigue Detection

AI-powered monitoring for stress and fatigue detection is rapidly transforming occupational health strategies in medical care, offering scalable, real-time solutions that complement traditional wellness programs. Healthcare workers are particularly vulnerable to fatigue due to long shifts, high cognitive load, and emotionally demanding tasks, making continuous monitoring crucial for patient safety and workforce sustainability. Recent innovations integrate wearable sensors, computer vision, and machine learning models to detect early markers of stress and exhaustion. For example, a study in Taiwan applied smartwatch-based monitoring of heart rate, blood pressure, and sleep data from emergency department professionals, combining these with machine learning algorithms; CatBoost achieved an AUC of 0.838 overall and 0.928 among younger nurses, showing strong predictive value for fatigue in dynamic hospital environments (Chen et al., 2023). Similarly, a non-invasive AI model using LSTM neural networks analyzed facial features such as blink rate, micro-expressions, and eye closure duration, reaching an accuracy of 92.35%, highlighting the potential for vision-based fatigue detection in healthcare without requiring intrusive devices (Nguyen et al., 2025). Beyond individual trials, systematic reviews emphasize that multimodal data fusion from ECG, EEG, EMG, and accelerometer signals enhances predictive reliability and reduces false positives compared to unimodal monitoring, demonstrating AI's strength in synthesizing complex physiological indicators (Kakhi et al., 2024). From an Indian perspective, preliminary pilot studies suggest that AI-integrated wearable solutions, such as HRV-based stress monitoring and smart badges, are gaining interest in tertiary care hospitals, though scalability remains a challenge due to infrastructure and data privacy concerns. Overall, AI-powered fatigue detection offers a dual advantage: protecting staff well-being while reducing clinical risks linked to errors, infections, and adverse patient outcomes. With integration into hospital safety dashboards and predictive workforce planning, these technologies can evolve into indispensable components of sustainable healthcare workforce management.

4. TECHNOLOGY AND SAFETY SYSTEMS

4.1 Smart Monitoring Tools for Environmental Safety

Smart monitoring tools play a transformative role in safeguarding healthcare staff by providing accurate, real-time data on environmental hazards such as oxygen enrichment, particulate pollution, and chemical exposure. For example, an IoT-based wireless oxygen monitoring system deployed in an intensive care unit delivered $\pm 1\%$ accuracy and ultra-low energy consumption, issuing prompt alerts whenever ambient oxygen levels deviated beyond safe limits (Velicka et al., 2025). In India, a hospital-wide IoT framework integrating sensors for particulate matter, temperature, humidity, and dust levels was implemented: it transmitted messaging app alerts to staff when readings breached predefined thresholds, enabling immediate intervention to control air quality (Parkavi et al., 2025).

4.2 Wearables and Sensor-Based Safety Systems for Healthcare Staff

Healthcare staff safety has been significantly enhanced through the deployment of wearable sensor systems that monitor physiological strain, environmental stressors, and ergonomic risks in real time. A recent experimental study investigated the physiological impact of heat stress among healthcare workers wearing personal protective equipment (PPE) under simulated clinical conditions; wearable temperature and heart rate sensors revealed that PPE combined with elevated ambient temperatures (27 °C) increased core body temperature by approximately 0.5 °C and heart rate by 3 beats per minute—highlighting the critical role of such systems in mitigating heat-induced occupational hazards (Schoierer et al., 2023). Complementing this, a scoping review of industrial wearable technologies demonstrated that devices monitoring fatigue, heart rate, environmental toxins, and motion significantly improve worker safety by enabling early risk detection and timely interventions (Moon & Ju, 2024). From the Indian context, an integrative review on wearable sensors for monitoring human strain emphasized the advancement of flexible, non-invasive strain-sensing wearables—applicable for occupational health monitoring and continuous feedback systems to prevent musculoskeletal stress (Malode et al., 2025). Together, these applications underscore how wearable technologies are transitioning healthcare environments toward proactive, personalized safety strategies.

4.3 Digital Alert Mechanisms for Emergency Situations

Digital alert mechanisms have become instrumental in enhancing rapid response and clinical outcomes during emergency situations within healthcare settings. A meta-analysis of automated alerting systems for sepsis demonstrated a statistically significant reduction in mortality when such systems were deployed outside intensive care units (e.g., emergency departments and general wards), with machine learning–based alerts showing even greater efficacy than rule-based approaches (Zhang et al., 2022).

4.4 Data-Driven Approaches to Enhancing Staff Safety

The integration of data-driven strategies in healthcare has fundamentally altered the way staff safety is addressed, moving from reactive responses to proactive, predictive interventions. With the proliferation of electronic health records (EHRs), wearable devices, and smart hospital infrastructures, massive datasets are continuously being generated that can be leveraged to assess environmental hazards, staff fatigue, and workflow inefficiencies. For example, the TILES-2018 longitudinal dataset demonstrated how multimodal behavioral and physiological data collected from hospital workers could be used to model stress levels, cognitive load, and productivity, providing a data-driven foundation for developing tailored safety interventions (Mundnich et al., 2020). Such continuous monitoring allows hospitals to anticipate occupational hazards before they manifest into critical incidents, thereby improving both staff well-being and patient outcomes.

Beyond physiological monitoring, predictive analytics plays a crucial role in identifying staff safety risks in high-intensity units such as intensive care and emergency departments. Machine learning models applied to EHR and operational data have shown promise in predicting staff exposure to infection risks, particularly during pandemics, by analyzing patient-staff interaction networks (Jiang et al., 2022). This approach enables administrators to redesign shift schedules and redistribute workloads in a way that reduces infection exposure and burnout risk. Additionally, data-driven scheduling supported by artificial intelligence has been employed to optimize staff duty rosters, leading to a measurable reduction in fatigue-related errors and absenteeism in tertiary hospitals in India (Ramaswamy et al., 2023).

Another significant application is the use of IoT-based asset and personnel tracking systems to optimize operational efficiency and reduce unsafe delays. A recent study in Indian hospitals demonstrated that real-time data collected from Bluetooth beacons and RFID tags on staff uniforms reduced average inpatient transfer delays from 41% to 26.5%, simultaneously lowering physical strain on caregivers while improving patient throughput (Singh et al., 2024). Data from these systems can also be integrated into dashboards that provide hospital administrators with actionable insights into workflow inefficiencies, enabling interventions such as reallocating staff resources or reconfiguring ward layouts. Finally, process mining techniques applied to healthcare data offer deep insights into staff performance under varying workload conditions. By reconstructing actual care pathways from digital logs, healthcare organizations can pinpoint deviations that contribute to staff stress or errors and redesign processes for safety optimization (Cachazo et al., 2022). These advanced analytics techniques, when combined with behavioral sensing and IoT-based real-time monitoring, represent a comprehensive data-driven framework. Such systems not only mitigate occupational hazards but also foster a culture of continuous improvement, where staff well-being becomes an integral performance metric aligned with institutional safety and sustainability goals.

5. POLICY, GOVERNANCE, AND ETHICAL CONSIDERATIONS

5.1 Occupational Safety Standards and Global Best Practices

Occupational safety standards in healthcare are fundamental to safeguarding staff who are consistently exposed to biological, chemical, ergonomic, and psychosocial risks. Globally, regulatory frameworks such as the Occupational Safety and Health Administration (OSHA) guidelines in the United States and the European Union Directive on the protection of workers from biological agents form the basis of comprehensive staff protection strategies (Kang et al., 2022). These frameworks emphasize preventive controls including mandatory training, vaccination programs, protective gear, and incident reporting protocols. In India, the National Accreditation Board for Hospitals and Healthcare Providers (NABH) has integrated staff safety into its hospital accreditation criteria, requiring compliance with infection control protocols, biomedical waste management, and occupational exposure prevention measures (Rathi & Gupta, 2023). Such standardization ensures that healthcare staff safety becomes an institutional priority rather than an optional practice.

Best practices from global healthcare systems highlight the importance of embedding safety into organizational culture alongside compliance with standards. For example, Scandinavian countries have pioneered the use of participatory ergonomics and staff engagement in safety decision-making, leading to significantly lower rates of musculoskeletal injuries among healthcare workers (Arvidsson et al., 2022). Similarly, data-driven safety audits and risk assessments in Australian hospitals have reduced occupational accidents by aligning evidence-based monitoring with staff training initiatives (Ferguson et al., 2023). In the Indian context, research has shown that while formal standards exist, gaps in implementation persist due to under-reporting of occupational incidents and limited access to safety infrastructure in smaller hospitals (Desai et al., 2024). Bridging these gaps requires harmonizing international best practices with localized strategies that account for contextual challenges such as resource constraints.

A growing trend across global best practices is the incorporation of digital monitoring and predictive analytics into occupational safety frameworks. Hospitals in South Korea and Japan have introduced IoT-based systems to track staff exposure to airborne pathogens and noise levels, providing real-time alerts that help mitigate risks before they escalate (Lee & Kim, 2022). Indian pilot projects have experimented with integrating wearable exposure monitors and smartphone-based reporting apps for healthcare staff, enabling faster detection of occupational hazards and supporting compliance with NABH and WHO recommendations (Patel et al., 2023). Collectively, these approaches underscore that the future of occupational safety in healthcare lies in blending international standards with local realities, supported by technology-driven practices that create safer and more sustainable workplaces.

5.2 Legal and Ethical Dimensions of Staff Monitoring

The increasing use of monitoring technologies such as surveillance cameras, biometric systems, and wearable sensors in healthcare raises complex legal and ethical considerations. On the one hand, these systems enhance occupational safety by detecting hazards, preventing workplace violence, and ensuring compliance with infection control protocols. However, they also raise concerns about privacy, data ownership, and informed consent. Studies have shown that excessive surveillance without adequate safeguards may erode trust among healthcare staff, resulting in psychological stress and reduced job satisfaction (Agarwal et al., 2023). In the Indian context, the absence of a comprehensive occupational privacy framework and reliance on fragmented laws such as the Information Technology Act of 2000 and the emerging Digital Personal Data Protection Act of 2023 complicates the governance of staff monitoring practices (Sinha & Raj, 2024).

Ethical dilemmas often arise in balancing institutional responsibility for staff safety with individual rights to privacy and autonomy. For example, real-time monitoring of healthcare workers' exposure to airborne pathogens or fatigue levels may be justified as a preventive safety measure, but without clear boundaries on data usage, such practices could lead to profiling or punitive actions (McBride et al., 2021). Ethical frameworks such as the principles of beneficence and non-maleficence emphasize that monitoring should aim to promote worker well-being while minimizing potential harm. Moreover, transparent communication and participatory decision-making are critical in ensuring that staff perceive monitoring as supportive rather than coercive (Chattopadhyay & Mehta, 2022).

Globally, legal compliance is increasingly guided by standards such as the European Union's General Data Protection Regulation (GDPR) and the U.S. Health Insurance Portability and Accountability Act (HIPAA). These frameworks stress proportionality, necessity, and data minimization in employee monitoring. Evidence from comparative studies suggests that hospitals that integrate GDPR-compliant monitoring systems not only reduce legal liabilities but also strengthen employee confidence in institutional safety policies (Lopez et al., 2022). For Indian hospitals, aligning with these international best practices—while embedding them into local regulatory contexts—can create a more ethically robust monitoring ecosystem..

5.3 Psychological and Social Impacts of Monitoring

While staff monitoring technologies aim to enhance safety and operational efficiency, they can also produce unintended psychological and social consequences. Healthcare workers often perceive continuous surveillance—through CCTV, wearable sensors, or biometric tracking—as a signal of mistrust, which can reduce morale and increase workplace stress (Gupta & Sharma, 2023). Studies in Indian hospitals suggest that nurses and junior staff, who are subject to stricter supervisory protocols, frequently report feelings of anxiety and "being watched," which negatively affects concentration and performance (Rajesh & Nambiar, 2022). This phenomenon is consistent with the concept of "function creep," where technologies designed for safety gradually expand into performance evaluation, eroding professional autonomy and job satisfaction.

From a psychological perspective, monitoring can trigger heightened stress responses, sleep disturbances, and even burnout, especially when workers believe that data is being collected without their consent or transparency (Zhang et al., 2022). Social dynamics within healthcare teams may also shift, as constant monitoring can discourage peer-to-peer trust and collaborative decision-making. Instead, staff may engage in "surface compliance," prioritizing monitored behaviors over genuine patient-centered care (Fernández & Rivas, 2021). In cultures such as India's, where hierarchical structures already influence workplace interactions, surveillance may further reinforce power imbalances between management and frontline staff, reducing open communication and innovation (Mishra & Das, 2024).

On the other hand, evidence indicates that when monitoring is implemented transparently and framed as a supportive safety measure rather than a disciplinary tool, it can strengthen trust and promote a culture of care. For instance, digital fatigue monitoring systems that help allocate rest breaks are often perceived positively, as they align with staff well-being (Liang et al., 2023).

5.4 Policy Frameworks and Ethical Guidelines

The increasing reliance on digital monitoring in healthcare demands a robust policy and ethical framework to balance staff safety, organizational efficiency, and individual rights. Globally, regulatory bodies such as the World Health Organization (WHO) and the International Labour Organization (ILO) emphasize that monitoring technologies must uphold the principles of dignity, fairness, and proportionality (WHO, 2022). These guidelines stress that surveillance should be limited to legitimate safety concerns and that staff should be informed and involved in the decision-making process. In the European Union, the General Data Protection Regulation

(GDPR) has set strong precedents by requiring explicit consent, data minimization, and safeguards against misuse of personal information (Chassang, 2017).

In the Indian context, the Digital Personal Data Protection Act (2023) provides a legal foundation for handling sensitive employee data generated by hospital monitoring systems. However, enforcement in healthcare settings remains inconsistent, especially in public hospitals where resource constraints limit compliance (Kumar & Singh, 2024). Ethical dilemmas also arise from cultural factors—Indian healthcare institutions often operate within hierarchical structures where junior staff may not feel empowered to question surveillance practices. Without clear institutional guidelines, monitoring risks becoming punitive rather than supportive, potentially undermining trust between staff and administrators (Shukla & Menon, 2022).

To ensure ethical monitoring, healthcare organizations should adopt participatory governance models where policies are co-developed with staff representatives. Transparent communication, regular ethical audits, and grievance redressal mechanisms can prevent misuse while fostering acceptance. International best practices, such as Canada's "Privacy by Design" framework, suggest embedding ethical considerations into every stage of technology deployment, from procurement to day-to-day operations (Cavoukian, 2021).

6. CASE STUDIES AND BEST PRACTICES

6.1 Indian Case Studies on Staff Safety and Well-being

The Indian healthcare sector has faced unique challenges in ensuring staff safety and well-being, particularly during the COVID-19 pandemic, which exposed systemic gaps in occupational safety measures. One important example is the introduction of AI-enabled infection surveillance systems in select tertiary hospitals in Delhi, where surface contamination and air quality in COVID-19 wards were continuously monitored. This initiative not only reduced hospital-acquired infections but also strengthened staff confidence in workplace safety (Gupta et al., 2023). Similarly, the deployment of digital exposure-tracking applications in large government hospitals in Tamil Nadu helped monitor staff exposure to high-risk zones and provided timely alerts for quarantine and preventive testing. These technological innovations demonstrated how localized interventions could directly reduce infection risk among frontline healthcare workers (Rajesh & Menon, 2022).

Beyond infection control, Indian hospitals have increasingly adopted structured well-being programs that address psychological, ergonomic, and occupational risks. A case study at All India Institute of Medical Sciences (AIIMS), New Delhi, reported significant reductions in burnout and stress levels among nursing staff following the introduction of peer-support groups, counseling sessions, and mindfulness training (Sharma & Kaur, 2022). Private hospitals in Bengaluru have also integrated IoT-based monitoring of radiation exposure for radiology staff, thereby ensuring long-term occupational safety in high-risk environments. These initiatives reflect a gradual shift in both public and private hospitals toward institutionalizing staff well-being as part of sustainable healthcare practice.

However, disparities in the availability of such measures remain across India, particularly in rural and semi-urban healthcare centers. Limited resources and infrastructure often prevent these facilities from deploying advanced monitoring systems. In response, low-cost innovations such as mobile testing units for occupational hazards and community-led safety audits have been introduced with moderate success (Verma & Singh, 2021). These case studies emphasize the need for scalable models of staff safety that blend technological adoption with resource-sensitive practices, enabling healthcare institutions across diverse regions to enhance both staff well-being and patient care outcomes.

6.2 Global Examples of Sustainable Safety Initiatives in Healthcare

Globally, healthcare systems have increasingly adopted sustainable safety initiatives to protect staff while improving overall care delivery. In the United States, several hospitals have implemented IoT-based air quality monitoring systems in intensive care units to ensure safe working environments for medical staff, particularly during outbreaks of respiratory illnesses. A study at a Boston-based teaching hospital showed that real-time monitoring of airborne particulate matter helped reduce staff exposure to respiratory hazards by nearly 30 percent (Pereira et al., 2022). Similarly, Scandinavian countries such as Sweden and Denmark have institutionalized noise reduction programs in neonatal intensive care units, employing smart acoustic sensors and sound-absorbing materials to mitigate stress and fatigue among healthcare staff (Johansson & Larsson, 2021). These interventions highlight how technological solutions can be integrated into sustainable hospital design to safeguard worker well-being.

In Europe, radiation safety has received significant attention due to the extensive use of diagnostic imaging. Hospitals in Germany have deployed AI-based monitoring tools that track cumulative staff radiation exposure and provide predictive alerts for threshold exceedance, leading to measurable improvements in compliance with occupational safety standards (Klein et al., 2022). The introduction of wearable radiation detectors has also allowed healthcare professionals to make more informed decisions in high-exposure zones, reinforcing both staff protection and regulatory compliance. Beyond radiation, European health institutions are focusing on ergonomic safety through adjustable workstations and robotic assistance in surgical theaters, reducing musculoskeletal strain among doctors and nurses.

In low- and middle-income countries, global collaborations have played a vital role in strengthening safety initiatives. For instance, hospitals in Kenya and Uganda, supported by international health agencies, have deployed solar-powered IoT sensors for continuous monitoring of indoor air quality and water safety, ensuring that staff in resource-constrained settings are protected from environmental hazards (Okello et al., 2023). In addition, initiatives in Brazil and Chile have shown that integrating psychological support programs, including digital counseling platforms and peer-support networks, significantly reduces burnout and compassion fatigue among healthcare workers. These case studies collectively demonstrate that sustainable safety practices, whether technologically advanced or resource-sensitive, are critical to building resilient health systems and safeguarding staff well-being.

6.3 Lessons Learned and Replicable Models

The global and Indian experiences in implementing staff safety and well-being measures in healthcare have generated valuable lessons that can guide replicable models across diverse settings. One of the foremost lessons is the importance of integrating environmental monitoring systems into routine hospital operations rather than treating them as temporary measures. Research from European hospitals demonstrates that embedding IoT-based environmental monitoring systems for air quality and radiation into daily workflows leads to higher staff compliance and reduced occupational hazards (van Dijk et al., 2022). Similarly, in India, case studies from tertiary hospitals in Bengaluru and Delhi suggest that sustainable models require low-cost, scalable solutions such as sensor-based indoor air monitoring units and solar-powered backup systems to ensure feasibility in resource-limited environments (Rajkumar & Menon, 2023). This indicates that customization and affordability are essential for replicability in different healthcare contexts.

Another critical lesson is the role of leadership and institutional safety culture in ensuring staff protection. Hospitals that successfully institutionalized staff well-being programs emphasized participatory decision-making, continuous training, and peer-led safety audits, which significantly improved both staff morale and adherence to safety protocols (Anderson et al., 2021). Models from Nordic countries and Japan show that integrating psychological support systems like counseling, mindfulness programs, and AI-driven fatigue detection into workplace routines helps reduce burnout and compassion fatigue while maintaining long-term sustainability. These approaches highlight the need for a holistic framework that addresses both physical safety and mental well-being of staff.

7. FUTURE DIRECTIONS

7.1 AI and Predictive Analytics for Staff Well-being Monitoring

Artificial intelligence (AI) and predictive analytics are emerging as transformative tools in monitoring and enhancing the well-being of healthcare staff. Unlike traditional reactive approaches, AI enables early detection of stress, fatigue, and occupational hazards by analyzing diverse data sources, including wearable sensors, environmental monitors, and electronic health records. Studies have shown that AI-powered fatigue detection models using physiological parameters such as heart rate variability and sleep patterns can predict burnout among nurses with high accuracy, enabling proactive interventions (Chen et al., 2022). In the Indian context, pilot projects in metropolitan hospitals have used predictive analytics to monitor workload distribution and stress levels among healthcare workers, leading to improved scheduling and reduced absenteeism (Rajan & Thomas, 2023). These insights underscore the role of AI in shifting from treatment of burnout to prevention.

Another critical advantage of predictive analytics lies in its ability to correlate workplace environmental conditions with staff health outcomes. For instance, machine learning models analyzing air quality, noise levels, and ergonomic factors have successfully predicted occupational fatigue and related musculoskeletal disorders in intensive care staff (González et al., 2021). By integrating such systems into sustainable hospital infrastructures, healthcare organizations can reduce workplace hazards while enhancing overall staff performance. Moreover, predictive systems have proven useful in real-time staffing optimization, where AI-based scheduling tools balance staff availability, patient demand, and employee well-being metrics, ensuring safer and more sustainable workflows.

Importantly, predictive analytics also supports institutional decision-making by providing actionable insights into long-term workforce planning. Predictive dashboards can highlight patterns such as recurring peak-stress periods, burnout risk zones, and potential attrition trends, allowing administrators to implement preventive policies and wellness programs (Kumar & Sharma, 2023). These applications show that the integration of AI into staff well-being monitoring not only enhances individual resilience but also contributes to institutional sustainability, aligning with global occupational safety standards. With further advancements in natural language processing, AI systems may soon analyze communication patterns to detect early emotional distress, making well-being monitoring more comprehensive and human-centered.

7.2 Sustainable Infrastructure and Green Healthcare Facilities

Sustainable infrastructure plays a central role in ensuring staff safety and well-being within medical care systems. Green healthcare facilities, designed with eco-friendly architecture, energy-efficient systems, and ergonomic workplace layouts, create environments that not only conserve resources but also reduce occupational health risks. Research indicates that poor ventilation, noise pollution, and high energy demands in conventional hospital buildings contribute to stress and fatigue among staff (Ulrich et al., 2022). By contrast, sustainable hospital designs incorporating natural lighting, advanced air filtration, and low-emission construction materials significantly enhance indoor environmental quality, thereby reducing respiratory hazards and mental exhaustion among healthcare workers.

In India, several green-certified hospitals have begun adopting renewable energy systems and water recycling technologies, which not only reduce operational costs but also improve the work environment by stabilizing energy supply and minimizing environmental stressors (Ramesh & Rao, 2023). Globally, green infrastructure is increasingly aligned with staff well-being metrics, with studies showing that healthcare facilities designed according to Leadership in Energy and Environmental Design (LEED) standards report lower levels of staff absenteeism and improved job satisfaction (Gupta et al., 2022). Sustainable infrastructure thus bridges environmental responsibility with occupational safety, making it an essential pillar of resilient healthcare systems.

7.3 Role of Multi-Stakeholder Collaboration in Ensuring Staff Safety

The complexity of staff safety and well-being in healthcare demands active collaboration among multiple stakeholders, including hospital management, government agencies, professional associations, and technology providers. Multi-stakeholder collaboration ensures that safety strategies are not siloed but integrated into broader institutional and policy frameworks. Studies have shown that partnerships between hospital administrators and occupational health organizations can significantly reduce workplace hazards through shared safety audits, training programs, and policy implementation (Singh & Menon, 2023).

Technology providers also play a vital role by integrating digital monitoring tools, IoT-based hazard detection systems, and AI-driven predictive platforms into staff safety frameworks. For example, collaborations between Indian hospital networks and start-ups specializing in wearable health devices have enabled continuous monitoring of staff fatigue and exposure to harmful environments (Chatterjee et al., 2022). Governments and regulatory bodies further support this ecosystem by enforcing compliance with occupational health standards and incentivizing hospitals to adopt sustainable safety practices. Importantly, involving healthcare workers themselves in decision-making enhances the relevance and acceptance of safety interventions, creating a culture of shared responsibility and resilience.

7.4 Towards a Holistic Model of Sustainable Medical Care Workforce Safety

A holistic model of workforce safety in medical care extends beyond physical hazard mitigation to encompass mental health, environmental sustainability, and institutional resilience. Such a model integrates three dimensions: environmental design, technological innovation, and human-centered policies. On the environmental side, hospitals must adopt green infrastructure and ergonomic workplace planning. On the technological front, AI and IoT systems provide predictive insights into hazards and stress levels, allowing preventive action. Finally, at the policy level, healthcare institutions must adopt inclusive well-being programs, flexible work schedules, and long-term occupational health strategies (Patel & Verma, 2024).

Globally, healthcare systems that have embraced holistic workforce safety models report improved staff retention, reduced burnout, and enhanced quality of care (Bai et al., 2023). In India, emerging initiatives that combine environmental monitoring with employee wellness programs are creating early examples of such integrative approaches. The holistic model also emphasizes the importance of equity, ensuring that all healthcare workers, including support staff and frontline personnel, have access to safe working conditions. This systemic approach positions staff safety not as a standalone priority but as a cornerstone of sustainable healthcare delivery, directly linking workforce well-being with patient safety and organizational resilience.

8. CONCLUSION

Staff safety and well-being emerge as indispensable pillars of sustainable healthcare, directly influencing the quality of patient care, workforce retention, and institutional resilience. Key takeaways highlight that staff safety goes beyond physical hazard mitigation, extending into mental health, ergonomic design, and organizational culture, all of which must be supported through continuous monitoring and proactive interventions. The integration of sustainable environment monitoring systems into medical care provides a transformative pathway, enabling early detection of risks, data-driven decision-making, and alignment with green healthcare infrastructure for healthier workplaces. Looking ahead, future research and innovation should focus on developing holistic workforce safety models that combine artificial intelligence, IoT-enabled predictive monitoring, and policy frameworks tailored to diverse healthcare contexts, particularly in emerging economies. By embedding sustainability and staff well-being into the core of healthcare systems, medical institutions can create a resilient workforce capable of delivering high-quality care in an increasingly complex and resource-constrained world.

REFERENCES

Agarwal, R., Singh, M., & Kumar, S. (2023). Surveillance, privacy, and occupational well-being: Perceptions of healthcare workers in Indian hospitals. *Indian Journal of Medical Ethics*, *8*(2), 112–119. DOI: 10.20529/IJME.2023.028

Anderson, M., Wilson, J., & Patel, R. (2021). Building a culture of safety in health-care: Leadership and participatory approaches. *Journal of Healthcare Management*, *66*(5), 329–339. DOI: 10.1097/JHM-D-20-00167

Arvidsson, I., Balogh, I., Hansson, G.-Å., & Lindegård, A. (2022). Participatory ergonomics and staff involvement as strategies for reducing musculoskeletal disorders in healthcare. *Applied Ergonomics*, *101*, 103694. DOI: 10.1016/j.apergo.2021.103694

Bai, X., Li, Z., & Zhou, H. (2023). Integrated occupational safety models in sustainable healthcare systems. *International Journal of Environmental Research and Public Health*, *20*(18), 6789. DOI: 10.3390/ijerph20186789

Bedi, R., Sharma, A., & Gupta, N. (2022). Ergonomic risk factors and prevalence of musculoskeletal disorders among laboratory health care workers in North India. *Indian Journal of Occupational and Environmental Medicine*, *26*(1), 45–51. DOI: 10.4103/ijoem.ijoem_190_21

Bhutani, J., Bhutani, S., Balhara, Y. P. S., & Kalra, S. (2012). Compassion fatigue and burnout amongst clinicians: A medical exploratory study. *Indian Journal of Psychological Medicine*, *34*(4), 332–337. DOI: 10.4103/0253-7176.108206

Cachazo, R., González, M., & Valero, M. (2022). Process mining in healthcare: A data-driven methodology for staff performance and safety optimization. *Health Informatics Journal*, *28*(2), 1–15. DOI: 10.1177/14604582221091733

Cannaby, A., Connell, L., Viehweger, E., & Hignett, S. (2021). Feasibility and validity of real-time locating systems to measure nurses' movement and workflow in hospitals: An observational study. *Journal of Research in Nursing : JRN*, *26*(6), 571–586. DOI: 10.1177/17449871211016169

Cavoukian, A. (2021). Privacy by design: From rhetoric to reality. *Health Management*, *21*(3), 112–118. DOI: 10.1007/s10729-021-09587-2

Chassang, G. (2017). The impact of the EU general data protection regulation on medical research. *Journal of Medical Internet Research*, *19*(6), e193. DOI: 10.2196/jmir.7108

Chatterjee, A., Sinha, R., & Deshmukh, P. (2022). Wearable health technologies and occupational safety in Indian healthcare settings. *Health and Technology, 12*(5), 1001–1012. DOI: 10.1007/s12553-022-00691-2

Chattopadhyay, S., & Mehta, K. (2022). Ethics of digital monitoring in healthcare workplaces: Balancing safety and autonomy. *Journal of Medical Ethics, 48*(11), 789–794. DOI: 10.1136/medethics-2021-107871

Chen, H.-L., Lin, C.-Y., & Chang, W.-C. (2022). Patient safety culture and staff well-being in Taiwan: An organizational resource perspective. *Journal of Patient Safety, 18*(8), 663–670. DOI: 10.1097/PTS.0000000000000947

Chen, Y., Wang, X., & Li, J. (2022). Artificial intelligence-driven fatigue detection in healthcare professionals: A machine learning approach. *Journal of Biomedical Informatics, 130*, 104089. DOI: 10.1016/j.jbi.2022.104089

Chen, Y.-Y., Chien, W.-C., Lee, M.-S., Chen, L.-H., Chan, T.-C., & Lee, C.-H. (2023). Applying a smartwatch to predict work-related fatigue for emergency healthcare professionals: Machine learning method. *Journal of Medical Internet Research, 25*, e30405. DOI: 10.2196/30405

Desai, P., Kumar, V., & Singh, A. (2024). Occupational safety challenges among healthcare workers in Indian hospitals: An implementation gap analysis. *Indian Journal of Occupational and Environmental Medicine, 28*(1), 45–52. DOI: 10.4103/ijoem.ijoem_14_24

Dufera, M., Tuly, L., & Mwale, L.. (2023). Occupational-related injuries and associated risk factors among healthcare workers working in developing countries: A systematic review. *Journal of Occupational Health, 65*(1), e12455. DOI: 10.1002/joh2.12455

Dyrbye, L. N., Shanafelt, T. D., Sinsky, C. A., Cipriano, P. F., Bhatt, J., Ommaya, A., West, C. P., & Meyers, D. (2020). Burnout among healthcare professionals: A call to explore and address this underrecognized threat to safe, high-quality care. *National Academy of Medicine, 99*(1), 11–20. DOI: 10.31478/202001a

Ferguson, C., Yu, M., & Bismark, M. (2023). Data-driven safety audits in healthcare: Reducing occupational hazards through real-time monitoring. *Journal of Healthcare Risk Management, 42*(2), 23–33. DOI: 10.1002/jhrm.22156

Fernández, J., & Rivas, A. (2021). The social consequences of workplace monitoring in healthcare: From compliance to resistance. *Social Science & Medicine, 285*, 114262. DOI: 10.1016/j.socscimed.2021.114262

Galvão, D. M.. (2023). Hospital sustainability indicators and reduction of socio-environmental impacts: A scoping review. *Revista da Escola de Enfermagem da USP*, *57*, e20220364. DOI: 10.1590/1980-220X-REEUSP-2022-0364en

George, C. E., Varghese, J., & Ravi, D. (2020). Burnout among nurses and its impact on patient care in South India: A cross-sectional study. *Indian Journal of Occupational and Environmental Medicine*, *24*(3), 202–207. DOI: 10.4103/ijoem.IJOEM_257_19

González, M., Rivera, P., & López, C. (2021). Predictive modeling of occupational fatigue among intensive care staff using machine learning. *Safety and Health at Work*, *12*(4), 443–450. DOI: 10.1016/j.shaw.2021.09.002

Green Paper, E. S. I. C. M. (2018). Environmental sustainability in intensive care: The path forward. *Intensive Care Medicine*. Advance online publication. DOI: 10.1007/s00134-018-5111-9

Gupta, R., Chatterjee, S., & Nair, A. (2023). AI-enabled monitoring for infection control in Indian hospitals: A COVID-19 case study. *International Journal of Healthcare Management*, *16*(2), 85–94. DOI: 10.1080/20479700.2023.2178452

Gupta, V., & Sharma, P. (2023). Surveillance and workplace stress among Indian healthcare workers: An emerging concern. *Indian Journal of Occupational and Environmental Medicine*, *27*(1), 15–21. DOI: 10.4103/ijoem.ijoem_89_22

Hall, L. H., Johnson, J., Watt, I., Tsipa, A., & O'Connor, D. B. (2016). Healthcare staff wellbeing, burnout, and patient safety: A systematic review. *PLoS One*, *11*(7), e0159015. DOI: 10.1371/journal.pone.0159015

Ho, S. S., Sosina, W., DePierro, J. M., Perez, S., Khan, A., Starkweather, S., Marin, D. B., Sharma, V., Ripp, J. A., Peccoralo, L. A., & Charney, D. S. (2024). Promoting resilience in healthcare workers: A preventative mental health education program. *International Journal of Environmental Research and Public Health*, *21*(10), 1365. DOI: 10.3390/ijerph21101365

Jiang, Y., Xu, J., & Wang, X. (2022). Machine learning for predicting occupational risks of healthcare workers during infectious disease outbreaks. *Journal of Biomedical Informatics*, *128*, 104048. DOI: 10.1016/j.jbi.2022.104048

Johansson, A., & Larsson, P. (2021). Smart acoustic monitoring for occupational safety in neonatal intensive care units: A Swedish case study. *Journal of Environmental Health Science & Engineering*, *19*(4), 425–433. DOI: 10.1007/s40201-021-00650-3

Johnson, C. T., & Hessels, A. J. (2023). Associations between negative patient safety climate and infection prevention practices. *American Journal of Infection Control, 52*(9), 1102–1104. DOI: 10.1016/j.ajic.2024.06.010

Joseph, B., Ramesh, N., & Sreejith, N. (2021). Prevalence and risk factors of work-related musculoskeletal disorders among nurses in South India. *International Journal of Occupational Safety and Ergonomics, 27*(4), 1036–1043. DOI: 10.1080/10803548.2019.1645309

Kakhi, K., Jagatheesaperumal, S. K., Khosravi, A., Alizadehsani, R., & Acharya, U. R. (2024). Fatigue monitoring using wearables and AI: Trends, challenges, and future opportunities. *Sensors (Basel), 24*(1), 112. DOI: 10.3390/s24010112

Kang, J., Cho, S., & Park, J. (2022). Global occupational safety standards in healthcare: A comparative review of OSHA and EU directives. *Safety Science, 148*, 105653. DOI: 10.1016/j.ssci.2022.105653

Klein, H., Bauer, F., & Richter, T. (2022). Artificial intelligence-based monitoring of radiation exposure in European hospitals: Advancing occupational safety. *European Journal of Radiology, 149*, 110229. DOI: 10.1016/j.ejrad.2021.110229

Kumar, A., & Singh, R. (2024). Data protection and staff surveillance in Indian healthcare: Challenges of implementation. *Journal of Health Management, 26*(1), 45–60. DOI: 10.1177/09720634241230215

Kumar, R., & Sharma, A. (2023). Predictive workforce analytics for healthcare staff well-being: An Indian hospital perspective. *Indian Journal of Occupational and Environmental Medicine, 27*(2), 85–92. DOI: 10.4103/ijoem.ijoem_154_23

Lakshmikanthcharan, S., Sivakumar, M. N., & Hisham, M. (2019). Stress and burnout among intensive care unit healthcare professionals in an Indian tertiary care hospital. *Indian Journal of Critical Care Medicine : Peer-Reviewed, Official Publication of Indian Society of Critical Care Medicine, 23*(10), 462–466. DOI: 10.5005/jp-journals-10071-23311

Lee, H., & Kim, J. (2022). IoT-enabled occupational safety monitoring for healthcare workers: A hospital-based study in South Korea. *International Journal of Environmental Research and Public Health, 19*(22), 15012. DOI: 10.3390/ijerph192215012

Li, J., Zhang, Y., & Wang, Q. (2022). Effectiveness of ergonomic interventions in reducing musculoskeletal disorders among hospital nurses: Evidence from a Chinese tertiary care hospital. *Journal of Advanced Nursing, 78*(2), 712–721. DOI: 10.1111/jan.15022

Liang, H., Zhou, J., & Chen, Y. (2023). Wearable fatigue monitoring in hospitals: Impacts on staff well-being and organizational culture. *Journal of Nursing Management, 31*(4), 785–795. DOI: 10.1111/jonm.13876

Lopez, M. J., García, J., & Ruiz, C. (2022). GDPR compliance in employee monitoring: Lessons for healthcare institutions. *Computer Law & Security Review, 45*, 105657. DOI: 10.1016/j.clsr.2022.105657

Malode, S. J., Alshehri, M. A., & Shetti, N. P. (2025). Revolutionizing human healthcare with wearable sensors for monitoring human strain. *Colloids and Surfaces. B, Biointerfaces, 246*, 114384. DOI: 10.1016/j.colsurfb.2024.114384

McBride, B., Carter, A., & Verma, R. (2021). Legal and ethical implications of wearable monitoring technologies in healthcare. *Health Policy and Technology, 10*(3), 100564. DOI: 10.1016/j.hlpt.2021.100564

Minhas, S., Kotwal, A., & Singh, M. (2011). Infection control in health care facilities. *Medical Journal, Armed Forces India, 67*(1), 7–8. DOI: 10.1016/S0377-1237(11)80003-1

Minikumary, C. K., & Pillai, J. S. K. (2023). A study on occupational safety and health among workers at a tertiary care hospital in south India. *International Journal of Community Medicine and Public Health, 10*(1), 254–257. DOI: 10.18203/2394-6040.ijcmph20223553

Mishra, R., & Das, K. (2024). Workplace hierarchy, digital surveillance, and employee well-being in Indian healthcare institutions. *Journal of Health Management, 26*(2), 167–182. DOI: 10.1177/09720634241234567

Moon, J., & Ju, B.-K. (2024). Wearable sensors for healthcare of industrial workers: A scoping review. *Electronics (Basel), 13*(19), 3849. DOI: 10.3390/electronics13193849

Moreno, A., (2025). Integrating environmental sustainability into hospitals performance management systems: A scoping review. *BMC Health Services Research, 25*, 12928. Advance online publication. DOI: 10.1186/s12913-025-12928-x

Mundnich, K., Booth, B. M., L'Hommedieu, M., Girault, B., Lerman, K., & Narayanan, S. (2020). TILES-2018: A longitudinal multimodal dataset of hospital staff for modeling behavioral and physiological factors. *Nature Scientific Data, 7*(354), 1–14. DOI: 10.1038/s41597-020-00676-y

Nguyen, T. P., Pham, D. T., & Tran, Q. L. (2025). Non-invasive fatigue detection and human–machine interaction using LSTM and multimodal AI: A case study. *Multimodal Technologies and Interaction, 9*(6), 63. DOI: 10.3390/mti9060063

Occupational Hazards among Healthcare Workers in Africa: A Systematic Review. (2018). *Annals of Global Health, 84*(3), 367–384. https://doi.org/DOI: 10.5334/aogh.2434

Okello, D., Namusoke, J., & Mwesige, C. (2023). Sustainable safety monitoring in East African hospitals: Solar-powered IoT innovations for healthcare staff. *International Journal of Environmental Research and Public Health, 20*(2), 1125. DOI: 10.3390/ijerph20021125

Parkavi, A., Sowmya, B. J., Alex, S. A., Supreeth, S., Shruthi, G., Rohith, S., Chatterjee, S., & Lingaraj, K. (2025). *Air quality and dust level monitoring systems in hospitals using IoT*. Discover Internet of Things., DOI: 10.1007/s43926-025-00120-w

Patel, S., Sharma, D., & Menon, R. (2023). Mobile technology and wearable monitors for occupational health surveillance in Indian healthcare. *Journal of Occupational Health, 65*(1), e12378. DOI: 10.1002/1348-9585.12378

Patel, S., & Verma, D. (2024). Towards holistic workforce safety in healthcare: Policies and practices for sustainable systems. *Journal of Health Policy and Management, 13*(1), 45–57. DOI: 10.34172/jhpm.2024.06

Patil, K. H., Tawar, N. S., & Kudale, A. M. (2024). A post-COVID-19 assessment of resilience of nurses and paramedical workers in municipal hospitals of urban Pune, India. *Journal of Family Medicine and Primary Care, 13*(4), 1460–1466. DOI: 10.4103/jfmpc.jfmpc_947_23

Pereira, L., Radovic, T., & Haykal, K. A. (2021). Peer support programs in the fields of medicine and nursing: A systematic search and narrative review. *Canadian Medical Education Journal, 12*(3), 113–125. DOI: 10.36834/cmej.71129

Pereira, R., Adams, J., & White, L. (2022). IoT-based air quality monitoring for occupational safety in US hospitals: A case study. *Journal of Occupational and Environmental Hygiene, 19*(6), 289–298. DOI: 10.1080/15459624.2022.2049364

Rajan, D., & Thomas, P. (2023). Artificial intelligence and staff scheduling: Reducing burnout risk in Indian healthcare systems. *Journal of Health Management, 25*(3), 321–333. DOI: 10.1177/09720634231102587

Rajesh, K., & Menon, V. (2022). Digital exposure monitoring for frontline workers in Indian healthcare settings: Lessons from COVID-19. *Journal of Health Research, 36*(4), 642–650. DOI: 10.1108/JHR-08-2021-0456

Rajesh, M., & Nambiar, S. (2022). Nurses under watch: Perceptions of monitoring technologies in Indian hospitals. *International Journal of Healthcare Management, 15*(3), 189–197. DOI: 10.1080/20479700.2021.1998754

Rajkumar, S., & Menon, V. (2023). Scalable environmental monitoring for healthcare staff safety: Insights from Indian tertiary hospitals. *Indian Journal of Public Health Research & Development, 14*(1), 56–63. DOI: 10.37506/ijphrd.v14i1.18491

Ramaswamy, P., Sahu, A., & Krishnan, R. (2023). AI-enabled workforce scheduling for improving occupational safety of healthcare staff in Indian tertiary hospitals. *Indian Journal of Occupational and Environmental Medicine, 27*(3), 175–183. DOI: 10.4103/ijoem.ijoem_126_23

Ramesh, V., & Rao, P. (2023). Sustainable hospital design in India: Implications for staff safety and environmental health. *Indian Journal of Occupational and Environmental Medicine, 27*(3), 145–153. DOI: 10.4103/ijoem.ijoem_182_23

Rao, M., & Kumar, A. (2021). Well-being of healthcare workers and its impact on patient care in India: A review. *Journal of Health Management, 23*(2), 317–329. DOI: 10.1177/0972063421994945

Rathi, N., & Gupta, R. (2023). Evaluating NABH standards for occupational safety in Indian hospitals: Compliance and challenges. *Journal of Health Management, 25*(3), 345–359. DOI: 10.1177/09720634231120245

Saraswat, P. P., & Tiwari, R. R.. (2021). Hospital-acquired infection awareness and control practices among healthcare staff: An evaluation. *British Journal of Health Care Management, 27*(11), 296–302. DOI: 10.12968/bjhc.2020.0037

Sarker, H., Hossain, M., & Choudhury, T., & al. (2022). A field trial of a smartphone-based sensing platform for understanding clinician stress in a hospital setting. *Scientific Data, 9*, 332. DOI: 10.1038/s41597-022-01361-y

Schoierer, J., Dorman, L., & Havenith, G. (2023). Effects of heat and personal protective equipment on thermal strain in healthcare workers: Part B—application of wearable sensors to observe heat strain among healthcare workers under controlled conditions. *International Archives of Occupational and Environmental Health.* Advance online publication. DOI: 10.1007/s00420-023-02022-2

Senthil, A., Anandh, B., Jayachandran, P., Thangavel, G., Josephin, D., & Kalpana, B. (2015). Perception and prevalence of work-related health hazards among health care workers in public health facilities in southern India. *International Journal of Occupational and Environmental Health, 21*(1), 74–81. DOI: 10.1179/2049396714Y.0000000096

Senthil, A., Anandh, B., Jayachandran, P., Thangavel, G., Josephin, D., & Kalpana, B. (2015). Perception and prevalence of work-related health hazards among health care workers in public health facilities in southern India. *International Journal of Occupational and Environmental Health, 21*(1), 74–81. DOI: 10.1179/2049396714Y.0000000096

Serranheira, F., Sousa-Uva, M., & Sousa-Uva, A. (2020). Hospital nurses' working conditions in relation to musculoskeletal disorders: A systematic review. *Applied Ergonomics, 87*, 103114. DOI: 10.1016/j.apergo.2020.103114

Sharma, P., & Kaur, G. (2022). Addressing burnout among nurses in Indian tertiary care hospitals: A case-based intervention study. *Indian Journal of Occupational and Environmental Medicine, 26*(3), 174–181. DOI: 10.4103/ijoem.ijoem_189_22

Sharma, S., Khandelwal, V., & Mishra, G. (2019). Video surveillance of hand hygiene: A better tool for monitoring and ensuring hand hygiene adherence. *Indian Journal of Critical Care Medicine : Peer-Reviewed, Official Publication of Indian Society of Critical Care Medicine, 23*(5), 224–226. DOI: 10.5005/jp-journals-10071-23165

Shukla, P., & Menon, S. (2022). Ethical implications of digital surveillance in Indian hospitals. *Indian Journal of Medical Ethics, 7*(2), 93–99. DOI: 10.20529/IJME.2022.024

Simms, L., Ottman, K. E., Griffith, J. L., Knight, M. G., Norris, L., Karakcheyeva, V., & Kohrt, B. A. (2023). Psychosocial peer support to address mental health and burnout of health care workers affected by COVID-19: A qualitative evaluation. *International Journal of Environmental Research and Public Health, 20*(5), 4536. DOI: 10.3390/ijerph20054536

Singh, R., Mehta, K., & Sharma, P. (2024). IoT-based real-time staff and patient tracking for enhancing hospital safety and efficiency. *Sensors (Basel), 24*(1), 2020. DOI: 10.3390/s24012020

Singh, R., & Menon, S. (2023). Collaborative frameworks for healthcare workforce safety: An Indian perspective. *Journal of Occupational Health, 65*(2), e12345. DOI: 10.1002/1348-9585.12345

Sinha, T., & Raj, A. (2024). Staff monitoring, data protection, and legal gaps in Indian healthcare: An analysis of evolving frameworks. *Journal of Health Law and Policy, 6*(1), 25–39. DOI: 10.1177/23992026241234567

Sulosaari, V., Unal, E., & Cinar, F. I. (2022). The effectiveness of mindfulness-based interventions on the psychological well-being of nurses: A systematic review. *Applied Nursing Research, 64*, 151565. DOI: 10.1016/j.apnr.2022.151565

Thazha, S. K., & Cruz, J. P.. (2022). Infection prevention and control awareness, attitudes, and practices among healthcare professionals in South India. *BMC Health Services Research, 22*(1), 272. DOI: 10.1186/s12913-022-07673-4

Ulrich, R., Zimring, C., & Quan, X. (2022). The impact of healthcare design on staff well-being: A review of evidence. *Health Environments Research & Design Journal, 15*(4), 75–92. DOI: 10.1177/19375867221103256

van Dijk, J., Meijer, A., & Schmidt, K. (2022). Embedding IoT-based monitoring systems for staff safety in European hospitals. *Safety Science, 153*, 105792. DOI: 10.1016/j.ssci.2022.105792

Velicka, J., Pies, M., Hajovsky, R., Barnova, K., & Martinek, R. (2025). Smart oxygen monitoring in hospitals: A pilot study during COVID-19. *Scientific Reports*. Advance online publication. DOI: 10.1038/s41598-025-87665-6

Verma, S., & Singh, A. (2021). Low-cost workplace safety interventions in rural Indian hospitals: A pilot study. *Indian Journal of Public Health, 65*(2), 123–128. DOI: 10.4103/ijph.IJPH_1058_20

Vonderlin, R., Biermann, M., Bohus, M., & Lyssenko, L. (2020). Mindfulness-based programs in the workplace: A meta-analysis of randomized controlled trials. *Mindfulness, 11*(3), 2020. DOI: 10.1007/s12671-019-01391-5

World Health Organization. (2022). *Ethical considerations for digital health monitoring in workplaces*. WHO Press., DOI: 10.26719/9789240053456

Zhang, T., Wang, L., & Hu, X. (2022). Psychological stress and burnout in healthcare workers under digital monitoring systems. *BMC Health Services Research, 22*(1), 945. DOI: 10.1186/s12913-022-08456-3

Zhang, Y., Chen, X., Lao, Y., Qiu, X., Liu, K., Zhuang, Y., Gong, X., & Wang, P. (2023). Effects of the implementation of intelligent technology for hand hygiene in hospitals: Systematic review and meta-analysis. *Journal of Medical Internet Research, 25*, e37249. DOI: 10.2196/37249

Zhang, Z., Chen, L., Xu, P., Wang, Q., Zhang, J., Chen, K., Clements, C. M., Celi, L. A., Herasevich, V., & Hong, Y. (2022). Effectiveness of automated alerting system compared to usual care for the management of sepsis. *NPJ Digital Medicine, 5*, 134. Advance online publication. DOI: 10.1038/s41746-022-00650-5

Chapter 10
Psychological Impacts of Natural Disasters:
Recent Understandings and Future Directions

Guddo
https://orcid.org/0000-0002-0322-5606
Lovely Professional University, Punjab, India

Belinda Nyarkoh
https://orcid.org/0009-0002-8891-6330
Lovely Professional University, Punjab, India

Shikha Pandey
https://orcid.org/0009-0007-4443-5662
University of Lucknow, India

ABSTRACT

This chapter examines the complex psychological impact of natural disasters on individuals and communities across different contexts and populations. Drawing on interdisciplinary research from clinical psychology, public health, disaster management, and social sciences, the chapter provides an integrative analysis of the psychological sequelae of natural disasters, ranging from immediate stress responses to long-term mental health outcomes. Particular attention is given to vulnerable populations, factors influencing psychological resilience, current intervention frameworks, and cultural variations in psychological responses. The chapter identifies critical gaps in current understanding, highlighting the need for more culturally responsive, trauma-informed approaches to disaster mental health. Finally, it proposes evidence-based recommendations for strengthening psychological

DOI: 10.4018/979-8-3373-5636-5.ch010

resilience at individual, community, and systems levels, emphasising the importance of integrating mental health considerations into broader disaster preparedness, response, and recovery frameworks.

INTRODUCTION

Natural disasters represent some of the most devastating disruptions to human life, affecting millions of people annually through earthquakes, hurricanes, floods, wildfires, tsunamis, and droughts. While the physical destruction from these events is immediately visible and quantifiable, the psychological aftermath often remains hidden yet profoundly impactful, sometimes persisting for decades (Goldmann & Galea, 2014). The World Health Organization estimates that between 30-50% of populations severely affected by disasters may experience some form of negative psychological outcome (WHO, 2019). These impacts extend beyond individual mental health to affect family systems, community cohesion, economic productivity, and long-term societal stability.

The psychological dimension of natural disasters has gained increasing attention in recent decades, particularly following high-profile events such as the 2004 Indian Ocean tsunami, Hurricane Katrina in 2005, the 2010 Haiti earthquake, and the 2011 Tohoku earthquake and tsunami in Japan. Research has demonstrated that beyond physical injury and loss of life, natural disasters can profoundly disrupt psychological well-being through multiple pathways: direct trauma exposure, loss of loved ones, destruction of homes and communities, displacement, disruption of social networks, economic insecurity, and breakdown of essential services (Norris et al., 2002). The global increase in frequency and intensity of natural disasters associated with climate change further heightens the urgency of understanding and addressing their psychological impacts.

METHODOLOGY

This chapter uses a narrative review method to critically examine and conceptualise the key inquiries surrounding the psychological dimensions of natural disasters. It will systematically synthesise existing literature on the psychosocial effects of these disasters, focusing on distinct phases of disaster response and long-term recovery. Furthermore, it will identify factors contributing to differential vulnerability and resilience in disaster-induced psychological distress. It will also develop empirically supported strategies to enhance psychological resilience across multiple levels, including individual, community, and institutional frameworks.

LITERATURE REVIEW

This literature review critically examines existing research on the psychological consequences of natural disasters, synthesising key findings on trauma, resilience, and recovery patterns across affected populations. It explores the differential psychological responses observed during immediate disaster impact, short-term adaptation, and long-term recovery phases. Special emphasis is placed on identifying risk factors (pre-existing mental health conditions, socioeconomic disparities) and protective mechanisms (social support, community cohesion) that influence post-disaster mental health outcomes. Additionally, the review highlights gaps in current knowledge, particularly concerning culturally sensitive interventions and the long-term psychosocial effects of climate-related disasters. Finally, it proposes future research directions, emphasising the need for longitudinal studies, cross-cultural comparisons, and integrated policy frameworks to enhance psychological resilience in disaster-prone regions.

Disaster and Mental Health

The study of psychological impacts of natural disasters has evolved through several conceptual frameworks. Early approaches primarily emphasised individual psychopathology, focusing on diagnosable conditions such as Post-Traumatic Stress Disorder (PTSD) and Major Depressive Disorder (MDD) (Norris et al., 2002). More recent frameworks have adopted ecological and systems perspectives that consider multiple levels of influence on disaster outcomes, from individual characteristics to family dynamics, community resources, cultural factors, and institutional responses (Hoffman & Kruczek, 2011).

The Conservation of Resources (COR) theory (Hobfoll, 1989) has been particularly influential, positing that psychological distress results from actual resource loss, threatened resource loss, or failure to gain resources following resource investment. In disaster contexts, these resources include material possessions (homes, belongings), personal characteristics (self-efficacy, optimism), conditions (employment, health), and energies (time, knowledge). The Psychological First Aid framework, developed by the National Child Traumatic Stress Network and the National Center for PTSD, provides practical guidelines for supporting immediate psychological needs following disasters (Brymer et al., 2006). Subsequently, the concept of resilience has gained prominence, shifting focus from deficits and vulnerabilities to strengths and adaptive capacities at individual and community levels (Bonanno et al., 2010), which has led to increased attention to post-traumatic growth–the positive psychological changes that can emerge from struggling with highly challenging life circumstances (Tedeschi & Calhoun, 2004).

Psychological Impacts Across Disaster Phases

The psychological responses evolve across different phases of disasters. The impact phase is characterised by shock, disbelief, fear, and panic reactions. The immediate post-impact phase often involves heightened arousal, hypervigilance, and numbing, alongside practical concerns for safety and survival. As immediate threats recede, psychological responses may include acute stress reactions, grief, anxiety, and initial trauma symptoms (North & Pfefferbaum, 2013). Similarly, recovery phase of disaster brings different psychological challenges, including displacement stress, loss of community, uncertainty about the future, and the emotional toll of rebuilding lives. Long-term outcomes vary considerably, with estimates suggesting that while most disaster survivors demonstrate psychological resilience, approximately 10-30% may develop clinically significant conditions such as PTSD, depression, anxiety disorders, substance use disorders, and complicated grief (Goldmann & Galea, 2014; Neria et al., 2008).

Factors Influencing Psychological Outcomes

Many studies have delineated critical risk and protective factors that shape psychological trajectories following natural disasters. These determinants operate across multiple ecological levels, mediating the severity and persistence of mental health consequences.

Risk Factors

Risk factors are conditions or characteristics that increase susceptibility to adverse psychological outcomes following natural disasters. These include disaster severity, high exposure, and pre-existing vulnerabilities such as low socioeconomic status or prior mental health conditions (Norris et al., 2002). Such factors heighten the likelihood of post-traumatic stress, depression, and prolonged grief.

- *Disaster-related characteristics:* Event severity including magnitude, duration, and unpredictability, physical destruction scale, and secondary adversities (Norris et al., 2002).
- *Exposure level:* Direct life threat, physical proximity to the disaster epicenter, traumatic exposure like witnessing casualties, and personal bereavement (Brewin et al., 2000).
- *Socio-demographic vulnerabilities:* Heightened risk among women, children, elderly populations, economically disadvantaged groups, and marginalized communities (Norris et al., 2002).

Protective Factors

Protective factors are individual, social, or institutional resources that mitigate psychological distress and foster resilience after disasters. These encompass personal traits, strong social support networks, and effective institutional responses (Bonanno et al., 2010; Kaniasty & Norris, 2009). They buffer against trauma and facilitate adaptive recovery, even in high-risk populations.

- *Individual-level resources:* Innate resilience capacities, adaptive coping strategies, perceived self-efficacy, and existential or spiritual grounding (Bonanno et al., 2010).
- *Social and community-level buffers:* Robust interpersonal support systems, collective solidarity, and culturally embedded protective practices (Kaniasty & Norris, 2009).
- *Structural and institutional enablers:* Effective disaster preparedness systems, accessible mental health services, and post-disaster socioeconomic stabilization measures (Patel et al., 2017).

Vulnerable Populations

Some demographic groups like children, women, elderly and people with disability exhibit increased susceptibility to adverse psychological outcomes in the aftermath of natural disasters. Children represent a particularly vulnerable population, often manifesting trauma through developmental regression, separation anxiety, and behavioural disturbances that may have long-term implications for their psychosocial development (La Greca et al., 2013). Elderly individuals confront distinct challenges stemming from age-related physical limitations, the psychological toll of forced relocation, diminished autonomy, and interruptions to essential medical services (Fernandez et al., 2002).

Similarly, populations with pre-existing psychiatric conditions face significant risks of symptom exacerbation and treatment discontinuity during disaster scenarios (Ursano et al., 2003). Socioeconomically disadvantaged groups experience compounded vulnerabilities due to inadequate housing infrastructure, financial constraints limiting evacuation capacity, and systemic barriers to post-disaster mental healthcare access (Fothergill & Peek, 2004). Indigenous communities present a unique case of cumulative vulnerability, where contemporary disaster impacts intersect with historical trauma, cultural dislocation, and the breakdown of traditional healing networks (Kirmayer et al., 2014). Therefore, this difference in people's vulnerability underscores the necessity for targeted, population-specific interventions in disaster mental health planning and response.

PSYCHOLOGICAL RESPONSES TO NATURAL DISASTERS

Natural disasters elicit profound psychological distress, with survivors frequently experiencing acute stress, anxiety, and PTSD, which can persist long after the event (Galea et al., 2005). The severity of these reactions often correlates with the magnitude of the disaster and individual susceptibility, manifesting in grief, depression, and PTSD (Norris et al., 2002). However, psychological resilience and strong social support systems can significantly buffer these adverse effects, promoting adaptive coping (Bonanno et al., 2010). Consequently, timely interventions such as trauma-focused counseling and community rehabilitation initiatives are critical in fostering recovery and reducing chronic mental health impairments (Watson et al., 2011).

Short-term Psychological Responses

The immediate psychological reactions to natural disasters stem from the acute activation of the human stress response system when confronted with life-threatening situations (Lazarus & Folkman, 1984). Common short-term responses include intense fear, shock, and hypervigilance, often accompanied by dissociation or emotional numbness (Bryant, 2011). Survivors may also exhibit cognitive impairment, such as confusion and difficulty concentrating, due to overwhelming stress (Arnberg et al., 2015). While these reactions are typically adaptive in the short term, prolonged distress can signal the onset of more severe conditions like acute stress disorder (American Psychiatric Association, 2013). Understanding these responses is critical for implementing timely psychological first aid and crisis interventions (World Health Organization, 2011). The typical acute psychological responses are discussed below;

Fear and Anxiety: In the immediate aftermath of disasters, survivors typically experience intense fear responses mediated by amygdala hyperactivity and sympathetic nervous system activation (Shin & Liberzon, 2010). While evolutionarily adaptive, these reactions frequently progress into pathological anxiety when threat perceptions persist beyond the danger period (Bryant, 2011). Research indicates approximately 25-35% of survivors develop disaster-specific phobias or panic symptoms, particularly when the event involved unpredictable threats or loss of control (Garakani et al., 2020). Neuroimaging studies reveal these responses correlate with decreased prefrontal cortex regulation of limbic system activity, creating a neural basis for chronic anxiety disorders if left unaddressed (Jovanovic & Norrholm, 2011).

Acute Stress Reactions: Many survivors exhibit transient dissociative symptoms like emotional numbing or derealization, representing the brain's protective mechanism against overwhelming trauma (Lanius et al., 2010). These responses involve temporary disruptions in thalamocortical connectivity and prefrontal inhibition of emotional processing (Cardeña & Carlson, 2011). However, when dissociation persists beyond two weeks, it predicts significantly higher risks for PTSD development, with neurobiological studies showing associated hippocampal volume reduction (Wolf et al., 2012). Approximately 15-25% of survivors meet criteria for acute stress disorder, particularly those with prior trauma exposure or limited social support post-disaster (Bryant, 2019).

Grief Responses: Disaster-related bereavement often produces complicated grief reactions due to the sudden, violent nature of deaths and frequent inability to recover remains (Kristensen et al., 2012). Neurobiological research demonstrates sustained activation in the brain's attachment systems (nucleus accumbens, ventral tegmental area) coupled with stress response hyperactivity (O'Connor et al., 2008). These dual activations explain the characteristic symptoms of persistent yearning and difficulty accepting the loss, which affects 10-20% of bereaved survivors (Arizmendi et al., 2016). Cultural disruptions in mourning rituals further exacerbate these responses by removing traditional coping mechanisms that facilitate grief resolution (Stroebe et al., 2017).

Cognitive Impairments: The extreme stress of disasters induces temporary but significant cognitive deficits, particularly in working memory and executive functioning (Arnsten, 2015). Cortisol-mediated suppression of hippocampal activity and prefrontal cortex dysfunction underlie these impairments, typically manifest as concentration difficulties and decision-making challenges (Starcke & Brand, 2012). Studies show these effects peak in the first month post-disaster, with 30-40% of survivors reporting noticeable cognitive impacts (Hermans et al., 2014). While usually transient, prolonged stress exposure can lead to lasting neurocognitive changes through mechanisms like reduced neurogenesis and synaptic plasticity (Brewin, 2011).

Physiological Arousal: Nearly all survivors experience heightened physiological arousal immediately following disasters, characterized by sleep disturbances, hypervigilance, and exaggerated startle responses (Shin & Liberzon, 2010). These symptoms reflect sustained activation of the hypothalamic-pituitary-adrenal axis and sympathetic nervous system, with measurable increases in cortisol and catecholamine levels (Arnsten, 2015). While normative in the acute phase, persistent arousal beyond one month signals increased risk for chronic stress disorders, affecting approximately 20-30% of exposed populations without intervention (Bryant, 2019).

Long-term Psychological Consequences

While many survivors demonstrate resilience, natural disasters can produce continuous psychological impacts for a significant minority. Chronic post-traumatic stress disorder (PTSD), depression, and anxiety disorders frequently persist years after the event, particularly among those with limited social support or pre-existing vulnerabilities (Neria et al., 2008). Survivors may also develop complex grief, substance abuse disorders, or somatic symptoms linked to prolonged distress (Kessler et al., 2008). The severity of long-term outcomes often correlates with disaster exposure intensity, economic losses, and inadequate mental health interventions (Norris et al., 2002). These findings underscore the need for sustained, culturally sensitive mental health services to mitigate chronic psychological burdens (Bonanno et al., 2010).

Post-Traumatic Stress Disorder (PTSD): Neria et al. (2008) reveal that PTSD prevalence among disaster survivors ranges from 10-30%, with variability strongly influenced by disaster type, exposure severity, and pre-existing vulnerabilities. The disorder's diagnostic criteria—including intrusive recollections, persistent avoidance, negative cognitive alterations, and hyperarousal—collectively impair functioning when symptoms endure beyond one month. These manifestations often reflect neurobiological changes in threat processing systems, particularly heightened amygdala reactivity coupled with prefrontal cortex dysfunction (Shalev et al., 2017).

Depression and Complicated Grief: Major depression affects 15-25% of survivors, frequently co-occurring with PTSD due to shared environmental triggers and genetic predispositions (Sung et al., 2011). Complicated grief, present in 10-15% of bereaved survivors, represents a distinct clinical entity characterised by prolonged... by prolonged yearning and impaired acceptance of loss that persists beyond typical mourning periods (Kristensen et al., 2012). This condition demonstrates unique neural correlates, including sustained activity in the nucleus accumbens, suggesting pathological maintenance of attachment bonds (O'Connor et al., 2008).

Anxiety Disorders: Beyond PTSD, disasters precipitate generalised anxiety (8-20% prevalence) through sustained activation of the hypothalamic-pituitary-adrenal axis, with phobic responses often conditioned to disaster-related stimuli (McFarlane et al., 2009). The development of these disorders reflects failures in fear extinction processes, particularly impaired safety signal learning in the ventromedial prefrontal cortex (Milad et al., 2012).

Substance Use Disorders: Post-disaster substance misuse surges by 25-50%, serving dual roles as both a maladaptive coping mechanism and independent psychopathological outcome (Cerda et al., 2011; Alexander et. al., 2018). Neurobiological research implicates dysregulation of the mesolimbic dopamine system in this phenomenon, where trauma-induced stress potentiates reward-seeking behaviors (Koob & Volkow, 2016).

POPULATION-SPECIFIC IMPACTS

Disasters affect demographic groups differently, with children often exhibiting regressive behaviors and attachment disorders due to disrupted developmental processes (Peek, 2008). Older adults face compounded risks from pre-existing health conditions and social isolation, frequently experiencing prolonged grief and depression (Fernandez et al., 2015). First responders demonstrate unique vulnerability to moral injury and compassion fatigue, while marginalized communities show heightened distress due to systemic inequities in recovery resources (Bonanno et al., 2010). Cultural minorities may experience cultural bereavement when disasters destroy heritage sites or disrupt traditional practices (Norris et al., 2002). These variations underscore the necessity for tailored mental health interventions that account for intersectional identities and pre-disaster vulnerabilities (Galea et al., 2005). The difference in population's experiences and the nature of their response to disaster-related psychological stress are discussed below:

- ***Children and Adolescents***: Young people are particularly vulnerable to disaster impacts due to developmental factors, dependence on adults, and limited coping resources. Common responses include regression, separation anxiety, sleep disturbances, and behavioral problems in younger children, and risk-taking behaviors, substance use, and academic difficulties in adolescents (La Greca et al., 2013). Research following Hurricane Katrina found that 37% of children who experienced the hurricane developed clinical-level symptoms of PTSD (McLaughlin et al., 2009). However, children also demonstrate remarkable resilience, particularly when caregivers provide stability and support.
- ***Older Adults***: The impact of disasters on older adults varies considerably based on pre-disaster health, social integration, and economic security. While some older adults show greater resilience due to life experience and coping skills, others face heightened vulnerability due to physical limitations, chronic health conditions, sensory impairments, and potential social isolation (Fernandez et al., 2002). Studies following the 1995 Great Hanshin Earthquake in Japan documented increased mortality among elderly survivors due to "disaster-related death," including suicide and stress-induced health deterioration (Krug et al., 1998).
- ***Individuals with Pre-existing Mental Health Conditions***: Pre-existing conditions can be exacerbated by disaster exposure, and treatment disruption can lead to decompensation. Studies indicate that individuals with prior mental health conditions are 2-3 times more likely to develop severe psychological distress following disasters (Ursano et al., 2003). However, prior treatment experience and established therapeutic relationships can also be protective factors if continuity of care is maintained.
- ***First Responders and Relief Workers***: Those who respond to disasters face distinct psychological risks, including vicarious traumatisation, compassion

fatigue, moral injury when unable to help all victims, and burnout from prolonged exposure to suffering (Benedek et al., 2007). Studies indicate that 10-20% of first responders develop PTSD following disaster response, with risk increased by factors including exposure to human remains, identification with victims, and lack of organizational support (Berger et al., 2012).

CULTURAL DIMENSIONS OF PSYCHOLOGICAL RESPONSE

The psychological impact of disasters is not uniform but is intensely mediated by cultural frameworks (Hoffman & Kruger, 2021). These frameworks shape how individuals perceive, interpret, and cope with traumatic events, influencing both personal and collective responses (Norris et al., 2020). Cultural norms dictate emotional expression, help-seeking behaviours, and community resilience strategies, thereby constructing distinct pathways for disaster recovery (Kirmayer, 2022). Understanding these variations is critical for developing culturally sensitive interventions (Marsella et al., 2008). This analysis explores the interplay between cultural contexts and psychological adaptation in disaster-affected populations.

Cultural Variations in Symptom Expression: The manifestation of psychological distress varies across cultural contexts, with some populations showing predominantly somatic symptoms (e.g., "attaques de nervios" in Latino communities) rather than the emotional and cognitive symptoms emphasized in Western psychiatric frameworks (Hinton & Lewis-Fernandez, 2011). Following the 2008 Sichuan earthquake in China, survivors commonly reported "heart pain" (xin teng) as an expression of emotional suffering.

Culturally-Specific Syndromes: Some cultures recognize specific patterns of post-disaster distress not captured in standard psychiatric nosology, such as "hikikomori" (social withdrawal) observed following disasters in Japan or "khyal attacks" (wind-based anxiety symptoms) reported by Cambodian disaster survivors (Hinton et al., 2010).

Meaning-Making and Interpretive Frameworks: Cultural and religious beliefs provide interpretive frameworks that shape psychological responses. For example, interpretations of disasters as divine punishment may intensify guilt and shame, while frameworks emphasising fate acceptance may promote certain forms of coping. Further, during 2004 Indian Ocean Tsunami found that religious interpretations could either support coping through meaning-making or exacerbate distress through attributions of divine punishment (Aten et al., 2019).

Collective Trauma and Cultural Identity: Beyond individual impacts, disasters can affect collective identities and cultural continuity, particularly for indigenous and minority communities. The destruction of cultural sites, disruption of traditional practices, and forced relocation can produce collective trauma that transcends individual experiences (Kirmayer et al., 2014). Following Hurricane Katrina, research documented impacts on cultural continuity in Gulf Coast Native American communities, with implications for both psychological well-being and cultural resilience (Simms, 2016).

INTERVENTION FRAMEWORKS

Various intervention frameworks have been developed to mitigate the psychological consequences of disasters, each targeting distinct phases of disaster response and recovery. These frameworks are grounded in empirical research, incorporating evidence-based strategies to address acute trauma and long-term mental health challenges (Smith et al., 2020). Van Vliet (2018) emphasise the importance of phase-specific interventions, distinguishing between immediate crisis response, short-term stabilisation, and sustained rehabilitation. Additionally, existing literature highlights the efficacy of multidisciplinary approaches, integrating psychological, social, and community-based support systems. These frameworks not only enhance resilience but also ensure culturally sensitive and scalable interventions in diverse disaster contexts (Patel et al., 2022). The effective interventions that address disaster-related psychological impacts across different phases are discussed below:

Psychological First Aid (PFA): This evidence-informed approach aims to reduce initial distress and support adaptive functioning through principles including: ensure safety, promote calm, enhance self-efficacy, maintain connectedness, and instill hope (Brymer et al., 2006). While intuitively compelling and widely adopted, empirical evaluation of PFA's efficacy remains limited due to methodological challenges in studying acute-phase interventions (Fox et al., 2012).

Trauma-Focused Cognitive Behavioral Therapy (TF-CBT): For those who develop clinical-level symptoms, evidence-based trauma treatments include TF-CBT, which has demonstrated efficacy across diverse disaster contexts (Murray et al., 2015). Adaptations for different cultural contexts and age groups show promising results, though implementation challenges remain in resource-limited settings.

Technology-Based Interventions: Digital mental health interventions offer promising approaches to overcoming access barriers, particularly in resource-limited settings. Mobile applications, telemedicine, and internet-based cognitive behavioral therapy have shown preliminary efficacy following disasters (Ruggiero et al., 2015), though digital divides must be addressed to prevent exacerbating disparities.

CASE STUDY

This section of the chapter deals with a few case studies related to natural disasters that imposed profound psychological consequences, often leaving lasting scars on survivors' mental health and well-being. These case studies examine the multifaceted psychological impacts—from acute trauma to chronic distress—while critically evaluating current intervention frameworks and their efficacy to identify gaps in disaster mental health research.

Haiti Earthquake-2010: Psychological Impacts and Cultural Considerations

The 2010 Haiti earthquake, which killed over 200,000 people and displaced approximately 1.5 million, illustrates the complex interplay of multiple factors influencing psychological outcomes in a resource-limited setting with distinct cultural characteristics. In the earthquake's aftermath, acute psychological responses were shaped by both universal trauma reactions and culturally specific expressions of distress. Research documented high rates of PTSD symptoms (37.8%) and depression (41.7%) among survivors (Derivois et al., 2014). However, these manifestations were often expressed through culturally specific idioms of distress, including "overthinking," "heart heaviness", and spiritual interpretations involving "spirits" (Kaiser et al., 2014).

Psychological impacts were compounded by massive displacement, with approximately 1.5 million people living in temporary camps that created ongoing stressors, including overcrowding, gender-based violence, inadequate sanitation, and uncertainty about the future. A longitudinal study found that displacement duration was a stronger predictor of persistent psychological symptoms than initial trauma exposure (Derivois et al., 2014).

Intervention efforts revealed both the importance and challenges of cultural adaptation. Initial responses by international organisations often reflected Western models that inadequately addressed local understanding of suffering and healing. More effective approaches emerged through collaboration with local healers (hougan and mambo), religious leaders, and community organisations, integrating mental health support with spiritual practices and community rebuilding efforts (Schafer, 2010). The Haiti experience highlights critical lessons about disaster mental health in culturally diverse, resource-limited contexts:

- The necessity of understanding local idioms of distress and healing traditions
- The importance of addressing ongoing displacement-related stressors as part of mental health response

- The value of building on existing community resources and cultural strengths
- The challenges of coordinating mental health services in settings with limited pre-existing infrastructure

Great East Japan Earthquake, Tsunami, and Nuclear Disaster-2011

The 2011 Great East Japan Earthquake and subsequent tsunami and Fukushima nuclear accident represent a catastrophic triple disaster that generated complex, multi-layered psychological consequences. This compounding disaster resulted in over 15,000 fatalities, mass displacement exceeding 300,000 individuals, and persistent psychological distress stemming from radiation-related uncertainties (Oe et al., 2016). Empirical studies reveal distinct patterns of psychological impact across affected groups:

- Bereaved survivors exhibited elevated rates of complicated grief (18.5%) and post-traumatic stress disorder (16.7%), with prolonged mourning processes exacerbated by the sudden, violent nature of losses (Maeda et al., 2018).
- Nuclear evacuees demonstrated unique distress profiles characterised by trauma from forced relocation, community disintegration, and persistent anxiety about radiation exposure (Bromet, 2014).
- First responders reported severe occupational stress, with many experiencing moral injury from triage decisions and radiation risk dilemmas during rescue operations (Shigemura et al., 2012).
- Pediatric populations showed significant developmental disruptions, with 26.8% exhibiting behavioral problems and attachment disorders linked to disrupted caregiving systems (Yabe et al., 2014).

This stratification of psychological outcomes following Japan's triple disaster highlights the critical need for differentiated mental health interventions that account for specific disaster exposures and population vulnerabilities (Maeda & Oe, 2017). Japan's mental health response revealed both systemic strengths and limitations that offer important lessons for disaster preparedness:

- ***System Preparedness:*** The rapid mobilization of existing community mental health teams demonstrated the efficacy of pre-established disaster response protocols (Kato et al., 1996). This preparedness enabled early psychological first aid, though primarily for acute rather than chronic needs.
- ***Cultural Resilience Factors:*** Traditional collective coping mechanisms, particularly through community gathering spaces (yoriai), facilitated organ-

ic psychosocial support networks that complemented formal interventions (Kawachi et al., 2020). These culturally embedded systems proved particularly effective for middle-aged and elderly populations.

- ***Structural Barriers:*** Persistent mental health stigma, especially among older demographics, created significant treatment gaps (Shultz et al., 2016). This was compounded by generational differences in help-seeking behaviors and mental health literacy.
- ***System Limitations:*** The unprecedented compound nature of the disaster exposed critical capacity limitations, particularly in addressing prolonged, complex trauma and radiation-related anxiety disorders (Bromet et al., 2011). Resource allocation challenges emerged in balancing immediate needs with long-term mental health care demands.

This case study suggests that while Japan's disaster mental health framework demonstrated notable strengths in acute response and cultural adaptation, it revealed the need for enhanced capacity to address stigma and prolonged psychological sequelae in future complex disasters.

Hurricane Maria in Puerto Rico-2017: Cascading Collapse of Mental Health Systems

The catastrophic impact of Hurricane Maria on Puerto Rico in 2017 illustrates how disasters can trigger systemic failures in mental health infrastructure, exacerbating pre-existing vulnerabilities (Kishore et al., 2018). Prior to the hurricane, Puerto Rico's mental health system was already strained, characterised by high rates of common mental disorders and inadequate service accessibility (Sánchez-Cardona et al., 2020). The hurricane amplified these challenges through multiple pathways:

- ***Direct Psychological Trauma***: Widespread exposure to life-threatening situations and bereavement created acute trauma (Orengo-Aguayo et al., 2019).
- ***Systemic Collapse:*** Extended disruptions to electricity, water, and healthcare infrastructure (lasting up to 11 months in some areas) undermined basic coping resources (García-López et al., 2021).
- ***Demographic Instability:*** A mass exodus of over 130,000 residents fractured community support networks (Meléndez et al., 2018).
- ***Economic Shock:*** The devastation of local economies compounded financial stressors, a known risk factor for depression and suicidality (Ramos et al., 2020).

Further, Ramos et al., (2020) and Orengo-Aguayo et al., (2019) studies documented alarming mental health consequences, including a 49.5% prevalence of probable PTSD symptoms at six months post-disaster and a 29% increase in suicide rates. Importantly, the mental health system itself became a casualty of the disaster. The mental healthcare system faced severe disruptions due to multiple compounding factors. Workforce depletion significantly impaired service capacity, with Rivera and Rolke (2019) documenting a 15% emigration rate among mental health professionals. Concurrently, infrastructure damage rendered over 70 community mental health facilities nonoperational (DHHS, 2018), drastically reducing service availability. These challenges were exacerbated by prolonged psychotropic medication shortages caused by supply chain failures (Santos-Lozada et al., 2020), which compromised treatment continuity. Furthermore, Gutierrez et al. (2021) identified telecommunications breakdowns as a critical barrier, impeding effective crisis coordination during this period of systemic vulnerability. These interconnected factors created a cascading effect that undermined the mental health infrastructure's stability and responsiveness.

Additionally, in response to systemic challenges, innovative and culturally informed solutions emerged to address gaps in mental health support. Sánchez et al. (2021) highlight the adaptation of community-based models, where churches and neighborhood centers served as critical hubs for psychological first aid, ensuring accessibility in resource-limited settings. Further integrating services, Halpern, J., & Vermeulen (2017) demonstrate the effectiveness of co-locating mental health support with material aid distribution, streamlining assistance for vulnerable populations. Capitalizing on cultural strengths, Bonilla-Silva (2020) documents the success of peer networks rooted in apoyo mutuo (mutual aid), leveraging collectivistic traditions to foster resilience. Additionally, Robles et al. (2021) emphasize the role of mobile outreach teams in delivering adapted mental health care to remote areas, overcoming geographic and infrastructural barriers. These approaches collectively illustrate how culturally embedded strategies can enhance service delivery in crisis contexts.

This case underscores two critical insights for disaster mental health planning- the necessity of hardening mental health infrastructure against systemic shocks, and the value of pre-positioning community-based alternatives that can function when formal systems fail (U.S. GAO, 2019).

CRITICAL CHALLENGES IN DISASTER MENTAL HEALTH

Disaster mental health response faces persistent challenges that complicate effective intervention. A key tension exists between implementing universal psychological frameworks and adapting to culturally specific needs, raising questions about efficacy and relevance. Additionally, structural vulnerabilities—such as pre-existing inequities and resource disparities—often exacerbate post-disaster mental health crises. Further complicating efforts and implementation barriers, including logistical constraints and workforce shortages, hinder timely and equitable care delivery. Addressing these interconnected issues requires a nuanced, systems-level approach to disaster mental health planning. Some of the persistent challenges are discussed below;

- ***Balancing Universal and Culturally Specific Approaches***: While certain aspects of trauma response appear relatively universal, effective interventions must balance evidence-based practices with cultural adaptation (Killikelly et al., 2018). It remains challenging in international disaster response, where external responders may lack cultural competence while local capacity is overwhelmed.
- ***Addressing Structural Vulnerabilities***: Disasters disproportionately affect marginalized communities due to pre-existing inequities in resource distribution, infrastructure quality, and service access (Fothergill & Peek, 2004). Yet mental health interventions often focus on individual symptoms without addressing these structural vulnerabilities, potentially reinforcing existing disparities.
- ***Sustainability and Capacity Building***: Short-term disaster mental health responses often fail to build sustainable local capacity, creating dependency on external resources that inevitably withdraw (WHO, 2013). Models that prioritise knowledge transfer, workforce development, and integration with existing systems show more promising long-term outcomes.
- ***Implementation Barriers***: Even when effective interventions exist, implementation barriers include resource limitations, workforce shortages, coordination challenges among responding organizations, and gaps between research and practice (Becker et al., 2014).

EMERGING DIRECTIONS AND INNOVATIONS IN DISASTER MENTAL HEALTH

Recent advancements in disaster mental health demonstrate a paradigm shift toward more holistic and adaptive interventions. Trauma-informed systems approaches are increasingly being implemented to address psychological distress while preventing re-traumatisation in vulnerable populations. Concurrently, technology-enabled solutions, such as telehealth platforms and AI-driven screening tools, are expanding access to care in resource-constrained settings. Indigenous and community-led models are gaining recognition for their culturally grounded efficacy. At the same time, integrating mental health support with climate change adaptation strategies reflects a growing acknowledgement of compounding environmental crises. These innovations collectively signal a transformative movement toward more resilient, equitable, and scalable disaster mental health frameworks.

- ***Trauma-Informed Systems Approaches***: Moving beyond individual clinical interventions, trauma-informed approaches aim to build organizational and community systems that recognize trauma impacts, avoid re-traumatization, and support recovery through all points of contact (Fallot & Harris, 2009).
- ***Technology-Enabled Solutions***: Digital mental health applications, telemedicine, and social media platforms offer innovative approaches to expanding reach, particularly in resource-limited or geographically isolated settings (Ruggiero et al., 2015). The COVID-19 pandemic accelerated adoption of these approaches across disaster contexts.
- ***Indigenous and Community-Led Models***: Growing recognition of the limitations of externally imposed interventions has led to greater emphasis on community-led approaches that build on cultural strengths, traditional practices, and local knowledge systems (Wexler et al., 2015).
- ***Integration with Climate Change Adaptation***: As climate-related disasters increase, integrating mental health considerations with climate change adaptation strategies offers opportunities for more comprehensive, forward-looking approaches to disaster resilience (Berry et al., 2018).

Strengthening Psychological Resilience to Natural Disasters

To strengthen psychological resilience in the face of natural disasters, it is essential to adopt trauma-informed systems that foster community support and recovery. Emphasising technology-enabled solutions can expand mental health access, particularly in underserved areas. Integrating indigenous and community-led models with climate change adaptation strategies will enhance preparedness and contribute to more effective recovery efforts. Based on the existing studies, the following recommendations are proposed to enhance disaster mental health preparedness, response, and recovery efforts:

Disaster Preparedness and Planning

- *Integrate mental health considerations into all phases of disaster management*, ensuring adequate resource allocation and clearly defined roles for mental health professionals.

- *Develop community-based psychosocial preparedness programs* to bolster individual and collective coping mechanisms, strengthen social support networks, and enhance psychological resilience prior to disaster events.
- *Implement workforce development initiatives* to expand the pool of disaster mental health practitioners, with specialized training in trauma-informed care, cross-cultural competencies, and lived experience in disaster contexts.

Acute Disaster Response

- *Deliver evidence-based psychological first aid (PFA)* through trained community members and first responders to mitigate acute distress and foster stabilization.
- *Establish culturally sensitive psychological screening protocols* to identify at-risk individuals while accounting for culturally specific expressions of distress.
- *Integrate mental health support with material aid distribution* to address both psychological and immediate survival needs, recognizing their interdependent influence on recovery.

Recovery and Long-Term Support

- *Adopt stepped-care intervention models* that tailor mental health services based on symptom severity, ensuring efficient resource allocation while maintaining accessibility.
- *Sustain community-based mental health services* beyond the immediate post-disaster phase to address lingering psychological effects and prevent chronic mental health conditions.
- *Develop targeted interventions for secondary stressors*, such as displacement, housing instability, and financial hardship, which compound psychological distress and impede long-term recovery.

These recommendations underscore the necessity of a multi-tiered, culturally responsive, and sustained approach to disaster mental health intervention, bridging immediate crisis response with long-term psychosocial recovery strategies.

CONCLUSION

The existing literature underscores several critical insights regarding the psychological consequences of natural disasters and their mitigation. First, disasters generate a continuum of mental health impacts—from temporary distress to chronic disorders—mediated by an intricate interplay of event severity, individual vulnerabilities, and socioecological factors. Second, while resilience predominates in affected populations, a clinically significant subset, particularly children, older adults, individuals with pre-existing conditions, and marginalised groups, requires tailored, sustained support. Third, cultural frameworks fundamentally shape disaster experiences and recovery trajectories, demanding interventions harmonising empirical rigour with cultural competence. Ultimately, an effective mental health response necessitates multi-tiered strategies that integrate prevention, acute care, and long-term rehabilitation while addressing systemic inequities across individual, familial, communal, and societal spheres. These findings collectively advocate for a nuanced, culturally grounded, and systems-oriented paradigm in disaster mental health practice and policy.

REFERENCES

Alexander, A. C., & Ward, K. D. (2018). Understanding Postdisaster Substance Use and Psychological Distress Using Concepts from the Self-Medication Hypothesis and Social Cognitive Theory. *Journal of Psychoactive Drugs*, *50*(2), 177–186. DOI: 10.1080/02791072.2017.1397304 PMID: 29125424

American Psychiatric Association, DSM-5 Task Force. (2013). *Diagnostic and statistical manual of mental disorders: DSM-5* (5th ed.). American Psychiatric Publishing, Inc., DOI: 10.1176/appi.books.9780890425596

Arnberg, F. K., Gudmundsdóttir, R., Butwicka, A., Fang, F., Lichtenstein, P., Hultman, C. M., & Valdimarsdóttir, U. A. (2015). Psychiatric disorders and suicide attempts in Swedish survivors of the 2004 southeast Asia tsunami: A 5-year matched cohort study. *The Lancet. Psychiatry*, *2*(9), 817–824. PMID: 26236006

Arnsten, A. F. (2015). Stress weakens prefrontal networks: Molecular insults to higher cognition. *Nature Neuroscience*, *18*(10), 1376–1385. DOI: 10.1038/nn.4087 PMID: 26404712

Aten, J. D., Smith, W. R., Davis, E. B., Van Tongeren, D. R., Hook, J. N., Davis, D. E., Shannonhouse, L., DeBlaere, C., Ranter, J., O'Grady, K., & Hill, P. C. (2019). The psychological study of religion and spirituality in a disaster context: A systematic review. *Psychological Trauma: Theory, Research, Practice, and Policy*, *11*(6), 597–613. PMID: 30730187

Becker, S. M., Middleton, S. A., & Becker, A. E. (2014). Barriers to treatment for mental health problems in disaster settings: Lessons from Haiti. *Prehospital and Disaster Medicine*, *29*(5), 528–533.

Benedek, D. M., Fullerton, C., & Ursano, R. J. (2007). First responders: Mental health consequences of natural and human-made disasters for public health and public safety workers. *Annual Review of Public Health*, *28*, 55–68. PMID: 17367284

Berger, W., Coutinho, E. S., Figueira, I., Marques-Portella, C., Luz, M. P., Neylan, T. C., Marmar, C. R., & Mendlowicz, M. V. (2012). Rescuers at risk: A systematic review and meta-regression analysis of the worldwide current prevalence and correlates of PTSD in rescue workers. *Social Psychiatry and Psychiatric Epidemiology*, *47*(6), 1001–1011. DOI: 10.1007/s00127-011-0408-2 PMID: 21681455

Berry, P., Enright, P. M., Shumake-Guillemot, J., Villalobos Prats, E., & Campbell-Lendrum, D. (2018). Assessing health vulnerabilities and adaptation to climate change: A review of international progress. *International Journal of Environmental Research and Public Health*, *15*(12), 2626. PMID: 30477122

. Bonanno, G. A., Brewin, C. R., Kaniasty, K., & La Greca, A. M. (2010). Weighing the costs of disaster: Consequences, risks, and resilience in individuals, families, and communities. *Psychological Science in the Public Interest: a journal of the American Psychological Society, 11*(1), 1–49. https://doi.org/.DOI: 10.1177/1529100610387086

Bonilla-Silva, E. (2020). Mutual aid and community resilience: Lessons from Puerto Rico post-Hurricane Maria. *Journal of Community Psychology, 48*(5), 1435–1449.

Brewin, C. R. (2011). The nature and significance of memory disturbance in post-traumatic stress disorder. *Annual Review of Clinical Psychology, 7*, 203–227. DOI: 10.1146/annurev-clinpsy-032210-104544 PMID: 21219190

Brewin, C. R., Andrews, B., & Valentine, J. D. (2000). Meta-analysis of risk factors for posttraumatic stress disorder in trauma-exposed adults. *Journal of Consulting and Clinical Psychology, 68*(5), 748–766. DOI: 10.1037//0022-006x.68.5.748 PMID: 11068961

Bromet, E. J. (2014). Emotional consequences of nuclear power plant disasters. *Health Physics, 106*(2), 206–210. DOI: 10.1097/HP.0000000000000012 PMID: 24378494

Bromet, E. J., Havenaar, J. M., & Guey, L. T. (2011). A 25-year retrospective review of the psychological consequences of the Chernobyl accident. *Clinical oncology (Royal College of Radiologists (Great Britain)), 23*(4), 297–305. https://doi.org/ DOI: 10.1016/j.clon.2011.01.501

Bryant, R. A. (2019). Post-traumatic stress disorder: A state-of-the-art review of evidence and challenges. *World Psychiatry; Official Journal of the World Psychiatric Association (WPA), 18*(3), 259–269. DOI: 10.1002/wps.20656 PMID: 31496089

Bryant, R. A., Friedman, M. J., Spiegel, D., Ursano, R., & Strain, J. (2011). A review of acute stress disorder in DSM-5. *Depression and Anxiety, 28*(9), 802–817. PMID: 21910186

Brymer, M., Jacobs, A., Layne, C., Pynoos, R., Ruzek, J., Steinberg, A., Vernberg, E., & Watson, P. (2006). *Psychological first aid: Field operations guide* (2nd ed.). National Child Traumatic Stress Network and National Center for PTSD.

Cardeña, E., & Carlson, E. (2011). Acute stress disorder revisited. *Annual Review of Clinical Psychology, 7*, 245–267. PMID: 21275643

. Cerda, G., Pérez, C., & Melipillán, R. (2011). Test de inteligencia Lógica superior (TILS). *Manual de aplicación.*

Derivois, D., Mérisier, G. G., Cenat, J. M., & Castelot, V. (2014). Symptoms of posttraumatic stress disorder and social support among children and adolescents after the 2010 Haitian earthquake. *Journal of Loss and Trauma*, *19*(3), 202–212. DOI: 10.1080/15325024.2013.789759

. Fallot, R. D., Harris, M. (2009). Creating Cultures of Trauma-Informed Care (CCTIC): A Self-Assessment and Planning Protocol. *Community Connections* 2.2/ 7-09

Fernandez, L. S., Byard, D., Lin, C. C., Benson, S., & Barbera, J. A. (2002). Frail elderly as disaster victims: Emergency management strategies. *Prehospital and Disaster Medicine*, *17*(2), 67–74. DOI: 10.1017/S1049023X14001435 PMID: 12500729

Fothergill, A., & Peek, L. A. (2004). Poverty and Disasters in the United States: A Review of Recent Sociological Findings. *Natural Hazards*, *32*, 89–110. DOI: 10.1023/B:NHAZ.0000026792.76181.d9

Fox, J. H., Burkle, F. M., Bass, J., Pia, F. A., Epstein, J. L., & Markenson, D. (2012). The effectiveness of psychological first aid as a disaster intervention tool: Research analysis of peer-reviewed literature from 1990-2010. *Disaster Medicine and Public Health Preparedness*, *6*(3), 247–252. PMID: 23077267

Galea, S., Nandi, A., & Vlahov, D. (2005). The epidemiology of post-traumatic stress disorder after disasters. *Epidemiologic Reviews*, *27*(1), 78–91. DOI: 10.1093/ epirev/mxi003 PMID: 15958429

Garakani, A., Murrough, J. W., Freire, R. C., Thom, R. P., Larkin, K., Buono, F. D., & Iosifescu, D. V. (2020). Pharmacotherapy of anxiety disorders: Current and emerging treatment options. *Frontiers in Psychiatry*, *11*, 595584. DOI: 10.3389/ fpsyt.2020.595584 PMID: 33424664

García-López, G. A., Pérez-Báez, C., & Rosado, M. (2021). The impact of infrastructure collapse on mental health: Puerto Rico after Hurricane Maria. *Disasters*, *45*(3), 593–615.

Goldmann, E., & Galea, S. (2014). Mental health consequences of disasters. *Annual Review of Public Health*, *35*, 169–183. DOI: 10.1146/annurev-publhealth-032013-182435 PMID: 24159920

Gutierrez, J. M., Koralnik, I. J., & Teener, J. W. (2021). Communication failures in disaster response: The Puerto Rico experience. *The New England Journal of Medicine*, *384*(12), 1183–1185.

Halpern, J., & Vermeulen, K. (2017). *Disaster mental health interventions: Core principles and practices*. Routledge.

Hermans, E. J., Henckens, M. J., Joëls, M., & Fernández, G. (2014). Dynamic adaptation of large-scale brain networks in response to acute stressors. *Trends in Neurosciences*, *37*(6), 304–314. DOI: 10.1016/j.tins.2014.03.006 PMID: 24766931

Hinton, D. E., & Lewis-Fernández, R. (2011). The cross-cultural validity of post-traumatic stress disorder: Implications for DSM-5. *Depression and Anxiety*, *28*(9), 783–801. DOI: 10.1002/da.20753 PMID: 21910185

Hobfoll, S. E. (1989). Conservation of resources: A new attempt at conceptualizing stress. *The American Psychologist*, *44*(3), 513. PMID: 2648906

Hoffman, M. A., & Kruczek, T. (2011). A bioecological model of mass trauma: Individual, community, and societal effects. *The Counseling Psychologist*, *39*(8), 1087–1127. DOI: 10.1177/0011000010397932

Hoffman, Y., & Kruger, T. (2021). *Culture and disaster response: A psychological perspective*. Oxford University Press.

Jovanovic, T., & Norrholm, S. D. (2011). Neural mechanisms of impaired fear inhibition in posttraumatic stress disorder. *Frontiers in Behavioral Neuroscience*, *5*, 44. DOI: 10.3389/fnbeh.2011.00044 PMID: 21845177

Kaiser, B. N., McLean, K. E., Kohrt, B. A., Hagaman, A. K., Wagenaar, B. H., Khoury, N. M., & Keys, H. M. (2014). Reflechi twòp—thinking too much: Description of a cultural syndrome in Haiti's Central Plateau. *Culture, Medicine and Psychiatry*, *38*(3), 448–472. PMID: 25038935

. Kaniasty, K., & Norris, F. H. (2009). Distinctions that matter: Received social support, perceived social support, and social embeddedness after disasters. *Mental health and disasters*, 2009, 175-200.

Kato, H., Asukai, N., Miyake, Y., Minakawa, K., & Nishiyama, A. (1996). Post-traumatic symptoms among younger and elderly evacuees in the early stages following the 1995 Hanshin-Awaji earthquake in Japan. *Acta Psychiatrica Scandinavica*, *93*(6), 477–481. DOI: 10.1111/j.1600-0447.1996.tb10680.x PMID: 8831865

Kawachi, I., Subramanian, S. V., & Kim, D. (2020). Global Perspective in Social capital and health. In *Social capital and health* (pp. 1–26). Springer., DOI: 10.1007/978-1-4614-7464-7_1

Kessler, R. C., Galea, S., Gruber, M. J., Sampson, N. A., Ursano, R. J., & Wessely, S. (2008). Trends in mental illness and suicidality after Hurricane Katrina. *Molecular Psychiatry*, *13*(4), 374–384. PMID: 18180768

Killikelly, C., Bauer, S., & Maercker, A. (2018). The assessment of grief in refugees and post-conflict survivors: A narrative review of etic and emic research. *Frontiers in Psychology*, *9*, 1957. PMID: 30405474

Kirmayer, L. J. (2022). Suicide in cultural context: An ecosocial approach. *Transcultural Psychiatry*, *59*(1), 3–12. DOI: 10.1177/13634615221076424 PMID: 35179066

Kirmayer, L. J., Gone, J. P., & Moses, J. (2014). Rethinking historical trauma. *Transcultural Psychiatry*, *51*(3), 299–319. PMID: 24855142

Kishore, N., Marqués, D., Mahmud, A., Kiang, M. V., Rodriguez, I., Fuller, A., & Buckee, C. O. (2018). Mortality in Puerto Rico after Hurricane Maria. *The New England Journal of Medicine*, *379*(2), 162–170. DOI: 10.1056/NEJMsa1803972 PMID: 29809109

Koob, G. F., & Volkow, N. D. (2016). Neurobiology of addiction: A neurocircuitry analysis. *The Lancet. Psychiatry*, *3*(8), 760–773. DOI: 10.1016/S2215-0366(16)00104-8 PMID: 27475769

Kristensen, P., Weisæth, L., & Heir, T. (2012). Bereavement and mental health after sudden and violent losses: *A review. Psychiatry*, *75*(1), 76–97. https://guilfordjournals.com/doi/10.1521/psyc.2012.75.1.76 PMID: 22397543

Krug, E. G., Kresnow, M., Peddicord, J. P., Dahlberg, L. L., Powell, K. E., Crosby, A. E., & Annest, J. L. (1998). Suicide after natural disasters. *The New England Journal of Medicine*, *338*(6), 373–378. DOI: 10.1056/NEJM199802053380607 PMID: 9449732

La Greca, A. M., Lai, B. S., Joormann, J., Auslander, B. B., & Short, M. A. (2013). Children's risk and resilience following a natural disaster: Genetic vulnerability, posttraumatic stress, and depression. *Journal of Affective Disorders*, *151*(3), 860–867. DOI: 10.1016/j.jad.2013.07.024 PMID: 24035489

Lanius, R. A., Vermetten, E., Loewenstein, R. J., Brand, B., Schmahl, C., Bremner, J. D., & Spiegel, D. (2010). Emotion modulation in PTSD: Clinical and neurobiological evidence for a dissociative subtype. *The American Journal of Psychiatry*, *167*(6), 640–647. DOI: 10.1176/appi.ajp.2009.09081168 PMID: 20360318

Lazarus, R., & Folkman, S. (1984). *Stress, Appraisal, and Coping*. Springer.

Maeda, M., & Oe, M. (2017). Mental health consequences and social issues after the Fukushima disaster. *Asia-Pacific Journal of Public Health*, *31*(2, suppl), 36S–46S. PMID: 28330398

Maeda, M., Oe, M., Lee, M., & Miyazaki, M. (2018). Mental health consequences of the Great East Japan Earthquake. In *Mental Health and Disasters* (pp. 217–231). Cambridge University Press.

Marsella, A. J., Johnson, J. L., Watson, P., & Gryczynski, J. (Eds.). (2008). *Ethnocultural perspectives on disaster and trauma: Foundations, issues, and applications*. Springer Science + Business Media. https://doi.org/DOI: 10.1007/978-0-387-73285-5

McFarlane, A. C., & Van Hooff, M. (2009). Impact of childhood exposure to a natural disaster on adult mental health: 20-year longitudinal follow-up study. *The British Journal of Psychiatry*, *195*(2), 142–148. DOI: 10.1192/bjp.bp.108.054270 PMID: 19648546

McLaughlin, K. A., Fairbank, J. A., Gruber, M. J., Jones, R. T., Lakoma, M. D., Pfefferbaum, B., Sampson, N. A., & Kessler, R. C. (2009). Serious emotional disturbance among youths exposed to Hurricane Katrina 2 years post disaster. *Journal of the American Academy of Child and Adolescent Psychiatry*, *48*(11), 1069–1078. PMID: 19797983

Meléndez, E., Hinojosa, J., & Roman, N. (2018). Puerto Rico's post-Maria outmigration. *Centro Journal*, *30*(3), 54–85.

Milad, M. R., & Quirk, G. J. (2012). Fear extinction as a model for translational neuroscience: Ten years of progress. *Annual Review of Psychology*, *63*, 129–151. DOI: 10.1146/annurev.psych.121208.131631 PMID: 22129456

Murray, L. K., Skavenski, S., Kane, J. C., Mayeya, J., Dorsey, S., Cohen, J. A., Michalopoulos, L. T., Imasiku, M., & Bolton, P. A. (2015). Effectiveness of Trauma-Focused Cognitive Behavioral Therapy Among Trauma-Affected Children in Lusaka, Zambia: A Randomized Clinical Trial. *JAMA Pediatrics*, *169*(8), 761–769. DOI: 10.1001/jamapediatrics.2015.0580 PMID: 26111066

Neria, Y., Nandi, A., & Galea, S. (2008). Post-traumatic stress disorder following disasters: A systematic review. *Psychological Medicine*, *38*(4), 467–480. PMID: 17803838

Norris, F. H., Friedman, M. J., Watson, P. J., Byrne, C. M., Diaz, E., & Kaniasty, K. (2002). 60,000 disaster victims speak: Part I. An empirical review of the empirical literature, 1981–2001. *Psychiatry*, *65*(3), 207–239. DOI: 10.1521/psyc.65.3.207.20173 PMID: 12405079

Norris, F. H., Stevens, S. P., Pfefferbaum, B., Wyche, K. F., & Pfefferbaum, R. L. (2020). Community resilience as a metaphor, theory, set of capacities, and strategy for disaster readiness. *American Journal of Community Psychology, 41*(1-2), 127–150. DOI: 10.1007/s10464-007-9156-6 PMID: 18157631

North, C. S., & Pfefferbaum, B. (2013). Mental health response to community disasters: A systematic review. *Journal of the American Medical Association, 310*(5), 507–518. DOI: 10.1001/jama.2013.107799 PMID: 23925621

O'Connor, M. F., Wellisch, D. K., Stanton, A. L., Eisenberger, N. I., Irwin, M. R., & Lieberman, M. D. (2008). Craving love? Enduring grief activates brain's reward center. *NeuroImage, 42*(2), 969–972. DOI: 10.1016/j.neuroimage.2008.04.256 PMID: 18559294

Oe, M., Maeda, M., Nagai, M., Yasumura, S., Yabe, H., Suzuki, Y., & Bromet, E. (2016). Predictors of severe psychological distress trajectory after nuclear disaster: Evidence from the Fukushima Health Management Survey. *BMJ Open, 6*(9), e013400. DOI: 10.1136/bmjopen-2016-013400 PMID: 27798033

Orengo-Aguayo, R., Stewart, R. W., de Arellano, M. A., Suárez-Kindy, J. L., & Young, J. (2019). Disaster exposure and mental health among Puerto Rican youths after Hurricane Maria. *JAMA Network Open, 2*(4), e192619. DOI: 10.1001/jamanetworkopen.2019.2619 PMID: 31026024

Patel, R., Green, L., & Kumar, S. (2022). *Culturally adaptive frameworks for disaster resilience: Global perspectives*. Oxford University Press.

Patel, S. S., Rogers, M. B., Amlôt, R., & Rubin, G. J. (2017). What do we mean by 'community resilience'? A systematic literature review of how it is defined in the literature. [ecurrents-dis.]. *PLoS Currents*, •••, 9. PMID: 29188132

Patel, S. S., Rogers, M. B., Amlôt, R., & Rubin, G. J. (2017). What Do We Mean by 'Community Resilience'? A Systematic Literature Review of How It Is Defined in the Literature. *PLoS Currents, 9*. Advance online publication. DOI: 10.1371/currents.dis.db775aff25efc5ac4f0660ad9c9f7db2 PMID: 29188132

Peek, L. (2008). Children and disasters: Understanding vulnerability, developing capacities, and promoting resilience—An introduction. *Children, Youth and Environments, 18*(1), 1–29. https://www.jstor.org/stable/10.7721/chilyoutenvi.18.1.0001

Ramos, G., Chardón, C. E., & Rivera, F. I. (2020). Suicide trends in Puerto Rico before and after Hurricane Maria. *Crisis, 41*(5), 347–352.

Rivera, F. I., & Rolke, L. (2019). Health care provider migration from Puerto Rico after Hurricane Maria. *Journal of Immigrant and Minority Health, 21*(3), 556–563.

Robles, R. R., Reyes, J. C., Colón, H. M., Sahai, H., Marrero, C. A., Matos, T. D., & Shepard, E. W. (2021). Community-based mobile health services in post-disaster Puerto Rico. *International Journal of Environmental Research and Public Health, 18*(4), 1675. PMID: 33572443

Ruggiero, K. J., Price, M., Adams, Z., Stauffacher, K., McCauley, J., Danielson, C. K., & Resnick, H. S. (2015). Web intervention for adolescents affected by disaster: Population-based randomized controlled trial. *Journal of the American Academy of Child and Adolescent Psychiatry, 54*(9), 709–717. PMID: 26299292

Sánchez, J., Román, J., & Martínez, K. (2021). Faith-based organizations in disaster mental health response. *Spirituality in Clinical Practice, 8*(1), 1–15.

Sánchez-Cardona, I., Ortega-Polanco, J. C., & Bernal, G. (2020). Mental health services in Puerto Rico before Hurricane Maria. *Puerto Rico Health Sciences Journal, 39*(2), 84–91.

Santos-Lozada, A. R., Howard, J. T., & Verdery, A. M. (2020). Medication shortages after Hurricane Maria. *Health Affairs, 39*(5), 847–855.

Schafer, A. (2010). Spirituality and mental health in humanitarian contexts: An exploration based on World Vision Haiti earthquake response. *Intervention (Amstelveen, Netherlands), 8*(2), 121–130.

Shalev, A., Liberzon, I., & Marmar, C. (2017). Post-traumatic stress disorder. *The New England Journal of Medicine, 376*(25), 2459–2469. DOI: 10.1056/NEJMra1612499 PMID: 28636846

Shigemura, J., Tanigawa, T., Saito, I., & Nomura, S. (2012). Psychological distress in workers at the Fukushima nuclear power plants. *Journal of the American Medical Association, 308*(7), 667–669. DOI: 10.1001/jama.2012.9699 PMID: 22893158

Shin, L. M., & Liberzon, I. (2010). The neurocircuitry of fear, stress, and anxiety disorders. *Neuropsychopharmacology : Official Publication of the American College of Neuropsychopharmacology, 35*(1), 169–191. DOI: 10.1038/npp.2009.83 PMID: 19625997

Shultz, J. M., Cela, T., Marcelin, L. H., Espinola, M., Heitmann, I., Sanchez, C., & Rechkemmer, A. (2016). The trauma signature of 2016 Hurricane Matthew and the psychosocial impact on Haiti. *Disaster Health, 3*(4), 121–138. DOI: 10.1080/21665044.2016.1263538 PMID: 28321360

Smith, T., Lee, C., & Zhang, W. (2020). Evidence-based psychological interventions in disaster settings. *Journal of Traumatic Stress, 33*(4), 512–525.

Starcke, K., & Brand, M. (2012). Decision making under stress: A selective review. *Neuroscience and Biobehavioral Reviews*, *36*(5), 1228–1248. DOI: 10.1016/j.neubiorev.2012.02.003 PMID: 22342781

Stroebe, M., Schut, H., & Boerner, K. (2017). Cautioning health-care professionals: Bereaved persons are misguided through the stages of grief. *Omega*, *74*(4), 455–473. DOI: 10.1177/0030222817691870 PMID: 28355991

Sung, S. C., Dryman, M. T., Marks, E., Shear, M. K., Ghesquiere, A., Fava, M., & Simon, N. M. (2011). Complicated grief among individuals with major depression: Prevalence, comorbidity, and associated features. *Journal of Affective Disorders*, *134*(1-3), 453–458. PMID: 21621849

Tedeschi, R. G., & Calhoun, L. G. (2004). TARGET ARTICLE: "Posttraumatic Growth: Conceptual Foundations and Empirical Evidence.". *Psychological Inquiry*, *15*(1), 1–18. DOI: 10.1207/s15327965pli1501_01

Ursano, R. J., Fullerton, C. S., & Norwood, A. E. (Eds.). (2003). *Terrorism and Disaster Paperback with CD-ROM: Individual and Community Mental Health Interventions*. Cambridge University Press.

U.S. Department of Health and Human Services. (2018). Mental health infrastructure assessment: Puerto Rico post-Hurricane Maria (Report No. 18-2100). https://www.hhs.gov/sites/default/files/puerto-rico-mental-health-report.pdf

U.S. Government Accountability Office. (2019). Disaster recovery: Lessons from Hurricane Maria for Puerto Rico's mental health system (GAO-19-576). https://www.gao.gov/products/gao-19-576

Van Vliet, N. I., Huntjens, R. J., Van Dijk, M. K., & De Jongh, A. (2018). Phase-based treatment versus immediate trauma-focused treatment in patients with childhood trauma-related posttraumatic stress disorder: Study protocol for a randomized controlled trial. *Trials*, *19*(1), 138. PMID: 29471855

Watson, P. J., Brymer, M. J., & Bonanno, G. A. (2011). Postdisaster psychological intervention since 9/11. *The American Psychologist*, *66*(6), 482–494. DOI: 10.1037/a0024806 PMID: 21823776

Wexler, L., White, J., & Trainor, B. (2015). Why an alternative to suicide prevention gatekeeper training is needed for rural Indigenous communities: Presenting an empowering community storytelling approach. *Critical Public Health*, *25*(2), 205–217. DOI: 10.1080/09581596.2014.904039 PMID: 36779086

Wolf, E. J., Lunney, C. A., Miller, M. W., Resick, P. A., Friedman, M. J., & Schnurr, P. P. (2012). The dissociative subtype of PTSD: A replication and extension. *Depression and Anxiety*, *29*(8), 679–688. DOI: 10.1002/da.21946 PMID: 22639402

World Health Organization. (2013). *Building back better: Sustainable mental health care after emergencies*. World Health Organization.

World Health Organization. (2019). *Mental health in emergencies*. World Health Organization.

Yabe, H., Suzuki, Y., Mashiko, H., Nakayama, Y., Hisata, M., Niwa, S. I., & Abe, M. (2014). Psychological distress after the Great East Japan Earthquake and Fukushima Daiichi Nuclear Power Plant accident: Results of a mental health and lifestyle survey through the Fukushima Health Management Survey in FY2011 and FY2012. *Fukushima Journal of Medical Science*, *60*(1), 57–67. DOI: 10.5387/fms.2014-1 PMID: 25030715

Compilation of References

10. Berry, P., Enright, P. M., Shumake-Guillemot, J., Villalobos Prats, E., & Campbell-Lendrum, D. (2018). Assessing health vulnerabilities and adaptation to climate change: A review of international progress. *International Journal of Environmental Research and Public Health, 15*(12), 2626. PMID: 30477122

11. Becker, S. M., Middleton, S. A., & Becker, A. E. (2014). Barriers to treatment for mental health problems in disaster settings: Lessons from Haiti. *Prehospital and Disaster Medicine, 29*(5), 528–533.

12. Benedek, D. M., Fullerton, C., & Ursano, R. J. (2007). First responders: Mental health consequences of natural and human-made disasters for public health and public safety workers. *Annual Review of Public Health, 28*, 55–68. PMID: 17367284

13. Berger, W., Coutinho, E. S., Figueira, I., Marques-Portella, C., Luz, M. P., Neylan, T. C., Marmar, C. R., & Mendlowicz, M. V. (2012). Rescuers at risk: A systematic review and meta-regression analysis of the worldwide current prevalence and correlates of PTSD in rescue workers. *Social Psychiatry and Psychiatric Epidemiology, 47*(6), 1001–1011. DOI: 10.1007/s00127-011-0408-2 PMID: 21681455

14. Bonanno, G. A., Brewin, C. R., Kaniasty, K., & La Greca, A. M. (2010). Weighing the costs of disaster: Consequences, risks, and resilience in individuals, families, and communities. *Psychological Science in the Public Interest: a journal of the American Psychological Society, 11*(1), 1–49. https://doi.org/.DOI: 10.1177/1529100610387086

15. Bonilla-Silva, E. (2020). Mutual aid and community resilience: Lessons from Puerto Rico post-Hurricane Maria. *Journal of Community Psychology, 48*(5), 1435–1449.

16. Bryant, R. A., Friedman, M. J., Spiegel, D., Ursano, R., & Strain, J. (2011). A review of acute stress disorder in DSM-5. *Depression and Anxiety, 28*(9), 802–817. PMID: 21910186

17. Bryant, R. A. (2019). Post-traumatic stress disorder: A state-of-the-art review of evidence and challenges. *World Psychiatry; Official Journal of the World Psychiatric Association (WPA), 18*(3), 259–269. DOI: 10.1002/wps.20656 PMID: 31496089

18. Brymer, M., Jacobs, A., Layne, C., Pynoos, R., Ruzek, J., Steinberg, A., Vernberg, E., & Watson, P. (2006). *Psychological first aid: Field operations guide* (2nd ed.). National Child Traumatic Stress Network and National Center for PTSD.

19. Cardeña, E., & Carlson, E. (2011). Acute stress disorder revisited. *Annual Review of Clinical Psychology, 7*, 245–267. PMID: 21275643

1. Alexander, A. C., & Ward, K. D. (2018). Understanding Postdisaster Substance Use and Psychological Distress Using Concepts from the Self-Medication Hypothesis and Social Cognitive Theory. *Journal of Psychoactive Drugs, 50*(2), 177–186. DOI: 10.1080/02791072.2017.1397304 PMID: 29125424

20. Cerda, G., Pérez, C., & Melipillán, R. (2011). Test de inteligencia Lógica superior (TILS). *Manual de aplicación.*

21. Derivois, D., Mérisier, G. G., Cenat, J. M., & Castelot, V. (2014). Symptoms of posttraumatic stress disorder and social support among children and adolescents after the 2010 Haitian earthquake. *Journal of Loss and Trauma, 19*(3), 202–212. DOI: 10.1080/15325024.2013.789759

22. Fallot, R. D., Harris, M. (2009). Creating Cultures of Trauma-Informed Care (CCTIC): A Self-Assessment and Planning Protocol. *Community Connections* 2.2/7-09

23. Fernandez, L. S., Byard, D., Lin, C. C., Benson, S., & Barbera, J. A. (2002). Frail elderly as disaster victims: Emergency management strategies. *Prehospital and Disaster Medicine, 17*(2), 67–74. DOI: 10.1017/S1049023X14001435 PMID: 12500729

24. Fothergill, A., & Peek, L. A. (2004). Poverty and Disasters in the United States: A Review of Recent Sociological Findings. *Natural Hazards, 32*, 89–110. DOI: 10.1023/B:NHAZ.0000026792.76181.d9

25. Fox, J. H., Burkle, F. M., Bass, J., Pia, F. A., Epstein, J. L., & Markenson, D. (2012). The effectiveness of psychological first aid as a disaster intervention tool: Research analysis of peer-reviewed literature from 1990-2010. *Disaster Medicine and Public Health Preparedness, 6*(3), 247–252. PMID: 23077267

26. Galea, S., Nandi, A., & Vlahov, D. (2005). The epidemiology of post-traumatic stress disorder after disasters. *Epidemiologic Reviews, 27*(1), 78–91. DOI: 10.1093/epirev/mxi003 PMID: 15958429

27. Garakani, A., Murrough, J. W., Freire, R. C., Thom, R. P., Larkin, K., Buono, F. D., & Iosifescu, D. V. (2020). Pharmacotherapy of anxiety disorders: Current and emerging treatment options. *Frontiers in Psychiatry, 11*, 595584. DOI: 10.3389/fpsyt.2020.595584 PMID: 33424664

28. Goldmann, E., & Galea, S. (2014). Mental health consequences of disasters. *Annual Review of Public Health, 35*, 169–183. DOI: 10.1146/annurev-publhealth-032013-182435 PMID: 24159920

29. García-López, G. A., Pérez-Báez, C., & Rosado, M. (2021). The impact of infrastructure collapse on mental health: Puerto Rico after Hurricane Maria. *Disasters, 45*(3), 593–615.

2. Aten, J. D., Smith, W. R., Davis, E. B., Van Tongeren, D. R., Hook, J. N., Davis, D. E., Shannonhouse, L., DeBlaere, C., Ranter, J., O'Grady, K., & Hill, P. C. (2019). The psychological study of religion and spirituality in a disaster context: A systematic review. *Psychological Trauma: Theory, Research, Practice, and Policy, 11*(6), 597–613. PMID: 30730187

30. Gutierrez, J. M., Koralnik, I. J., & Teener, J. W. (2021). Communication failures in disaster response: The Puerto Rico experience. *The New England Journal of Medicine, 384*(12), 1183–1185.

31. Halpern, J., & Vermeulen, K. (2017). *Disaster mental health interventions: Core principles and practices*. Routledge.

32. Hermans, E. J., Henckens, M. J., Joëls, M., & Fernández, G. (2014). Dynamic adaptation of large-scale brain networks in response to acute stressors. *Trends in Neurosciences, 37*(6), 304–314. DOI: 10.1016/j.tins.2014.03.006 PMID: 24766931

33. Hoffman, M. A., & Kruczek, T. (2011). A bioecological model of mass trauma: Individual, community, and societal effects. *The Counseling Psychologist, 39*(8), 1087–1127. DOI: 10.1177/0011000010397932

34. Hoffman, Y., & Kruger, T. (2021). *Culture and disaster response: A psychological perspective*. Oxford University Press.

35. Hobfoll, S. E. (1989). Conservation of resources: A new attempt at conceptualizing stress. *The American Psychologist, 44*(3), 513. PMID: 2648906

36. Jovanovic, T., & Norrholm, S. D. (2011). Neural mechanisms of impaired fear inhibition in posttraumatic stress disorder. *Frontiers in Behavioral Neuroscience, 5*, 44. DOI: 10.3389/fnbeh.2011.00044 PMID: 21845177

37. Hinton, D. E., & Lewis-Fernández, R. (2011). The cross-cultural validity of posttraumatic stress disorder: Implications for DSM-5. *Depression and Anxiety, 28*(9), 783–801. DOI: 10.1002/da.20753 PMID: 21910185

38. Kessler, R. C., Galea, S., Gruber, M. J., Sampson, N. A., Ursano, R. J., & Wessely, S. (2008). Trends in mental illness and suicidality after Hurricane Katrina. *Molecular Psychiatry, 13*(4), 374–384. PMID: 18180768

39. Kaiser, B. N., McLean, K. E., Kohrt, B. A., Hagaman, A. K., Wagenaar, B. H., Khoury, N. M., & Keys, H. M. (2014). Reflechi twòp—thinking too much: Description of a cultural syndrome in Haiti's Central Plateau. *Culture, Medicine and Psychiatry, 38*(3), 448–472. PMID: 25038935

3. American Psychiatric Association, DSM-5 Task Force. (2013). *Diagnostic and statistical manual of mental disorders: DSM-5* (5th ed.). American Psychiatric Publishing, Inc., DOI: 10.1176/appi.books.9780890425596

40. Krug, E. G., Kresnow, M., Peddicord, J. P., Dahlberg, L. L., Powell, K. E., Crosby, A. E., & Annest, J. L. (1998). Suicide after natural disasters. *The New England Journal of Medicine, 338*(6), 373–378. DOI: 10.1056/NEJM199802053380607 PMID: 9449732

41. Koob, G. F., & Volkow, N. D. (2016). Neurobiology of addiction: A neurocircuitry analysis. *The Lancet. Psychiatry, 3*(8), 760–773. DOI: 10.1016/S2215-0366(16)00104-8 PMID: 27475769

42. Kishore, N., Marqués, D., Mahmud, A., Kiang, M. V., Rodriguez, I., Fuller, A., & Buckee, C. O. (2018). Mortality in Puerto Rico after Hurricane Maria. *The New England Journal of Medicine, 379*(2), 162–170. DOI: 10.1056/NEJMsa1803972 PMID: 29809109

43. Killikelly, C., Bauer, S., & Maercker, A. (2018). The assessment of grief in refugees and post-conflict survivors: A narrative review of etic and emic research. *Frontiers in Psychology, 9*, 1957. PMID: 30405474

44. Kristensen, P., Weisæth, L., & Heir, T. (2012). Bereavement and mental health after sudden and violent losses: *A review. Psychiatry, 75*(1), 76–97. https://guilfordjournals.com/doi/10.1521/psyc.2012.75.1.76 PMID: 22397543

45. Kawachi, I., Subramanian, S. V., & Kim, D. (2020). Global Perspective in Social capital and health. In *Social capital and health* (pp. 1–26). Springer., DOI: 10.1007/978-1-4614-7464-7_1

46. Kato, H., Asukai, N., Miyake, Y., Minakawa, K., & Nishiyama, A. (1996). Post-traumatic symptoms among younger and elderly evacuees in the early stages following the 1995 Hanshin-Awaji earthquake in Japan. *Acta Psychiatrica Scandinavica, 93*(6), 477–481. DOI: 10.1111/j.1600-0447.1996.tb10680.x PMID: 8831865

47. Kirmayer, L. J., Gone, J. P., & Moses, J. (2014). Rethinking historical trauma. *Transcultural Psychiatry, 51*(3), 299–319. PMID: 24855142

48. Kirmayer, L. J. (2022). Suicide in cultural context: An ecosocial approach. *Transcultural Psychiatry, 59*(1), 3–12. DOI: 10.1177/13634615221076424 PMID: 35179066

49. Kaniasty, K., & Norris, F. H. (2009). Distinctions that matter: Received social support, perceived social support, and social embeddedness after disasters. *Mental health and disasters*, 2009, 175-200.

4. Arnsten, A. F. (2015). Stress weakens prefrontal networks: Molecular insults to higher cognition. *Nature Neuroscience, 18*(10), 1376–1385. DOI: 10.1038/nn.4087 PMID: 26404712

50. Lanius, R. A., Vermetten, E., Loewenstein, R. J., Brand, B., Schmahl, C., Bremner, J. D., & Spiegel, D. (2010). Emotion modulation in PTSD: Clinical and neurobiological evidence for a dissociative subtype. *The American Journal of Psychiatry, 167*(6), 640–647. DOI: 10.1176/appi.ajp.2009.09081168 PMID: 20360318

51. La Greca, A. M., Lai, B. S., Joormann, J., Auslander, B. B., & Short, M. A. (2013). Children's risk and resilience following a natural disaster: Genetic vulnerability, posttraumatic stress, and depression. *Journal of Affective Disorders, 151*(3), 860–867. DOI: 10.1016/j.jad.2013.07.024 PMID: 24035489

52. Lazarus, R., & Folkman, S. (1984). *Stress, Appraisal, and Coping*. Springer.

53. Murray, L. K., Skavenski, S., Kane, J. C., Mayeya, J., Dorsey, S., Cohen, J. A., Michalopoulos, L. T., Imasiku, M., & Bolton, P. A. (2015). Effectiveness of Trauma-Focused Cognitive Behavioral Therapy Among Trauma-Affected Children in Lusaka, Zambia: A Randomized Clinical Trial. *JAMA Pediatrics, 169*(8), 761–769. DOI: 10.1001/jamapediatrics.2015.0580 PMID: 26111066

54. Meléndez, E., Hinojosa, J., & Roman, N. (2018). Puerto Rico's post-Maria outmigration. *Centro Journal, 30*(3), 54–85.

55. McFarlane, A. C., & Van Hooff, M. (2009). Impact of childhood exposure to a natural disaster on adult mental health: 20-year longitudinal follow-up study. *The British Journal of Psychiatry, 195*(2), 142–148. DOI: 10.1192/bjp.bp.108.054270 PMID: 19648546

56. Marsella, A. J., Johnson, J. L., Watson, P., & Gryczynski, J. (Eds.). (2008). *Ethnocultural perspectives on disaster and trauma: Foundations, issues, and applications*. Springer Science + Business Media. https://doi.org/DOI: 10.1007/978-0-387-73285-5

57. Milad, M. R., & Quirk, G. J. (2012). Fear extinction as a model for translational neuroscience: Ten years of progress. *Annual Review of Psychology*, *63*, 129–151. DOI: 10.1146/annurev.psych.121208.131631 PMID: 22129456

58. McLaughlin, K. A., Fairbank, J. A., Gruber, M. J., Jones, R. T., Lakoma, M. D., Pfefferbaum, B., Sampson, N. A., & Kessler, R. C. (2009). Serious emotional disturbance among youths exposed to Hurricane Katrina 2 years post disaster. *Journal of the American Academy of Child and Adolescent Psychiatry*, *48*(11), 1069–1078. PMID: 19797983

59. Maeda, M., Oe, M., Lee, M., & Miyazaki, M. (2018). Mental health consequences of the Great East Japan Earthquake. In *Mental Health and Disasters* (pp. 217–231). Cambridge University Press.

5. Arnberg, F. K., Gudmundsdóttir, R., Butwicka, A., Fang, F., Lichtenstein, P., Hultman, C. M., & Valdimarsdóttir, U. A. (2015). Psychiatric disorders and suicide attempts in Swedish survivors of the 2004 southeast Asia tsunami: A 5-year matched cohort study. *The Lancet. Psychiatry*, *2*(9), 817–824. PMID: 26236006

60. Maeda, M., & Oe, M. (2017). Mental health consequences and social issues after the Fukushima disaster. *Asia-Pacific Journal of Public Health*, *31*(2, suppl), 36S–46S. PMID: 28330398

61. Neria, Y., Nandi, A., & Galea, S. (2008). Post-traumatic stress disorder following disasters: A systematic review. *Psychological Medicine*, *38*(4), 467–480. PMID: 17803838

62. North, C. S., & Pfefferbaum, B. (2013). Mental health response to community disasters: A systematic review. *Journal of the American Medical Association*, *310*(5), 507–518. DOI: 10.1001/jama.2013.107799 PMID: 23925621

63. Norris, F. H., Friedman, M. J., Watson, P. J., Byrne, C. M., Diaz, E., & Kaniasty, K. (2002). 60,000 disaster victims speak: Part I. An empirical review of the empirical literature, 1981–2001. *Psychiatry*, *65*(3), 207–239. DOI: 10.1521/psyc.65.3.207.20173 PMID: 12405079

64. Norris, F. H., Stevens, S. P., Pfefferbaum, B., Wyche, K. F., & Pfefferbaum, R. L. (2020). Community resilience as a metaphor, theory, set of capacities, and strategy for disaster readiness. *American Journal of Community Psychology*, *41*(1-2), 127–150. DOI: 10.1007/s10464-007-9156-6 PMID: 18157631

65. O'Connor, M. F., Wellisch, D. K., Stanton, A. L., Eisenberger, N. I., Irwin, M. R., & Lieberman, M. D. (2008). Craving love? Enduring grief activates brain's reward center. *NeuroImage*, *42*(2), 969–972. DOI: 10.1016/j.neuroimage.2008.04.256 PMID: 18559294

66. Orengo-Aguayo, R., Stewart, R. W., de Arellano, M. A., Suárez-Kindy, J. L., & Young, J. (2019). Disaster exposure and mental health among Puerto Rican youths after Hurricane Maria. *JAMA Network Open*, *2*(4), e192619. DOI: 10.1001/jamanetworkopen.2019.2619 PMID: 31026024

67. Oe, M., Maeda, M., Nagai, M., Yasumura, S., Yabe, H., Suzuki, Y., & Bromet, E. (2016). Predictors of severe psychological distress trajectory after nuclear disaster: Evidence from the Fukushima Health Management Survey. *BMJ Open*, *6*(9), e013400. DOI: 10.1136/bmjopen-2016-013400 PMID: 27798033

68. Patel, S. S., Rogers, M. B., Amlôt, R., & Rubin, G. J. (2017). What do we mean by 'community resilience'? A systematic literature review of how it is defined in the literature. [ecurrents-dis.]. *PLoS Currents*, •••, 9. PMID: 29188132

69. Patel, S. S., Rogers, M. B., Amlôt, R., & Rubin, G. J. (2017). What Do We Mean by 'Community Resilience'? A Systematic Literature Review of How It Is Defined in the Literature. *PLoS Currents*, *9*. Advance online publication. DOI: 10.1371/currents.dis.db775aff25efc5ac4f0660ad9c9f7db2 PMID: 29188132

6. Bromet, E. J. (2014). Emotional consequences of nuclear power plant disasters. *Health Physics*, *106*(2), 206–210. DOI: 10.1097/HP.0000000000000012 PMID: 24378494

70. Patel, R., Green, L., & Kumar, S. (2022). *Culturally adaptive frameworks for disaster resilience: Global perspectives*. Oxford University Press.

71. Peek, L. (2008). Children and disasters: Understanding vulnerability, developing capacities, and promoting resilience—An introduction. *Children, Youth and Environments*, *18*(1), 1–29. https://www.jstor.org/stable/10.7721/chilyoutenvi.18.1.0001

72. Rivera, F. I., & Rolke, L. (2019). Health care provider migration from Puerto Rico after Hurricane Maria. *Journal of Immigrant and Minority Health*, *21*(3), 556–563.

73. Ruggiero, K. J., Price, M., Adams, Z., Stauffacher, K., McCauley, J., Danielson, C. K., & Resnick, H. S. (2015). Web intervention for adolescents affected by disaster: Population-based randomized controlled trial. *Journal of the American Academy of Child and Adolescent Psychiatry, 54*(9), 709–717. PMID: 26299292

74. Ramos, G., Chardón, C. E., & Rivera, F. I. (2020). Suicide trends in Puerto Rico before and after Hurricane Maria. *Crisis, 41*(5), 347–352.

75. Robles, R. R., Reyes, J. C., Colón, H. M., Sahai, H., Marrero, C. A., Matos, T. D., & Shepard, E. W. (2021). Community-based mobile health services in post-disaster Puerto Rico. *International Journal of Environmental Research and Public Health, 18*(4), 1675. PMID: 33572443

76. Shin, L. M., & Liberzon, I. (2010). The neurocircuitry of fear, stress, and anxiety disorders. *Neuropsychopharmacology : Official Publication of the American College of Neuropsychopharmacology, 35*(1), 169–191. DOI: 10.1038/npp.2009.83 PMID: 19625997

77. Shalev, A., Liberzon, I., & Marmar, C. (2017). Post-traumatic stress disorder. *The New England Journal of Medicine, 376*(25), 2459–2469. DOI: 10.1056/NEJMra1612499 PMID: 28636846

78. Sánchez-Cardona, I., Ortega-Polanco, J. C., & Bernal, G. (2020). Mental health services in Puerto Rico before Hurricane Maria. *Puerto Rico Health Sciences Journal, 39*(2), 84–91.

79. Sánchez, J., Román, J., & Martínez, K. (2021). Faith-based organizations in disaster mental health response. *Spirituality in Clinical Practice, 8*(1), 1–15.

7. Bromet, E. J., Havenaar, J. M., & Guey, L. T. (2011). A 25-year retrospective review of the psychological consequences of the Chernobyl accident. *Clinical oncology (Royal College of Radiologists (Great Britain)), 23*(4), 297–305. https://doi.org/DOI: 10.1016/j.clon.2011.01.501

80. Starcke, K., & Brand, M. (2012). Decision making under stress: A selective review. *Neuroscience and Biobehavioral Reviews, 36*(5), 1228–1248. DOI: 10.1016/j.neubiorev.2012.02.003 PMID: 22342781

81. Sung, S. C., Dryman, M. T., Marks, E., Shear, M. K., Ghesquiere, A., Fava, M., & Simon, N. M. (2011). Complicated grief among individuals with major depression: Prevalence, comorbidity, and associated features. *Journal of Affective Disorders, 134*(1-3), 453–458. PMID: 21621849

82. Stroebe, M., Schut, H., & Boerner, K. (2017). Cautioning health-care professionals: Bereaved persons are misguided through the stages of grief. *Omega, 74*(4), 455–473. DOI: 10.1177/0030222817691870 PMID: 28355991

83. Shigemura, J., Tanigawa, T., Saito, I., & Nomura, S. (2012). Psychological distress in workers at the Fukushima nuclear power plants. *Journal of the American Medical Association, 308*(7), 667–669. DOI: 10.1001/jama.2012.9699 PMID: 22893158

84. Schafer, A. (2010). Spirituality and mental health in humanitarian contexts: An exploration based on World Vision Haiti earthquake response. *Intervention (Amstelveen, Netherlands), 8*(2), 121–130.

85. Smith, T., Lee, C., & Zhang, W. (2020). Evidence-based psychological interventions in disaster settings. *Journal of Traumatic Stress, 33*(4), 512–525.

86. Santos-Lozada, A. R., Howard, J. T., & Verdery, A. M. (2020). Medication shortages after Hurricane Maria. *Health Affairs, 39*(5), 847–855.

87. Shultz, J. M., Cela, T., Marcelin, L. H., Espinola, M., Heitmann, I., Sanchez, C., & Rechkemmer, A. (2016). The trauma signature of 2016 Hurricane Matthew and the psychosocial impact on Haiti. *Disaster Health, 3*(4), 121–138. DOI: 10.1080/21665044.2016.1263538 PMID: 28321360

88. Tedeschi, R. G., & Calhoun, L. G. (2004). TARGET ARTICLE: "Posttraumatic Growth: Conceptual Foundations and Empirical Evidence.". *Psychological Inquiry, 15*(1), 1–18. DOI: 10.1207/s15327965pli1501_01

89. Van Vliet, N. I., Huntjens, R. J., Van Dijk, M. K., & De Jongh, A. (2018). Phase-based treatment versus immediate trauma-focused treatment in patients with childhood trauma-related posttraumatic stress disorder: Study protocol for a randomized controlled trial. *Trials, 19*(1), 138. PMID: 29471855

8. Brewin, C. R. (2011). The nature and significance of memory disturbance in posttraumatic stress disorder. *Annual Review of Clinical Psychology, 7*, 203–227. DOI: 10.1146/annurev-clinpsy-032210-104544 PMID: 21219190

90. Ursano, R. J., Fullerton, C. S., & Norwood, A. E. (Eds.). (2003). *Terrorism and Disaster Paperback with CD-ROM: Individual and Community Mental Health Interventions*. Cambridge University Press.

91. U.S. Department of Health and Human Services. (2018). Mental health infrastructure assessment: Puerto Rico post-Hurricane Maria (Report No. 18-2100). https://www.hhs.gov/sites/default/files/puerto-rico-mental-health-report.pdf

92. U.S. Government Accountability Office. (2019). Disaster recovery: Lessons from Hurricane Maria for Puerto Rico's mental health system (GAO-19-576). https://www.gao.gov/products/gao-19-576

93. Wolf, E. J., Lunney, C. A., Miller, M. W., Resick, P. A., Friedman, M. J., & Schnurr, P. P. (2012). The dissociative subtype of PTSD: A replication and extension. *Depression and Anxiety*, *29*(8), 679–688. DOI: 10.1002/da.21946 PMID: 22639402

94. Watson, P. J., Brymer, M. J., & Bonanno, G. A. (2011). Postdisaster psychological intervention since 9/11. *The American Psychologist*, *66*(6), 482–494. DOI: 10.1037/a0024806 PMID: 21823776

95. Wexler, L., White, J., & Trainor, B. (2015). Why an alternative to suicide prevention gatekeeper training is needed for rural Indigenous communities: Presenting an empowering community storytelling approach. *Critical Public Health*, *25*(2), 205–217. DOI: 10.1080/09581596.2014.904039 PMID: 36779086

96. World Health Organization. (2013). *Building back better: Sustainable mental health care after emergencies*. World Health Organization.

97. World Health Organization. (2019). *Mental health in emergencies*. World Health Organization.

98. Yabe, H., Suzuki, Y., Mashiko, H., Nakayama, Y., Hisata, M., Niwa, S. I., & Abe, M. (2014). Psychological distress after the Great East Japan Earthquake and Fukushima Daiichi Nuclear Power Plant accident: Results of a mental health and lifestyle survey through the Fukushima Health Management Survey in FY2011 and FY2012. *Fukushima Journal of Medical Science*, *60*(1), 57–67. DOI: 10.5387/fms.2014-1 PMID: 25030715

9. Brewin, C. R., Andrews, B., & Valentine, J. D. (2000). Meta-analysis of risk factors for posttraumatic stress disorder in trauma-exposed adults. *Journal of Consulting and Clinical Psychology*, *68*(5), 748–766. DOI: 10.1037//0022-006x.68.5.748 PMID: 11068961

Abdulmalek, S., Nasir, A., Jabbar, W. A., Almuhaya, M. A. M., Bairagi, A. K., & Khan, Md. (2022). IoT-Based Healthcare-Monitoring System towards Improving Quality of Life: A Review. *Health Care*, *10*(10). Advance online publication. DOI: 10.3390/healthcare10101993 PMID: 36292441

Adel, H. M., Khaled, M., Yehya, M. A., Elsayed, R., Ali, R. S., & Ahmed, F. E. (2024). Nexus among artificial intelligence implementation, healthcare social innovation, and green image of hospitals' operations management in Egypt. *Cleaner Logistics and Supply Chain*, *11*, 100156.

Adibi, S., Rajabifard, A., Shojaei, D., & Wickramasinghe, N. (2024). Enhancing healthcare through sensor-enabled digital twins in smart environments: A comprehensive analysis. *Sensors (Basel), 24*(9), 2793. PMID: 38732899

Agarwal, R., Singh, M., & Kumar, S. (2023). Surveillance, privacy, and occupational well-being: Perceptions of healthcare workers in Indian hospitals. *Indian Journal of Medical Ethics, 8*(2), 112–119. DOI: 10.20529/IJME.2023.028

Ahmad, A. (2024). Enhancing Hospital Efficiency through IoT and AI: A Smart Healthcare System. [JOSAPEN]. *Journal of Computer Science Application and Engineering, 2*(2), 34–38.

Ahmadi, A. (2024). Artificial Intelligence Revolution: A Comprehensive Review of its Transformative Impact on Hospital Data Management in the Future. [IJBLS]. *International Journal of BioLife Sciences, 3*(3), 115–133.

AI Agents for Sustainable Enterprise: A Leader's Guide. (n.d.). GreenMetrica. https://www.greenmetrica.com/ai-agents

Albahar, S., Li, J., Al-Zoughool, M., Al-Hemoud, A., Gasana, J., Aldashti, H., & Alahmad, B. (2022). Air Pollution and Respiratory Hospital Admissions in Kuwait: The Epidemiological Applicability of Predicted PM2.5 in Arid Regions. *International Journal of Environmental Research and Public Health, 19*(10), 5998. DOI: 10.3390/ijerph19105998 PMID: 35627536

Al-Balushi, H. A., Singh, H., & Saleem, I. (2025). *Unlocking sustainable performance in the healthcare sector: the dynamic nexus of artificial intelligence, green innovation and green knowledge sharing*. Society and Business Review.

Al-Barazie, R., & Mohamed, A. (2025). Towards Sustainable Healthcare: Integrating Technology for Eco-friendly and Efficient Solutions. In *International conference on Environmental Design, Material Science, and Engineering Technologies* (pp. 301-310). Springer, Cham.

Allegranzi, B., Storr, J., Dziekan, G., Leotsakos, A., Donaldson, L., & Pittet, D. (2007). The first global patient safety challenge "clean care is safer care": From launch to current progress and achievements. *The Journal of Hospital Infection, 65*, 115–123.

Alotaibi, E., & Nassif, N. (2024). Artificial intelligence in environmental monitoring: In-depth analysis. *Discover Artificial Intelligence, 4*(1), 84. DOI: 10.1007/s44163-024-00198-1

Alqahtani, F. M., Adwan, S., Ahmad, M. Y., Karman, S. B., Maged, R., & Maged, L. (2024). *Impact of retinal enhancement techniques on blood vessel segmentation*. In *Proceedings of the 14th IEEE Symposium on Computer Applications & Industrial Electronics (ISCAIE)* (pp. 517–521). IEEE. DOI: 10.1109/ISCAIE61308.2024.10576581

Alreshidi, E., & Ahmad, M. (2020). Big data in healthcare: Management, analysis, and future prospects. *Journal of Big Data*, *6*(54). Advance online publication. DOI: 10.1186/s40537-019-0217-0

Anderson, D. M., Mahamane, E., Bauza, V., Mahamadou, K. O. B., Tantum, L., & Salzberg, A. (2023). Effects of environmental conditions on healthcare worker wellbeing and quality of care: A qualitative study in Niger. *PLOS Global Public Health*, *3*(12), e0002590. DOI: 10.1371/journal.pgph.0002590 PMID: 38117837

Anderson, M., Wilson, J., & Patel, R. (2021). Building a culture of safety in healthcare: Leadership and participatory approaches. *Journal of Healthcare Management*, *66*(5), 329–339. DOI: 10.1097/JHM-D-20-00167

Anicai, C., & Shakir, M. Z. (2025). A multimodal dataset of cardiac, electrodermal, and environmental signals. *Scientific Data*, *12*(1), 844. DOI: 10.1038/s41597-025-05051-3 PMID: 40404669

Anitha, M., & Kumar, L. S. (2023). Development of an IoT-enabled air pollution monitoring and air purifier system. *MAPAN*, *38*(3), 669–688.

Arvidsson, I., Balogh, I., Hansson, G.-Å., & Lindegård, A. (2022). Participatory ergonomics and staff involvement as strategies for reducing musculoskeletal disorders in healthcare. *Applied Ergonomics*, *101*, 103694. DOI: 10.1016/j.apergo.2021.103694

Arya, A., Bachheti, A., Bachheti, R. K., Singh, M., & Chandel, A. K. (2024). Role of artificial intelligence in minimizing carbon footprint: A systematic review of recent insights. *Biorefinery and Industry 4.0: Empowering Sustainability*, 365–386.

ASHRAE. (2019). HVAC Design Manual for Hospitals and Clinics (2nd ed.). American Society of Heating, Refrigerating and Air-Conditioning Engineers.

Asiri, M. A., Almutairi, A. D., Ozam, T. S., Al Ahmari, R. Y., Alhazmi, S. M., Almoudhi, A. A., & Alqahtani, N. M. (2024). AI-Driven Decision Support Systems: Transforming Hospital Management Strategies. [JICRCR]. *Journal of International Crisis & Risk Communication Research*, *7*(3).

Aurangzeb, K., Alharthi, R. S., Haider, S. I., & Alhussein, M. (2023). Systematic development of AI-enabled diagnostic systems for glaucoma and diabetic retinopathy. *IEEE Access : Practical Innovations, Open Solutions*, *11*, 105069–105081. DOI: 10.1109/ACCESS.2023.3317348

Bai, X., Li, Z., & Zhou, H. (2023). Integrated occupational safety models in sustainable healthcare systems. *International Journal of Environmental Research and Public Health*, *20*(18), 6789. DOI: 10.3390/ijerph20186789

Baker, M. L. (2021). Engaging stakeholders with healthcare data visualizations. *Journal of Healthcare Management*, *66*(1), 14–25. PMID: 33411481

Bala Dhandayuthapani, V. (2024). Advancing Healthcare: AI Integration, Interoperability and Sustainability Challenges. *Digital Health*, •••, 64.

Balpande, A., Moundekar, D., Kothari, R., Ashtikar, A., & Shelke, D. D. M. K. (2023). *Early detection of glaucoma using CNN architecture*. In *Proceedings of the International Conference for Advancement in Technology (ICONAT)* (pp. 1–8). IEEE. DOI: 10.1109/ICONAT57137.2023.10080853

Barbaro, A., Chiavassa, P., Fissore, V. I., Servetti, A., Raviola, E., Ramírez-Espinosa, G., Giusto, E., Montrucchio, B., Astolfi, A., & Fiori, F. (2024). Data Acquisition, Processing, and Aggregation in a Low-Cost IoT System for Indoor Environmental Quality Monitoring. *Applied Sciences (Basel, Switzerland)*, *14*(10), 4021. DOI: 10.3390/app14104021

Bashir, S.. (2023). *Exploring the impact of preprocessing techniques on retinal blood vessel segmentation using a study group learning scheme*. In *Proceedings of the IEEE Signal Processing in Medicine and Biology Symposium (SPMB)* (pp. 1–6). IEEE. DOI: 10.1109/SPMB59478.2023.10372702

Bedi, R., Sharma, A., & Gupta, N. (2022). Ergonomic risk factors and prevalence of musculoskeletal disorders among laboratory health care workers in North India. *Indian Journal of Occupational and Environmental Medicine*, *26*(1), 45–51. DOI: 10.4103/ijoem.ijoem_190_21

Bekbolatova, M., Mayer, J., Ong, C. W., & Toma, M. (2024). Transformative potential of AI in healthcare: Definitions, applications, and navigating the ethical landscape and public perspectives. *Health Care*, *12*(2), 125.

Bentameur, K., & Iguenane, B. (2023). Impact of Information Security on Online Operations: The Mediating Role of Risk Management. *International Journal of Computations* [IJCIM]. *Information and Manufacturing*, *3*(1), 27–34. DOI: 10.54489/ijcim.v3i1.224

Bhambri, P., & Khang, A. (2024). Managing and monitoring patient's healthcare using AI and IoT technologies. In *Driving Smart Medical Diagnosis Through AI-Powered Technologies and Applications* (pp. 1–23). IGI Global.

Bhamidipaty, V., Bhamidipaty, D. L., Guntoory, I., Bhamidipaty, K. D. P., Iyengar, K. P., Botchu, B., & Botchu, R. (2025). Revolutionizing Healthcare: The Impact of AI-Powered Sensors. *Generative Artificial Intelligence for Biomedical and Smart Health Informatics*, 355-373.

Bhutani, J., Bhutani, S., Balhara, Y. P. S., & Kalra, S. (2012). Compassion fatigue and burnout amongst clinicians: A medical exploratory study. *Indian Journal of Psychological Medicine*, *34*(4), 332–337. DOI: 10.4103/0253-7176.108206

Blinova, T., Singh Chauhan, S., Singla, T., Bansal, S., Mittal, A., & Yellanki, V. S. (2024). Performance Evaluation of IoT Sensors in Urban Air Quality Monitoring: Insights from the IoT Sensor Performance Test. *BIO Web of Conferences, 86*, 01088. https://doi.org/DOI: 10.1051/bioconf/20248601088

Bouzid, A., Gendy, M. E., & Leduc, L. (2020). Energy performance benchmarking for healthcare buildings in France. *Energy and Building*, *224*, 110241.

Bozic, V. (2023). Integrated Risk Management and Artificial Intelligence in Hospital. *Journal of AI*, *7*(1), 63–80. DOI: 10.61969/jai.1329224

Bradley, P. M., Journey, C. A., & Romanok, K. M.. (2020). Expanded target-chemical analysis reveals extensive mixed-organic-contaminant exposure in U.S. streams. *Environmental Science & Technology*, *54*(18), 11587–11598. PMID: 28401767

Brown, M. J., Forster, B. B., McInnes, M. D. F., Komar, M. A., Amin, P., Atwal, S., Chen, S., Hamwi, M., Ladak, R., Malik, A., McKee, H., Wang, M., Yang, J., Hamel, C., & Hanneman, K. (2025). Canadian Association of Radiologists Statement on Planetary Health Education in Radiology. *Canadian Association of Radiologists Journal*, *76*(2), 212–220. DOI: 10.1177/08465371241279359 PMID: 39313910

Building and managing an agentic AI workforce | McKinsey. (n.d.). Retrieved August 2, 2025, from https://www.mckinsey.com/capabilities/people-and-organizational-performance/our-insights/the-future-of-work-is-agentic

Buonanno, G., Stabile, L., Morawska, L., Giovinco, G., & Querol, X. (2017). Do air quality targets really represent safe limits for lung cancer risk? *The Science of the Total Environment*, *580*, 74–82.

Cachazo, R., González, M., & Valero, M. (2022). Process mining in healthcare: A data-driven methodology for staff performance and safety optimization. *Health Informatics Journal*, *28*(2), 1–15. DOI: 10.1177/14604582221091733

Cannaby, A., Connell, L., Viehweger, E., & Hignett, S. (2021). Feasibility and validity of real-time locating systems to measure nurses' movement and workflow in hospitals: An observational study. *Journal of Research in Nursing : JRN*, *26*(6), 571–586. DOI: 10.1177/17449871211016169

Cavoukian, A. (2021). Privacy by design: From rhetoric to reality. *Health Management*, *21*(3), 112–118. DOI: 10.1007/s10729-021-09587-2

Chanda, P., Gagan, J. H., Mallya, B. V., & Kumar, J. R. H. (2023). *Automatic optic cup segmentation using affine snakes in gradient vector field*. In *Proceedings of the IEEE 20th India Council International Conference (INDICON)* (pp. 1112–1115). IEEE. DOI: 10.1109/INDICON59947.2023.10440823

Chassang, G. (2017). The impact of the EU general data protection regulation on medical research. *Journal of Medical Internet Research*, *19*(6), e193. DOI: 10.2196/jmir.7108

Chatterjee, A., Sinha, R., & Deshmukh, P. (2022). Wearable health technologies and occupational safety in Indian healthcare settings. *Health and Technology*, *12*(5), 1001–1012. DOI: 10.1007/s12553-022-00691-2

Chattopadhyay, S., & Mehta, K. (2022). Ethics of digital monitoring in healthcare workplaces: Balancing safety and autonomy. *Journal of Medical Ethics*, *48*(11), 789–794. DOI: 10.1136/medethics-2021-107871

Chavan, R., & Pete, D. (2024). *Optic disc and blood vessel based diabetic disease detection using enhanced long-short-term memory*. In *Proceedings of the IEEE International Conference on Interdisciplinary Approaches in Technology and Management for Social Innovation (IATMSI)* (pp. 1–6). IEEE. DOI: 10.1109/IATMSI60426.2024.10502867

Chen, M. (n.d.). *Agentic AI: The Next Big Thing in Artificial Intelligence*. Retrieved August 2, 2025, from https://www.oracle.com/ro/artificial-intelligence/agentic-ai/

Chen, H.-L., Lin, C.-Y., & Chang, W.-C. (2022). Patient safety culture and staff well-being in Taiwan: An organizational resource perspective. *Journal of Patient Safety*, *18*(8), 663–670. DOI: 10.1097/PTS.0000000000000947

Chen, L.. (2022). Smart infection control in hospitals via decision support. *BMC Health Services Research*, *22*(1), 643. PMID: 35562697

Chen, Y., Wang, X., & Li, J. (2022). Artificial intelligence-driven fatigue detection in healthcare professionals: A machine learning approach. *Journal of Biomedical Informatics*, *130*, 104089. DOI: 10.1016/j.jbi.2022.104089

Chen, Y.-Y., Chien, W.-C., Lee, M.-S., Chen, L.-H., Chan, T.-C., & Lee, C.-H. (2023). Applying a smartwatch to predict work-related fatigue for emergency healthcare professionals: Machine learning method. *Journal of Medical Internet Research, 25*, e30405. DOI: 10.2196/30405

Chirchi, V., Chirchi, K. E., & Chirchi, E. (2024). IoT for health care: a sustainable approach. In *Sustainable IoT and Data Analytics Enabled Machine Learning Techniques and Applications* (pp. 109–126). Springer Nature Singapore.

Cilasun Kunduracı, A., & İvgin, S. (2022). Energy Saving Opportunities through Glazing and Shading Alternatives. *Iconarp International. Nihon Kenchiku Gakkai Keikaku-Kei Rombunshu.* Advance online publication. DOI: 10.15320/ICONARP.2022.211

Cleveland Clinic. (2024). *AI in surgical scheduling improves hospital efficiency.* https://clevelandclinic.org

Collaborative Intelligence: AI + Human Expertise for Sustainability. (2025, May 27). https://perspectives.se.com/blog-stream/collaborative-intelligence-ai-human-expertise-for-sustainability

Connor, A., Lillywhite, R., & Cooke, M. W. (2020). The carbon footprint of a renal service in the United Kingdom. *QJM: An International Journal of Medicine, 104*(9), 749–755. PMID: 20719900

Conti, M., Dehghantanha, A., Franke, K., & Watson, S. (2018). Internet of Things security and forensics: Challenges and opportunities. *Future Generation Computer Systems, 78*, 544–546. https://www.researchgate.net/publication/318715070_Internet_of_Things_Security_and_Forensics_Challenges_and_Opportunities

Cvitić, I., Peraković, D., Periša, M., & Husnjak, S. (2022). Boosting-based DDoS detection in Internet of Things systems. *IEEE Internet of Things Journal, 9*(2), 1172–1185. DOI: 10.1109/JIOT.2021.3079084

Danasekaran, R., Mani, G., & Annadurai, K. (2014). Prevention of healthcare-associated infections: Protecting patients, saving lives. *International Journal of Community Medicine and Public Health, 1*(1), 67–68.

Dangi, R. R., Sharma, A., & Vageriya, V. (2025). Transforming healthcare in low-resource settings with artificial intelligence: Recent developments and outcomes. *Public Health Nursing (Boston, Mass.), 42*(2), 1017–1030.

Data.org. (2023). Data and analytics in our work. (https://urbanhealth.org.uk/our-work/data)

Desai, P., Kumar, V., & Singh, A. (2024). Occupational safety challenges among healthcare workers in Indian hospitals: An implementation gap analysis. *Indian Journal of Occupational and Environmental Medicine, 28*(1), 45–52. DOI: 10.4103/ijoem.ijoem_14_24

Destoumieux-Garzón, D., Mavingui, P., Boetsch, G., Boissier, J., Darriet, F., Duboz, P., Fritsch, C., Giraudoux, P., Le Roux, F., Morand, S., Paillard, C., Pontier, D., Sueur, C., & Voituron, Y. (2018). The One Health Concept: 10 Years Old and a Long Road Ahead. *Frontiers in Veterinary Science, 5*. Advance online publication. DOI: 10.3389/fvets.2018.00014 PMID: 29484301

Devi, Y. A. S., & Chari, K. M. (2022). *Composite filtering and morphology for optic disc segmentation from retinal images*. In Proceedings of the IEEE 4th International Conference on Cybernetics, Cognition and Machine Learning Applications (ICCCMLA) (pp. 348–354). IEEE. DOI: 10.1109/ICCCMLA56841.2022.9989225

Dewasiri, N. J., Rathnasiri, M. S. H., & Karunarathna, K. S. S. N. (2025). Artificial Intelligence-Driven Technologies for Environmental Sustainability in the Healthcare Industry. In *Transforming Healthcare Sector Through Artificial Intelligence and Environmental Sustainability* (pp. 67–87). Springer Nature Singapore.

Dolcini, M., Ferrè, F., Brambilla, A., & Capolongo, S. (2025). Integrating environmental sustainability into hospitals performance management systems: A scoping review. *BMC Health Services Research, 25*(1), 764.

dos Santos, M., Howard, D., Kruger, P., Banos, A., & Kornik, S. (2019). Climate Change and Healthcare Sustainability in the Agincourt Sub-District, Kruger to Canyons Biosphere Region, South Africa. *Sustainability, 11*(2), 496. DOI: 10.3390/su11020496

Doss, R. (2022). *An optimized soft computing model using neural network with ant colony optimization algorithm for retinal image segmentation*. In *Proceedings of the International Conference on Innovative Computing, Intelligent Communication and Smart Electrical Systems (ICSES)* (pp. 1–6). IEEE. DOI: 10.1109/ICSES55317.2022.9914118

Dover, T. P. (2021, April). Evaluating Medical IoT (MIoT) device security using NISTIR-8228 expectations [Preprint]. arXiv. https://arxiv.org/abs/2104.03283

Dufera, M., Tuly, L., & Mwale, L.. (2023). Occupational-related injuries and associated risk factors among healthcare workers working in developing countries: A systematic review. *Journal of Occupational Health, 65*(1), e12455. DOI: 10.1002/joh2.12455

Dyrbye, L. N., Shanafelt, T. D., Sinsky, C. A., Cipriano, P. F., Bhatt, J., Ommaya, A., West, C. P., & Meyers, D. (2020). Burnout among healthcare professionals: A call to explore and address this underrecognized threat to safe, high-quality care. *National Academy of Medicine, 99*(1), 11–20. DOI: 10.31478/202001a

Ebi, K. L., & Bowen, K. (2022). Urban health and climate change. *Environmental Health Perspectives, 130*(12), 127001. DOI: 10.1289/EHP10113 PMID: 36454223

Edu, A. S. (2024). Configural paths for IoTs and big data analytics acceptance for healthcare improvement: A fuzzy-set qualitative comparative analysis. *Aslib Journal of Information Management, 76*(5), 800–821. DOI: 10.1108/AJIM-10-2022-0465

Elendu, C., Elendu, T. C., & Elendu, I. D. (2024). 5G-enabled smart hospitals: Innovations in patient care and facility management. *Medicine, 103*(20), e38239. PMID: 38758872

Energy and AI. (n.d.). International Energy Agency (IEA): New Report on Energy and AI | BUILD UP. Retrieved August 21, 2025, from https://build-up.ec.europa.eu/en/resources-and-tools/publications/international-energy-agency-iea-new-report-energy-and-ai

EPA. (2023). *Greenhouse Gas Equivalencies Calculator*. United States Environmental Protection Agency.

Epicenters, P. (2024). *Healthcare-associated infections (HAIs): Reports and Data*. https://www.cdc.gov/healthcare-associated-infections/php/data/index.html

Ernawati, K., Burhan, A., Syawqi Albar, A., Al-Khaliel, A. T., & Fawwaz Al-Fatich, A. S. (2024). Health Education for Sustainable E-Waste Management. In *International Journal of Engineering, Science and Information Technology* (Vol. 4, Issue 3, pp. 128–131). https://doi.org/DOI: 10.52088/ijesty.v4i3.556

Ernawati, K., Aslichan, A., Albar, A. S., Al Khaliel, A. T., & Al Fatich, A. S. F. (2025). *Green Leadership Strategy to Encourage Pro-Environmental Behavior*. IGI Global., DOI: 10.4018/979-8-3373-2106-6.ch006

Ernawati, K., Burhan, A., Albar, A. S., Al Khaliel, A. T., & Al Fatich, A. S. F. (2024). *Professional Development of Environmental Health Workers*., DOI: 10.4018/979-8-3693-4334-0.ch010

Ernawati, K., Hayurani, H., Karimulloh, K., Haryanti, S. C., & Utami, S. P. (2025). Development of a home health assessment application and website-based family disease registration. *International Journal of Innovative Research and Scientific Studies, 8*(3), 4471–4477. DOI: 10.53894/ijirss.v8i3.7538

Ernawati, K., Mardhiyah, D., Wulansari, R., Rifqatussaadah, R., & Utami, S. (2025). *AI's Role in Environmental Health and Tackling Ecological Impacts Through Multidimensional Views.*, DOI: 10.4018/979-8-3373-0680-3.ch005

Esmaeilzadeh, P. (2024). Challenges and strategies for wide-scale artificial intelligence (AI) deployment in healthcare practices: A perspective for healthcare organizations. *Artificial Intelligence in Medicine*, *151*, 102861.

European Commission. (2024). Digital health dashboards for decision-making to enable public health crises management. *JMIR Research Protocols*, *13*, e46810. DOI: 10.2196/46810

Fajar, M., Chandra, F. B., & Arfandy, H. (2023). Applying Use Case 2.0 Approach to The Development of IoT-Based Rainfall Monitoring System. [JANAPATI]. *Jurnal Nasional Pendidikan Teknik Informatika*, *12*(2), 244–252. DOI: 10.23887/janapati.v12i2.61529

Farraher, S. G. (2025, July 23). Agentic AI In Healthcare: A New Era Of Intelligent Automation. *Forrester*. https://www.forrester.com/blogs/agentic-ai-in-healthcare-a-new-era-of-intelligent-automation/

Ferguson, C., Yu, M., & Bismark, M. (2023). Data-driven safety audits in healthcare: Reducing occupational hazards through real-time monitoring. *Journal of Healthcare Risk Management*, *42*(2), 23–33. DOI: 10.1002/jhrm.22156

Fernández, J., & Rivas, A. (2021). The social consequences of workplace monitoring in healthcare: From compliance to resistance. *Social Science & Medicine*, *285*, 114262. DOI: 10.1016/j.socscimed.2021.114262

Fonseca, A., Abreu, I., Guerreiro, M. J., & Barros, N. (2022). Indoor air quality in healthcare units—A systematic literature review focusing recent research. *Sustainability*, *14*(2), 967.

Frimpong, B. A., Barbosa, C., & Raed A Abd, A. (2023). The Impact of the Internet of Things (IoT) on Healthcare Delivery: A Systematic Literature Review. *Journal of Techniques*, *5*(3), 84–91. DOI: 10.51173/jt.v5i3.1433

Galushchak, O., Burlaka, S., Kupchuk, I., Bondarenko, V., & Gontaruk, Y. (2023). Environmental indicators of the operation of a diesel generator running on a mixture of biofuels. *Polityka Energetyczna – Energy Policy Journal, 26*(4), 195–208. https://doi.org/DOI: 10.33223/epj/170759

Galvão, D. M.. (2023). Hospital sustainability indicators and reduction of socio-environmental impacts: A scoping review. *Revista da Escola de Enfermagem da USP*, *57*, e20220364. DOI: 10.1590/1980-220X-REEUSP-2022-0364en

Gani, V. K. U. A., & Shanmugasundaram, N. (2022). *Computerized framework used to detect glaucoma: A review*. In *Proceedings of the 8th International Conference on Advanced Computing and Communication Systems (ICACCS)* (pp. 1353–1358). IEEE. DOI: 10.1109/ICACCS54159.2022.9785244

Garcia, A., Saez, Y., Harris, I., Huang, X., & Collado, E. (2025). Advancements in air quality monitoring: A systematic review of IoT-based air quality monitoring and AI technologies. *Artificial Intelligence Review*, *58*(9), 275. DOI: 10.1007/s10462-025-11277-9

Garcia-Sanz-Calcedo, J., Al-Kassir, A., & Yusaf, T. (2018). Economic and environmental impact of energy saving in healthcare buildings. *Applied Energy*, *228*, 1354–1363.

Garg, P. P., Jayashree, J., & Vijayashree, J. (2025). Revolutionizing healthcare: The transformative role of artificial intelligence. In *Responsible and Explainable Artificial Intelligence in Healthcare* (pp. 1–23). Elsevier.

Gartner's Top 10 Strategic Technology Trends for 2025. (n.d.). Gartner. Retrieved August 2, 2025, from https://www.gartner.com/en/articles/top-technology-trends-2025

George, C. E., Varghese, J., & Ravi, D. (2020). Burnout among nurses and its impact on patient care in South India: A cross-sectional study. *Indian Journal of Occupational and Environmental Medicine*, *24*(3), 202–207. DOI: 10.4103/ijoem.IJOEM_257_19

Gohr, C., Rodríguez, G., Belomestnykh, S., Berg-Moelleken, D., Chauhan, N., Engler, J.-O., Heydebreck, L. V., Hintz, M. J., Kretschmer, M., Krügermeier, C., Meinberg, J., Rau, A.-L., Schwenck, C., Aoulkadi, I., Poll, S., Frank, E., Creutzig, F., Lemke, O., Maushart, M., & von Wehrden, H. (2025). Artificial intelligence in sustainable development research. *Nature Sustainability*, •••, 1–9. DOI: 10.1038/s41893-025-01598-6

González, A., García-Sanz-Calcedo, J., & Rodríguez Salgado, D. (2018). Evaluation of Energy Consumption in German Hospitals: Benchmarking in the Public Sector. *Energies*, *11*(9), 2279. DOI: 10.3390/en11092279

González, M., Rivera, P., & López, C. (2021). Predictive modeling of occupational fatigue among intensive care staff using machine learning. *Safety and Health at Work*, *12*(4), 443–450. DOI: 10.1016/j.shaw.2021.09.002

Gordon, L. B., Liu, K. T., Hudak, N. C., & Auerbach, A. (2023). Assessing hospitalists' opinions regarding the role of environmental health within the practice of hospital medicine. *Journal of Hospital Medicine*, *18*(7), 588–594. DOI: 10.1002/jhm.13098 PMID: 37039588

Green Paper, E. S. I. C. M. (2018). Environmental sustainability in intensive care: The path forward. *Intensive Care Medicine*. Advance online publication. DOI: 10.1007/s00134-018-5111-9

Gulraiz, A., Gulraiz, H., Zia, M., Badar, S., & Zaidi, S. S. H. (2024). Utilizing IoT and Cloud Computing for Weather-Health Monitoring Application. *International Journal of Electrical Engineering and Computer Science*, *6*, 152–158. DOI: 10.37394/232027.2024.6.18

Gupta, A. (2023). Smart air quality control in Indian hospitals. *Clean Technologies and Environmental Policy*, *25*, 122–130.

Gupta, R., Chatterjee, S., & Nair, A. (2023). AI-enabled monitoring for infection control in Indian hospitals: A COVID-19 case study. *International Journal of Healthcare Management*, *16*(2), 85–94. DOI: 10.1080/20479700.2023.2178452

Gupta, V., & Sharma, P. (2023). Surveillance and workplace stress among Indian healthcare workers: An emerging concern. *Indian Journal of Occupational and Environmental Medicine*, *27*(1), 15–21. DOI: 10.4103/ijoem.ijoem_89_22

Gürses, S., & Del Alamo, J. M. (2016). Privacy engineering: Shaping an emerging field of research and practice. *IEEE Security and Privacy*, *14*(2), 40–46. https://ieeexplore.ieee.org/abstract/document/7448344

Haddad, S., Smith, R., Johnson, P., & Lee, A. (2022). Disparity dashboards: An evaluation of the literature and applications. *Lancet Regional Health. Americas*. Advance online publication. DOI: 10.1016/j.lana.2022.100250

Hall, L. H., Johnson, J., Watt, I., Tsipa, A., & O'Connor, D. B. (2016). Healthcare staff wellbeing, burnout, and patient safety: A systematic review. *PLoS One*, *11*(7), e0159015. DOI: 10.1371/journal.pone.0159015

Hamdi, N., Oweis, R., Abu Zraiq, H., & Abu Sammour, D. (2012). An Intelligent Healthcare Management System: A New Approach in Work-order Prioritization for Medical Equipment Maintenance Requests. *Journal of Medical Systems*, *36*(2), 557–567. DOI: 10.1007/s10916-010-9501-4 PMID: 20703695

Han, S., Jeong, Y., Lee, K., & In, J. (2024). Environmental sustainability in health care: An empirical investigation of US hospitals. *Business Strategy and the Environment*, *33*(6), 6045–6065. DOI: 10.1002/bse.3790

Haque, M., Sartelli, M., McKimm, J., & Bakar, M. A. (2018). Health care-associated infections–an overview. *Infection and Drug Resistance*, •••, 2321–2333.

Haque, S. A., Aziz, S. M., & Rahman, M. (2014). Review of Cyber-Physical System in Healthcare. *International Journal of Distributed Sensor Networks, 10*(4), 217415. DOI: 10.1155/2014/217415

Harris, J. (2020). The Energy Burden of Medical Imaging: A Review. *Health Environments Research & Design Journal, 13*(4), 25–40.

Hasan, N., Bao, Y., Miah, S. J., & Fenton, A. (2023). Factors influencing the young physicians' intention to use Internet of Things (IoT) services in healthcare. *Information Development, 39*(4), 902–919. DOI: 10.1177/02666669211064114

Hasić, F., Beirens, B., & Serral, E. (2022). Maturity Model for IoT Adoption in Hospitals. *Computer Information, 41*(1), 213–232. DOI: 10.31577/cai_2022_1_213

Hassan, N. A., Hashim, Z., & Hashim, J. H. (2015). *Impact of Climate Change on Air Quality and Public Health in Urban Areas*. https://journals.sagepub.com/doi/10.1177/1010539515592951

Health Care-Associated Infections. (n.d.). Retrieved June 20, 2025, from https://www.ahrq.gov/professionals/quality-patient-safety/patient-safety-resources/resources/hais/index.html

Helminski, D., Roberts, J., Taylor, P., & Singh, M. (2024). Development, implementation, and evaluation methods for healthcare dashboards. JMIR Medical Informatics, 12(1), e59828.](https://doi.org/)DOI: 10.2196/59828

Hemalatha, R. J., Akila, D., Balaganesh, D., & Paul, A. (2022). *The internet of medical things (IoMT): Healthcare transformation*. John Wiley & Sons.

Hepsiba, J., & G, V. (2023). Effectiveness of Teaching Programme on Knowledge Regarding Hospital Waste Management a mong House Keeping Employees. *JOURNAL OF CLINICAL AND BIOMEDICAL SCIENCES, 13*(3), 81–84. https://doi.org/DOI: 10.58739/jcbs/v13i3.23.24

HIMSS. (2025). Davies Award of Excellence. (https://www.himss.org/initiatives/awards/davies-award-of-excellence/)

Hinostroza Fuentes, V. G., Karim, H. A., Tan, M. J. T., & AlDahoul, N. (2025). AI with agency: A vision for adaptive, efficient, and ethical healthcare. *Frontiers in Digital Health, 7*, 1600216.

Holmér, S., Nedlund, A.-C., Thomas, K., & Krevers, B. (2023). How health care professionals handle limited resources in primary care–an interview study. *BMC Health Services Research*, *23*(1), 6.

Holzinger, A., Biemann, C., Pattichis, C. S., & Kell, D. B. (2017). What do we need to build explainable AI systems for the medical domain? *arXiv Preprint arXiv:1712.09923.*

Horn Iwaya, L. H., Ahmad, A., & Babar, M. A. (2020, June). Security and privacy for mHealth and uHealth systems: A systematic mapping study [Preprint]. arXiv. https://arxiv.org/abs/2006.12069

Ho, S. S., Sosina, W., DePierro, J. M., Perez, S., Khan, A., Starkweather, S., Marin, D. B., Sharma, V., Ripp, J. A., Peccoralo, L. A., & Charney, D. S. (2024). Promoting resilience in healthcare workers: A preventative mental health education program. *International Journal of Environmental Research and Public Health*, *21*(10), 1365. DOI: 10.3390/ijerph21101365

Hossain, M. A., Arafat, M. S., Desai, K., Akter, S., & Asha, A. I. (2025). The Economic Impact of AI-Driven Remote Patient Monitoring: A Business Intelligence Perspective on Healthcare Cost Optimization. *International Interdisciplinary Business Economics Advancement Journal*, *6*(05), 39–67.

Hosseinzadeh, A., Reshadi, M. A. M., Nazaripour, M., & Rezaei, M. (2023). Medical Waste Management in Private Hospitals in Tehran. *Journal of Advances in Environmental Health Research*, *11*(3), 142–146. DOI: 10.34172/jaehr.1274

Houston Chronicle. (2025, June 14). Houston launches city data dashboard to track heat-related ER visits, health risks.](https://www.houstonchronicle.com/news/houston-weather/forecast/article/houston-unveils-new-heat-er-dashboard-20814042.php)

Huang, K. (2025). AI Agents in Healthcare. In *Agentic AI: Theories and Practices* (pp. 303–321). Springer.

Huang, C., Chen, Q., Lin, Z., Su, W., Zhang, Z., & Liu, S. (2024). The Economic Impact and Application Challenges of IoT Technology in Smart Home and Infrastructure. *Journal of Innovation and Development*, *6*(1), 35–39. DOI: 10.54097/y54jkp60

Ibrahim, M., Kebede, M., & Mengiste, B. (2023). Healthcare Waste Segregation Practice and Associated Factors among Healthcare Professionals Working in Public and Private Hospitals, Dire Dawa, Eastern Ethiopia. *Journal of Environmental and Public Health*, *2023*, 1–7. DOI: 10.1155/2023/8015856 PMID: 36747502

Internet of Things (IoT). (n.d.). 2021 Edition - IEEE Electronics Packaging Society. Retrieved August 9, 2025, from https://eps.ieee.org/technology/heterogeneous-integration-roadmap/2021-edition.html

Ishaq, A., Mohammad, S. J., Bello, A.-A. D., Wada, S. A., Adebayo, A., & Jagun, Z. T. (2023). Smart waste bin monitoring using IoT for sustainable biomedical waste management. *Environmental Science and Pollution Research International*. Advance online publication. DOI: 10.1007/s11356-023-30240-1 PMID: 37878175

Islam, M. M., Rahaman, A., & Islam, M. R. (2020). Development of smart healthcare monitoring system in IoT environment. *SN Computer Science*, *1*(3), 185.

Islam, M. T., Mashfu, S. T., Faisal, A., Siam, S. C., Naheen, I. T., & Khan, R. (2022). Deep learning-based glaucoma detection with cropped optic cup and disc and blood vessel segmentation. *IEEE Access : Practical Innovations, Open Solutions*, *10*, 2828–2841. DOI: 10.1109/ACCESS.2021.3139160

Jain, V., & Mitra, A. (2025). Artificial intelligence and machine learning for sustainable development: Enhancing health, equity, and environmental sustainability. In *Machine and Deep Learning Solutions for Achieving the Sustainable Development Goals* (pp. 107–124). IGI Global Scientific Publishing.

Jiang, Y., Xu, J., & Wang, X. (2022). Machine learning for predicting occupational risks of healthcare workers during infectious disease outbreaks. *Journal of Biomedical Informatics*, *128*, 104048. DOI: 10.1016/j.jbi.2022.104048

Johansson, A., & Larsson, P. (2021). Smart acoustic monitoring for occupational safety in neonatal intensive care units: A Swedish case study. *Journal of Environmental Health Science & Engineering*, *19*(4), 425–433. DOI: 10.1007/s40201-021-00650-3

Johnson, C. T., & Hessels, A. J. (2023). Associations between negative patient safety climate and infection prevention practices. *American Journal of Infection Control*, *52*(9), 1102–1104. DOI: 10.1016/j.ajic.2024.06.010

Jo, J., Jo, B., Kim, J., Kim, S., & Han, W. (2020). Development of an IoT-based indoor air quality monitoring platform. *Journal of Sensors*, *2020*(1), 8749764.

Joseph, B., Ramesh, N., & Sreejith, N. (2021). Prevalence and risk factors of work-related musculoskeletal disorders among nurses in South India. *International Journal of Occupational Safety and Ergonomics*, *27*(4), 1036–1043. DOI: 10.1080/10803548.2019.1645309

Joshi, U., et al., (2022). *IoT-Reg: An ontology-driven knowledge graph for governance in healthcare IoT.* UMBC Ebiquity. https://ebiquity.umbc.edu/get/a/publication/1282.pdf

Kaiser Permanente. (2024). *Sustainable healthcare infrastructure report.* https://about.kaiserpermanente.org

Kajornkasirat, S., Sawangwong, C., Puangsuwan, K., Chanapai, N., Phutthamongkhon, W., & Puttinaovarat, S. (2025). Integrating AI-driven predictive analytics in wearable IoT for real-time health monitoring in smart healthcare systems. *Applied Sciences (Basel, Switzerland)*, *15*(8), 4400.

Kakhi, K., Jagatheesaperumal, S. K., Khosravi, A., Alizadehsani, R., & Acharya, U. R. (2024). Fatigue monitoring using wearables and AI: Trends, challenges, and future opportunities. *Sensors (Basel)*, *24*(1), 112. DOI: 10.3390/s24010112

Kamangar, Z. U., Memon, R. A., Murtaza Memon, G., & Kamangar, U. A. (2023). Integration of Internet of Things and blockchain technology in healthcare domain: A systematic literature review. *International Journal of Communication Systems*, *36*(16). Advance online publication. DOI: 10.1002/dac.5582

Kang, J., Cho, S., & Park, J. (2022). Global occupational safety standards in healthcare: A comparative review of OSHA and EU directives. *Safety Science*, *148*, 105653. DOI: 10.1016/j.ssci.2022.105653

Karliner, J., Slotterback, S., Boyd, R., Ashby, B., & Steele, K. (2019). *Health care's climate footprint: How the health sector contributes to the global climate crisis and opportunities for action*. Health Care Without Harm.

Karrouk, Y., Debasa, F., & Sanchez, L. M. F. (2025). The Digital Transformation of Smart Hospitals: Challenges and Opportunities. *Utilizing AI of Medical Things for Healthcare Security and Sustainability*, 1–54.

Karunanayake, N. (2025). Next-generation agentic AI for transforming healthcare. *Informatics and Health*, *2*(2), 73–83.

Katal, N. (2024). Ai-driven healthcare services and infrastructure in smart cities. In *Smart Cities* (pp. 150–170). CRC Press.

Kaur, I., Mishra, R., Narwaria, M., & Saxena, S. (2023). Opportunities and Applications of Blockchain for Empowering Tele-Healthcare. In Khan, R., & Kumar, I. (Eds.), *Advancements in Bio-Medical Image Processing and Authentication in Telemedicine* (pp. 111–126). IGI Global Scientific Publishing., DOI: 10.4018/978-1-6684-6957-6.ch007

Kelly, F. J., & Fussell, J. C. (2015). Air pollution and public health: Emerging hazards and improved understanding of risk. *Environmental Geochemistry and Health*, *37*(4), 631–649. DOI: 10.1007/s10653-015-9720-1

Khaled, A. E. (2022). Internet of medical things (iomt): Overview, taxonomies, and classifications. *Journal of Computer and Communications*, *10*(8), 64–89.

Khalid, S., Haq, N., Sabiha, Z.-A., Latif, A., Khan, M. A., Iqbal, J., & Yousaf, N. (2021). Current practices of waste management in teaching hospitals and presence of incinerators in densely populated areas. *BMC Public Health*, *21*(1), 1340. DOI: 10.1186/s12889-021-11389-1 PMID: 34233645

Klein, H., Bauer, F., & Richter, T. (2022). Artificial intelligence-based monitoring of radiation exposure in European hospitals: Advancing occupational safety. *European Journal of Radiology*, *149*, 110229. DOI: 10.1016/j.ejrad.2021.110229

Klemeš, J. J., Fan, Y. V., Tan, R. R., & Jiang, P. (2020). Minimising the present and future plastic waste, energy and environmental footprints related to COVID-19. *Renewable & Sustainable Energy Reviews*, *127*, 109883. PMID: 34234614

Knight, E., Yolou, I., Li, J., Kockan, C., Jensen, M., & Gerstein, M. (2024). *Homomorphic Encryption: An Application to Polygenic Risk Scores*. https://doi.org/DOI: 10.1101/2024.05.26.595961

Kravchenko, J., Akushevich, I., Abernethy, A. P., Holman, S., Ross, W. G.Jr, & Lyerly, H. K. (2014). Long-term dynamics of death rates of emphysema, asthma, and pneumonia and improving air quality. *International Journal of Chronic Obstructive Pulmonary Disease*, •••, 613–627.

Krittanawong, C., Johnson, K. W., Rosenson, R. S., Wang, Z., Aydar, M., & Narayan, S. M. (2020). Artificial intelligence in cardiology. *JACC. Basic to Translational Science*, *5*(9), 1082–1093. DOI: 10.1016/j.jacbts.2020.06.006

Kumar, A. A., Suryadevara, R., Sowmyya, T., & Chanal, G. B. (2025). Exploring the Intersection of AI, Healthcare, and Environmental Sustainability: Future Trends and Challenges. *Transforming Healthcare Sector Through Artificial Intelligence and Environmental Sustainability*, 23-47.

Kumar, A., Masud, M., Alsharif, M. H., Gaur, N., & Nanthaamornphong, A. (2025). Integrating 6G technology in smart hospitals: Challenges and opportunities for enhanced healthcare services. *Frontiers in Medicine*, *12*, 1534551. PMID: 40255587

Kumar, A., & Singh, R. (2024). Data protection and staff surveillance in Indian healthcare: Challenges of implementation. *Journal of Health Management*, *26*(1), 45–60. DOI: 10.1177/09720634241230215

Kumar, P., Tripathi, S., & Gupta, B. B. (2022). Privacy-enhancing technologies in IoT-enabled healthcare: A review. *IEEE Access : Practical Innovations, Open Solutions*, *10*, 65311–65332. DOI: 10.1109/ACCESS.2022.3180082

Kumar, R., & Sharma, A. (2023). Predictive workforce analytics for healthcare staff well-being: An Indian hospital perspective. *Indian Journal of Occupational and Environmental Medicine*, *27*(2), 85–92. DOI: 10.4103/ijoem.ijoem_154_23

Kumar, R., & Singh, L. (2022). AI-powered decision support systems for medical sustainability. *Health Informatics Journal*, *28*(3), 220–230.

La Nauze, A., Parker, S., & Taylor, L. (2022). A review and reframing of participatory urban dashboards. Urban Studies. (https://www.researchgate.net/publication/335142206_A_review_and_reframing_of_participatory_urban_dashboards)

Lakshmikanthcharan, S., Sivakumar, M. N., & Hisham, M. (2019). Stress and burnout among intensive care unit healthcare professionals in an Indian tertiary care hospital. *Indian Journal of Critical Care Medicine : Peer-Reviewed, Official Publication of Indian Society of Critical Care Medicine*, *23*(10), 462–466. DOI: 10.5005/jp-journals-10071-23311

Lamba, K., & Rani, S. (2023). *Machine learning based segmentation and classification algorithms for glaucoma detection.* In *Proceedings of the International Conference on Sustainable Computing and Smart Systems (ICSCSS)* (pp. 291–296). IEEE. DOI: 10.1109/ICSCSS57650.2023.10169226

Landrigan, P. J., Fuller, R., Acosta, N. J., Adeyi, O., Arnold, R., Baldé, A. B., Bertollini, R., Bose-O'Reilly, S., Boufford, J. I., & Breysse, P. N. (2018). The Lancet Commission on pollution and health. *Lancet*, *391*(10119), 462–512.

Lee, H., & Kim, J. (2022). IoT-enabled occupational safety monitoring for healthcare workers: A hospital-based study in South Korea. *International Journal of Environmental Research and Public Health*, *19*(22), 15012. DOI: 10.3390/ijerph192215012

Lenzen, M., Malik, A., Li, M., Fry, J., Weisz, H., Pichler, P.-P., Chaves, L. S. M., Capon, A., & Pencheon, D. (2020). The environmental footprint of health care: A global assessment. *The Lancet. Planetary Health*, *4*(7), e271–e279.

Li, J., Lai, Y., Li, W., Ren, J., Zhang, M., Kang, X., Wang, S., Li, P., Zhang, Y.-Q., Ma, W., & Associates. (2024). Agent hospital: A simulacrum of hospital with evolvable medical agents. *arXiv Preprint arXiv:2405.02957.*

Liang, H., Zhou, J., & Chen, Y. (2023). Wearable fatigue monitoring in hospitals: Impacts on staff well-being and organizational culture. *Journal of Nursing Management*, *31*(4), 785–795. DOI: 10.1111/jonm.13876

Li, J., Zhang, Y., & Wang, Q. (2022). Effectiveness of ergonomic interventions in reducing musculoskeletal disorders among hospital nurses: Evidence from a Chinese tertiary care hospital. *Journal of Advanced Nursing*, *78*(2), 712–721. DOI: 10.1111/jan.15022

Lin, N., Paul, R., Guerra, S., Liu, Y., Doulgeris, J., Shi, M., Lin, M., Engeberg, E. D., Hashemi, J., & Vrionis, F. D. (2024). The frontiers of smart healthcare systems. *Health Care*, *12*(23), 2330.

Lopez, M. J., García, J., & Ruiz, C. (2022). GDPR compliance in employee monitoring: Lessons for healthcare institutions. *Computer Law & Security Review*, *45*, 105657. DOI: 10.1016/j.clsr.2022.105657

Luo, Y. (2021). Artificial intelligence for wearable healthcare: Applications, challenges, and future perspectives. *IEEE Internet of Things Journal*, *8*(12), 9605–9621. DOI: 10.1109/JIOT.2021.3074881

Mahajan, S. (2022). Design and development of an open-source framework for citizen-centric environmental monitoring and data analysis. *Scientific Reports*, *12*(1), 14416. DOI: 10.1038/s41598-022-18700-z PMID: 36002580

Mahesh, G., & Mishra, R. (2024). Implementing a Secured Blockchain-Based EHR Management System With Remix IDE. In Mishra, R., Dwivedi, V., & Saxena, S. (Eds.), *Computational Convergence and Interoperability in Electronic Health Records (EHR)* (pp. 265–276). IGI Global Scientific Publishing., DOI: 10.4018/979-8-3693-3989-3.ch014

Maleki Varnosfaderani, S., & Forouzanfar, M. (2024). The role of AI in hospitals and clinics: Transforming healthcare in the 21st century. *Bioengineering (Basel, Switzerland)*, *11*(4), 337.

Malode, S. J., Alshehri, M. A., & Shetti, N. P. (2025). Revolutionizing human healthcare with wearable sensors for monitoring human strain. *Colloids and Surfaces. B, Biointerfaces*, *246*, 114384. DOI: 10.1016/j.colsurfb.2024.114384

Mao, Z., Liu, C., Li, Q., Cui, Y., & Zhou, F. (2023). Intelligent intensive care unit: Current and future trends. *Intensive Care Research*, *3*(2), 182–188.

Ma, Q.. (2025). Blockchain-assisted puncturable signcryption for cloud and fog-hosted industrial cyber-physical systems. *IEEE Network*.

Mattjus, C. (2020). *Indoor air quality in various healthcare facilities and potential solutions for improving air quality.: A scoping review.*

McBride, B., Carter, A., & Verma, R. (2021). Legal and ethical implications of wearable monitoring technologies in healthcare. *Health Policy and Technology, 10*(3), 100564. DOI: 10.1016/j.hlpt.2021.100564

McCrory, M., Williams, R., Patel, H., & Kim, J. (2025). Evaluating Avacopan in the treatment of ANCA-associated vasculitis. Clinical Therapeutics. (https://www.ncbi.nlm.nih.gov/pubmed/39803605)

McGain, F., & Naylor, C. (2014). Environmental sustainability in hospitals – a systematic review and research agenda. *Journal of Health Services Research & Policy, 19*(4), 245–252. DOI: 10.1177/1355819614534836 PMID: 24813186

Mehta, S. R. (2022). Smart hospitals: Enabling eco-friendly patient care through analytics. *IEEE Transactions on Healthcare Systems, 18*(2), 134–140.

Miehling, E., Ramamurthy, K. N., Varshney, K. R., Riemer, M., Bouneffouf, D., Richards, J. T., Dhurandhar, A., Daly, E. M., Hind, M., & Sattigeri, P. (2025). Agentic ai needs a systems theory. *arXiv Preprint arXiv:2503.00237.*

Minhas, S., Kotwal, A., & Singh, M. (2011). Infection control in health care facilities. *Medical Journal, Armed Forces India, 67*(1), 7–8. DOI: 10.1016/S0377-1237(11)80003-1

Minikumary, C. K., & Pillai, J. S. K. (2023). A study on occupational safety and health among workers at a tertiary care hospital in south India. *International Journal of Community Medicine and Public Health, 10*(1), 254–257. DOI: 10.18203/2394-6040.ijcmph20223553

Mishbahuddin, A. A., Fadli, Justicia, A. K., & Ernawati, K. (2021). Understanding islamic commandments to maintain people's health and environment: A critical review on literature. In *International Journal of Health Sciences* (Vol. 5, Issue 2, pp. 202–211). Universidad Tecnica de Manabi. https://doi.org/DOI: 10.29332/ijhs.v5n2.1427

Mishra, R., Kaur, I., Sahu, S., & Saxena, S. -Malsa, N; Narwaria, M;(2023) Establishing three layer architecture to improve interoperability in Medicare using smart and strategic API led integration,SoftwareX,Volume 22,2023,101376,ISSN 2352-7110, https://doi.org/DOI: 10.1016/j.softx.2023.101376

Mishra, R., & Das, K. (2024). Workplace hierarchy, digital surveillance, and employee well-being in Indian healthcare institutions. *Journal of Health Management, 26*(2), 167–182. DOI: 10.1177/09720634241234567

Mittal, P. (2019). A Survey on Internet of Things (IoT) Based Healthcare Monitoring System. *International Journal of Advanced Trends in Computer Science and Engineering*, *6*(4), 1646–1653. DOI: 10.30534/ijatcse/2019/90842019

Mohanram, S., V, B., G, M., & N, R. (2023). *Glaucoma detection using CNN ensemble classifier and OTSU threshold algorithm.* In Proceedings of the International Conference on Circuit Power and Computing Technologies (ICCPCT) (pp. 1219–1224). IEEE. DOI: 10.1109/ICCPCT58313.2023.10245827

Moldovan, F., Moldovan, L., & Bataga, T. (2023). The Environmental Sustainability Assessment of an Orthopedics Emergency Hospital Supported by a New Innovative Framework. *Sustainability*, *15*(18), 13402. DOI: 10.3390/su151813402

Mominkhan, D., Alamri, F. A., Balharith, M., Alharbi, M., Alshebli, A., Alshareef, S. Y., Khairaldain, A., Almutairi, N., Abusit, A., Almuzaini, Y., Alahmari, A. A., & Alabdulaali, M. K. (2023). The current state and potential evolution of carbon emissions in the healthcare sector: A narrative review article. *Frontiers in Sustainable Energy Policy*, *2*. Advance online publication. DOI: 10.3389/fsuep.2023.1230253

Montuori, P., Russo, I., De Rosa, E., Di Duca, F., De Simone, B., & Triassi, M. (2024). Air Monitoring in Operating Rooms: Results from a Comprehensive Study in the Campania Region. *Atmosphere*, *15*(7), 859.

Monye, S. N., Monye, S. I., Afolalu, S. A., Okokpujie, I. P., Adetunla, A. O., Ikumapayi, O. M., Aderemi, K. B., Nwankwo, S. O., & Okpako, E. A. (2024). A Conceptual Framework for the Adoption of IoT in the Energy Sector: Technology-Organization-Environment Framework Approach. *2024 International Conference on Science, Engineering and Business for Driving Sustainable Development Goals (SEB4SDG)*, 1–6. https://doi.org/DOI: 10.1109/SEB4SDG60871.2024.10629924

Moon, J., & Ju, B.-K. (2024). Wearable sensors for healthcare of industrial workers: A scoping review. *Electronics (Basel)*, *13*(19), 3849. DOI: 10.3390/electronics13193849

Moritz, M., Topol, E., & Rajpurkar, P. (2025). Coordinated AI agents for advancing healthcare. *Nature Biomedical Engineering*, •••, 1–7.

Mundnich, K., Booth, B. M., L'Hommedieu, M., Girault, B., Lerman, K., & Narayanan, S. (2020). TILES-2018: A longitudinal multimodal dataset of hospital staff for modeling behavioral and physiological factors. *Nature Scientific Data*, *7*(354), 1–14. DOI: 10.1038/s41597-020-00676-y

Nabha, R., Laouiti, A., & Samhat, A. E. (2025). Internet of Things-based healthcare systems: An overview of privacy-preserving mechanisms. *Applied Sciences (Basel, Switzerland)*, *15*(7), 3629. https://www.mdpi.com/2076-3417/15/7/3629

Naga Rani Bandaru, V., Gayatri Sarman Kaligotla, V. S. H., Dhana Satya Prathap Varma, U., Prasadaraju, K., & Sugumaran, S. (2024). A Enhancing Data Security Solutions for Smart Energy Systems in IoT-Enabled Cloud Computing Environments through Lightweight Cryptographic Techniques. *IOP Conference Series. Earth and Environmental Science*, *1375*(1), 012003. DOI: 10.1088/1755-1315/1375/1/012003

Nguyen, M. T., & Morris, J. A. (2021). Digital transformation for sustainable health care. *International Journal of Healthcare Technology and Management*, *21*(3), 215–229.

Nguyen, T. P., Pham, D. T., & Tran, Q. L. (2025). Non-invasive fatigue detection and human–machine interaction using LSTM and multimodal AI: A case study. *Multimodal Technologies and Interaction*, *9*(6), 63. DOI: 10.3390/mti9060063

Nižetić, S., & Šolić, P., López-de-Ipiña González-de-Artaza, D., & Patrono, L. (2020). Internet of Things (IoT): Opportunities, issues and challenges towards a smart and sustainable future. *Journal of Cleaner Production*, *274*, 122877. DOI: 10.1016/j.jclepro.2020.122877 PMID: 32834567

Noaman, M., Khan, M. S., Abrar, M. F., Ali, S., Alvi, A., & Saleem, M. A. (2022). Challenges in integration of heterogeneous internet of things. *Scientific Programming*, *2022*(1), 8626882.

Nurmalia, D., & Khoirinnissa, N. (2021). Persepsi Perawat Tentang Integrasi Perangkat Berbasis Teknologi Internet of Things (IoT) Dalam Pelayanan Kesehatan Di Rumah Sakit. *Jurnal Kepemimpinan Dan Manajemen Keperawatan*, *4*(2), 199–206. DOI: 10.32584/jkmk.v4i2.1074

NVIDIA and GE HealthCare Collaborate to Advance the Development of Autonomous Diagnostic Imaging With Physical AI. (n.d.). NVIDIA Newsroom. Retrieved August 9, 2025, from https://nvidianews.nvidia.com/news/nvidia-and-ge-healthcare-collaborate-to-advance-the-development-of-autonomous-diagnostic-imaging-with-physical-ai

Nwokedi, T. V. (2025). A Conceptual Framework for AI-Driven Healthcare Optimization and Predictive Analytics. *Multidisciplinary Journal of Engineering. Technology and Sciences*, *2*, 1–22.

O'Donnell, J., & Crownhart, C. (2025, May). We did the math on AI's energy footprint. Here's the story you haven't heard. *MIT Technology Review*.

O'Sullivan-Dale, U. (2024, May 30). *'World's first' AI hospital with virtual doctors opens in China*. https://www.roboticsandautomationmagazine.co.uk/news/healthcare/worlds-first-ai-hospital-with-virtual-doctors-opens-in-china.html

Obubu, M., Chuku, N., Ananaba, A., Sadiq, F. U. S., Sambo, E., Kolade, O., Oyekanmi, T., Olaosebikan, K., & Serrano, O. (2023). Lagos State Hospital Waste Management Practices: A Descriptive Overview with Stakeholders' Role and Key Recommendations. *Journal of Environmental Protection, 14*(02), 108–125. DOI: 10.4236/jep.2023.142008

Occupational Hazards among Healthcare Workers in Africa: A Systematic Review. (2018). *Annals of Global Health, 84*(3), 367–384. https://doi.org/DOI: 10.5334/aogh.2434

Okafor, N., Ingle, R., Saunders, M., & Delaney, D. (2024). *Assessing and Improving the Quality of IoT Sensor Data in Environmental Monitoring Networks: A Focus on Peatlands*. https://doi.org/DOI: 10.36227/techrxiv.170905846.67456956/v1

Okello, D., Namusoke, J., & Mwesige, C. (2023). Sustainable safety monitoring in East African hospitals: Solar-powered IoT innovations for healthcare staff. *International Journal of Environmental Research and Public Health, 20*(2), 1125. DOI: 10.3390/ijerph20021125

Olawade, D. B., Wada, O. Z., David-Olawade, A. C., Fapohunda, O., Ige, A. O., & Ling, J. (2024). Artificial intelligence potential for net zero sustainability: Current evidence and prospects. *Next Sustainability, 4*, 100041.

Olawade, D. B., Wada, O. Z., Ige, A. O., Egbewole, B. I., Olojo, A., & Oladapo, B. I. (2024). Artificial intelligence in environmental monitoring: Advancements, challenges, and future directions. *Hygiene and Environmental Health Advances, 12*, 100114.

Omidvarborna, H., Kumar, P., Hayward, J., Gupta, M., & Nascimento, E. G. S. (2021). Low-cost air quality sensing towards smart homes. *Atmosphere, 12*(4), 453.

Ozcelik, M. M., Kok, I., & Ozdemir, S. (2025). A Survey on Internet of Medical Things (IoMT): Enabling Technologies, Security and Explainability Issues, Challenges, and Future Directions. *Expert Systems: International Journal of Knowledge Engineering and Neural Networks, 42*(5), e70010.

Pajouh, H. H.. (n.d.). A two-layer dimension reduction and two-tier classification model for anomaly-based intrusion detection in IoT backbone networks. *IEEE Transactions on Emerging Topics in Computing*.

Pal, S., Hitchens, M., Varadharajan, V., & Rabehaja, T. (2018). Fine-Grained Access Control for Smart Healthcare Systems in the Internet of Things. *EAI Endorsed Transactions on Industrial Networks and Intelligent Systems, 4*(13), 154370. DOI: 10.4108/eai.20-3-2018.154370

Panta, G., Richardson, A. K., Shaw, I. C., & Coope, P. A. (2020). Compliance of primary and secondary care public hospitals with standard practices for reprocessing and steam sterilization of reusable medical devices in Nepal: Findings from nation-wide multicenter clustered audits. *BMC Health Services Research*, *20*(1), 923. DOI: 10.1186/s12913-020-05788-0 PMID: 33028325

Pariso, P., Picariello, M., & Marino, A. (2025). AI integration in energy management: Enhancing efficiency in Italian hospitals. *Health Economics Review*, *15*(1), 1–10. PMID: 40388050

Parkavi, A., Sowmya, B. J., Alex, S. A., Supreeth, S., Shruthi, G., Rohith, S., Chatterjee, S., & Lingaraj, K. (2025). *Air quality and dust level monitoring systems in hospitals using IoT*. Discover Internet of Things., DOI: 10.1007/s43926-025-00120-w

Parker, S., Brown, J., Taylor, K., & Smith, D. (2024). Clinical and economic impact of digital dashboards on health service quality. *Journal of Medical Internet Research*, *26*, e12296400. DOI: 10.2196/12296400

Park, Y. M., Sousan, S., Streuber, D., & Zhao, K. (2021). GeoAir—A Novel Portable, GPS-Enabled, Low-Cost Air-Pollution Sensor: Design Strategies to Facilitate Citizen Science Research and Geospatial Assessments of Personal Exposure. *Sensors (Basel)*, *21*(11), 3761. DOI: 10.3390/s21113761 PMID: 34071590

Patel, K., & Banerjee, A. (2022). Waste management in healthcare using AI. *Journal of Cleaner Production*, *312*, 127732.

Patel, S., Sharma, D., & Menon, R. (2023). Mobile technology and wearable monitors for occupational health surveillance in Indian healthcare. *Journal of Occupational Health*, *65*(1), e12378. DOI: 10.1002/1348-9585.12378

Patel, S., & Verma, D. (2024). Towards holistic workforce safety in healthcare: Policies and practices for sustainable systems. *Journal of Health Policy and Management*, *13*(1), 45–57. DOI: 10.34172/jhpm.2024.06

Patil, K. H., Tawar, N. S., & Kudale, A. M. (2024). A post-COVID-19 assessment of resilience of nurses and paramedical workers in municipal hospitals of urban Pune, India. *Journal of Family Medicine and Primary Care*, *13*(4), 1460–1466. DOI: 10.4103/jfmpc.jfmpc_947_23

Peng, J., Wu, X., Wang, R., Li, C., Zhang, Q., & Wei, D. (2020). Medical waste management practice during the 2019-2020 novel coronavirus pandemic: Experience in a general hospital. *American Journal of Infection Control*, *48*(8), 918–921. DOI: 10.1016/j.ajic.2020.05.035 PMID: 32504761

Pereira, L., Radovic, T., & Haykal, K. A. (2021). Peer support programs in the fields of medicine and nursing: A systematic search and narrative review. *Canadian Medical Education Journal, 12*(3), 113–125. DOI: 10.36834/cmej.71129

Pereira, R., Adams, J., & White, L. (2022). IoT-based air quality monitoring for occupational safety in US hospitals: A case study. *Journal of Occupational and Environmental Hygiene, 19*(6), 289–298. DOI: 10.1080/15459624.2022.2049364

Pichler, P.-P., Jaccard, I. S., Weisz, U., & Weisz, H. (2019). International comparison of health care carbon footprints. *Environmental Research Letters, 14*(6), 064004.

Pradeep, M., Kumari, S., Tyagi, A. K., & Tiwari, S. (2024). Smart Hospital in Smart Cities. *Digital Twin and Blockchain for Smart Cities*, 579-603.

Qadri, Y. A., Nauman, A., Zikria, Y. B., Vasilakos, A. V., & Kim, S. W. (2020). The future of healthcare internet of things: A survey of emerging technologies. *IEEE Communications Surveys and Tutorials, 22*(2), 1121–1167.

Qi, Y. (2025). A conceptual framework for developing dashboards for big data applications. *Cartography and Geographic Information Science, 52*(1), 1–15. DOI: 10.1080/15230406.2023.2190164

Rajan, D., & Thomas, P. (2023). Artificial intelligence and staff scheduling: Reducing burnout risk in Indian healthcare systems. *Journal of Health Management, 25*(3), 321–333. DOI: 10.1177/09720634231102587

Rajesh, K., & Menon, V. (2022). Digital exposure monitoring for frontline workers in Indian healthcare settings: Lessons from COVID-19. *Journal of Health Research, 36*(4), 642–650. DOI: 10.1108/JHR-08-2021-0456

Rajesh, M., & Nambiar, S. (2022). Nurses under watch: Perceptions of monitoring technologies in Indian hospitals. *International Journal of Healthcare Management, 15*(3), 189–197. DOI: 10.1080/20479700.2021.1998754

Rajkumar, S., & Menon, V. (2023). Scalable environmental monitoring for healthcare staff safety: Insights from Indian tertiary hospitals. *Indian Journal of Public Health Research & Development, 14*(1), 56–63. DOI: 10.37506/ijphrd.v14i1.18491

Rajput, Y., Tarif, T., Wolfe, A., Dawson, E., & Fox, K. (2024). AI in Point-of-Care-A Sustainable Healthcare Revolution at the Edge. In *Biocomputing 2025: Proceedings of the Pacific Symposium* (pp. 734-747).

Ramaswamy, P., Sahu, A., & Krishnan, R. (2023). AI-enabled workforce scheduling for improving occupational safety of healthcare staff in Indian tertiary hospitals. *Indian Journal of Occupational and Environmental Medicine*, *27*(3), 175–183. DOI: 10.4103/ijoem.ijoem_126_23

Ramesh, V., & Rao, P. (2023). Sustainable hospital design in India: Implications for staff safety and environmental health. *Indian Journal of Occupational and Environmental Medicine*, *27*(3), 145–153. DOI: 10.4103/ijoem.ijoem_182_23

Rangarajan, D., Rangarajan, A., Reddy, C. K. K., & Doss, S. (2025). Exploring the Next-Gen Transformations in Healthcare Through the Impact of AI and IoT. In *Intelligent Systems and IoT Applications in Clinical Health* (pp. 73–98). IGI Global.

Rao, M., & Kumar, A. (2021). Well-being of healthcare workers and its impact on patient care in India: A review. *Journal of Health Management*, *23*(2), 317–329. DOI: 10.1177/0972063421994945

Rao, P., & Iyer, B. (2022). AI-enhanced inventory optimization for healthcare sustainability. *Expert Systems with Applications*, *208*, 118108.

Rathi, N., & Gupta, R. (2023). Evaluating NABH standards for occupational safety in Indian hospitals: Compliance and challenges. *Journal of Health Management*, *25*(3), 345–359. DOI: 10.1177/09720634231120245

Rath, K. C., Khang, A., Rath, S. K., Satapathy, N., Satapathy, S. K., & Kar, S. (2024). Artificial intelligence (AI)-enabled technology in medicine-advancing holistic healthcare monitoring and control systems. In *Computer Vision and AI-Integrated IoT Technologies in the Medical Ecosystem* (pp. 87–108). CRC Press.

Rattal, S., Badri, A., Moughit, M., Ar-Reyouchi, E. M., & Ghoumid, K. (2025). AI-Driven Optimization of Low-Energy IoT Protocols for Scalable and Efficient Smart Healthcare Systems. *IEEE Access : Practical Innovations, Open Solutions*.

Rehman, A.. (2022, September). A secure healthcare 5.0 system based on blockchain technology entangled with federated learning technique [Preprint]. arXiv. https://arxiv.org/abs/2209.09642

Riedl, C., & De Cremer, D. (2025). AI for collective intelligence. *Collective Intelligence*, *4*(2), 26339137251328909.

Rocha, A., Monteiro, M., Mattos, C., Dias, M., Soares, J., Magalhaes, R., & Macedo, J. (2024). Edge AI for Internet of Medical Things: A literature review. *Computers & Electrical Engineering*, *116*, 109202.

Russell, S. J., & Norvig, P. (2021). *Artificial Intelligence: A Modern Approach* (Global Edition 4e).

Russell, S., Norvig, P., & Intelligence, A. (1995). A modern approach. *Artificial Intelligence. Prentice-Hall. Egnlewood Cliffs*, *25*(27), 79–80.

Ryan, S. M., & Nielsen, C. J. (2010). Global warming potential of inhaled anesthetics: Application to clinical use. *Anesthesia and Analgesia*, *111*(1), 92–98. PMID: 20519425

Salahuddin, M. A., Al-Fuqaha, A., & Guizani, M. (2018, May). Softwarization of Internet of Things infrastructure for secure and smart healthcare [Preprint]. arXiv. https://arxiv.org/abs/1805.11011

Salman, O., & Ahmad, I. (2023). Security and privacy in IoT-based healthcare systems: A review. *ResearchGate*. https://www.researchgate.net/publication/369913866

Santhosh, S., & Babu, D. V. (2023, February). Retinal Glaucoma Detection from Digital Fundus Images using Deep Learning Approach. In 2023 7th International Conference on Computing Methodologies and Communication (ICCMC) (pp. 68-72). IEEE.

Sapkota, R., Roumeliotis, K. I., & Karkee, M. (2025). Ai agents vs. Agentic ai: A conceptual taxonomy, applications and challenges. *arXiv Preprint arXiv:2505.10468*.

Saraswat, P. P., & Tiwari, R. R.. (2021). Hospital-acquired infection awareness and control practices among healthcare staff: An evaluation. *British Journal of Health Care Management*, *27*(11), 296–302. DOI: 10.12968/bjhc.2020.0037

Sarker, H., Hossain, M., & Choudhury, T., & al. (2022). A field trial of a smartphone-based sensing platform for understanding clinician stress in a hospital setting. *Scientific Data*, *9*, 332. DOI: 10.1038/s41597-022-01361-y

Sarnat, J. A., & Holguin, F. (2007). Asthma and air quality. *Current Opinion in Pulmonary Medicine*, *13*(1), 63–66.

Sathyamoorthy, S., Matthew, U. O., Adekunle, T. S., & Okafor, N. U. (2024). Advances and Challenges in IoT Sensors Data Handling and Processing in Environmental Monitoring Networks. *HAFED POLY Journal of Science. Management and Technology*, *5*(2), 40–60. DOI: 10.4314/hpjsmt.v5i2.3

Schoierer, J., Dorman, L., & Havenith, G. (2023). Effects of heat and personal protective equipment on thermal strain in healthcare workers: Part B—application of wearable sensors to observe heat strain among healthcare workers under controlled conditions. *International Archives of Occupational and Environmental Health.* Advance online publication. DOI: 10.1007/s00420-023-02022-2

Sehulster, L., Chinn, R. Y., Arduino, M. J., Carpenter, J., Donlan, R., Ashford, D., Besser, R., Fields, B., McNeil, M. M., & Whitney, C. (2003). Guidelines for environmental infection control in health-care facilities. *Morbidity and Mortality Weekly Report Recommendations and Reports RR, 52*(10).

Senbekov, M., Saliev, T., Bukeyeva, Z., Almabayeva, A., Zhanaliyeva, M., Aitenova, N., Toishibekov, Y., & Fakhradiyev, I. (2020). The Recent Progress and Applications of Digital Technologies in Healthcare: A Review. *International Journal of Telemedicine and Applications, 2020*, 1–18. DOI: 10.1155/2020/8830200 PMID: 33343657

Senthil, A., Anandh, B., Jayachandran, P., Thangavel, G., Josephin, D., & Kalpana, B. (2015). Perception and prevalence of work-related health hazards among health carc workers in public health facilities in southern India. *International Journal of Occupational and Environmental Health, 21*(1), 74–81. DOI: 10.1179/2049396714Y.0000000096

Senturk, S., Kok, I., & Senturk, F. (2022). Internet of nano, bio-nano, biodegradable and ingestible things: A survey. *arXiv Preprint arXiv:2202.12409.*

Serranheira, F., Sousa-Uva, M., & Sousa-Uva, A. (2020). Hospital nurses' working conditions in relation to musculoskeletal disorders: A systematic review. *Applied Ergonomics, 87*, 103114. DOI: 10.1016/j.apergo.2020.103114

Shah, A., & Ho, S. (2024). Developing public health surveillance dashboards. *Public Health, 235*, 152–160. DOI: 10.1016/j.puhe.2023.09.010

Sharma, M. Samriti, & Singh, G. (2019). Need and design of smart and secure energy-efficient IoT-based healthcare framework. In *Energy Conservation for IoT Devices: Concepts, Paradigms and Solutions* (pp. 259–281). Springer.

Sharma, D., & Cotton, M. (2023). Overcoming the barriers between resource constraints and healthcare quality. [). SAGE Publications Sage UK: London, England.]. *Tropical Doctor, 53*(3), 341–343.

Sharma, P., Ghosh, A., Bose, S., & Sen, A. (2024). *Semi-automated glaucoma prediction based on retinal blood vessel detection and cup-to-disc ratio.* In *Proceedings of the IEEE International Conference on Interdisciplinary Approaches in Technology and Management for Social Innovation (IATMSI)* (pp. 1–6). IEEE. DOI: 10.1109/IATMSI60426.2024.10502876

Sharma, P., & Kaur, G. (2022). Addressing burnout among nurses in Indian tertiary care hospitals: A case-based intervention study. *Indian Journal of Occupational and Environmental Medicine*, *26*(3), 174–181. DOI: 10.4103/ijoem.ijoem_189_22

Sharma, P., Moparthi, N. R., Namasudra, S., Shanmuganathan, V., & Hsu, C. (2022). Blockchain-based iot architecture to secure healthcare system using identity-based encryption. *Expert Systems: International Journal of Knowledge Engineering and Neural Networks*, *39*(10). Advance online publication. DOI: 10.1111/exsy.12915

Sharma, S., Khandelwal, V., & Mishra, G. (2019). Video surveillance of hand hygiene: A better tool for monitoring and ensuring hand hygiene adherence. *Indian Journal of Critical Care Medicine : Peer-Reviewed, Official Publication of Indian Society of Critical Care Medicine*, *23*(5), 224–226. DOI: 10.5005/jp-journals-10071-23165

Sharma, T.. (2023). Optimizing HVAC performance using AI in hospitals. *Sustainable Cities and Society*, *86*, 104029.

Shaw, S. K., & Dey, J. L. (2023). Emergence of IoT in Healthcare Industry: Towards Sustainable Digital Health Systems. In *Advances in Business Informatics empowered by AI & Intelligent Systems* (pp. 108–125). CSMFL Publications., DOI: 10.46679/978819573220308

Shukla, P., & Menon, S. (2022). Ethical implications of digital surveillance in Indian hospitals. *Indian Journal of Medical Ethics*, *7*(2), 93–99. DOI: 10.20529/IJME.2022.024

Simms, L., Ottman, K. E., Griffith, J. L., Knight, M. G., Norris, L., Karakcheyeva, V., & Kohrt, B. A. (2023). Psychosocial peer support to address mental health and burnout of health care workers affected by COVID-19: A qualitative evaluation. *International Journal of Environmental Research and Public Health*, *20*(5), 4536. DOI: 10.3390/ijerph20054536

Singh, D. P. (2025, April 3). Agentic AI: A Catalyst for Achieving Sustainability Goals. *Daily Host News*. https://www.dailyhostnews.com/agentic-ai-a-catalyst-for-achieving-sustainability-goals

Singh, R., Mehta, K., & Sharma, P. (2024). IoT-based real-time staff and patient tracking for enhancing hospital safety and efficiency. *Sensors (Basel)*, *24*(1), 2020. DOI: 10.3390/s24012020

Singh, R., & Menon, S. (2023). Collaborative frameworks for healthcare workforce safety: An Indian perspective. *Journal of Occupational Health*, *65*(2), e12345. DOI: 10.1002/1348-9585.12345

Sinha, T., & Raj, A. (2024). Staff monitoring, data protection, and legal gaps in Indian healthcare: An analysis of evolving frameworks. *Journal of Health Law and Policy*, *6*(1), 25–39. DOI: 10.1177/23992026241234567

Sivakumar, R., Singh, N., Kumar, C. J., & Prasath, N. (2023). *Blood vessel segmentation for retinal fundus disease detection*. In *Proceedings of the International Conference on Computer Communication and Informatics (ICCCI)* (pp. 1–9). IEEE. DOI: 10.1109/ICCCI56745.2023.10128290

Song, H., Srinivasan, K., Sookoor, T., & Jeschke, S. (2015). Security of the Internet of Things: Vulnerabilities, attacks, and countermeasures. *IEEE Communications Surveys and Tutorials*, *17*(2), 982–1004. DOI: 10.1109/COMST.2014.2365950

Soni, T., Gupta, S., & Kumar, K. S. (2025). *Exploring retinal vessel segmentation: Deep learning models and their applications*. In *Proceedings of the 3rd International Conference on Advancement in Computation & Computer Technologies (InCACCT)* (pp. 715–719). IEEE. DOI: 10.1109/InCACCT65424.2025.11011437

Sorouri, S., Ahmari Tehran, H., Parhoon, M., & Saeidi, M. (2025). Air Pollution in Hospitals: A Critical Public Health Emergency and Strategies for Improving Indoor Air Quality and Patient Safety. *Health Providers*, *5*(1), 15–34.

Sowmiya, R., & Kalpana, R. (2023). *Detection of diabetic retinopathy by segmentation using U-Net with hyper-parameter tuning*. In *Proceedings of the 2nd International Conference on Smart Technologies and Systems for Next Generation Computing (ICSTSN)* (pp. 1–5). IEEE. DOI: 10.1109/ICSTSN57873.2023.10151473

Springer. (2025). Machine learning-driven framework for real-time air quality monitoring. Scientific Reports, 15, 14214. https://doi.org/)DOI: 10.1038/s41598-025-14214-6

Sreejith, S., Panigrahy, A. K., Ajayan, J., Radhika, J. M., Reddy, N. V. R., Reddy, N. V. U., & Umamaheswaran, S. (2025). IoT sensor-based systems in real-time monitoring of health and environment: A review. *Journal of the Korean Physical Society*, *87*(1), 1–27. DOI: 10.1007/s40042-025-01378-7

Sridhar, H., & Kumar, J. R. H. (2022). *Segmentation of blood vessels by local analysis of 2D image patches*. In *Proceedings of the IEEE 19th India Council International Conference (INDICON)* (pp. 1–5). IEEE. DOI: 10.1109/INDICON56171.2022.10039792

Stergiou, C. L., Psannis, K. E., & Gupta, B. B. (2021, December). Blockchain-assisted secure fine-grained searchable encryption for a cloud-based healthcare cyber-physical system. *IEEE/CAA Journal of Automatica Sinica*. https://www.ieee-jas.net/article/doi/10.1109/JAS.2021.1004003

Sudarvizhi, T., Chandran, A. A., Gowtham, L., & Poomainthan, M. (2025). Smart Air Quality Monitoring With Model Context Protocol for Environmental Safety Technology. *2025 3rd International Conference on Inventive Computing and Informatics (ICICI)*, 01–07. https://doi.org/DOI: 10.1109/ICICI65870.2025.11069802

Suherman, R., Nataraja, P. K., Pratama, A., & Kahfi, A. H. (2023). Electricity management system with technology internet of things. *Jurnal Techno Nusa Mandiri*, *20*(2), 95–101. DOI: 10.33480/techno.v20i2.4520

Sulosaari, V., Unal, E., & Cinar, F. I. (2022). The effectiveness of mindfulness-based interventions on the psychological well-being of nurses: A systematic review. *Applied Nursing Research*, *64*, 151565. DOI: 10.1016/j.apnr.2022.151565

Sunarno, S., Purwanto, P., & Suryono, S. (2020). The Monitoring System of Sulfur Dioxide Gas Using a Web-based Wireless Sensor. *Proceedings of the Proceedings of the 13th International Interdisciplinary Studies Seminar, IISS 2019*, 30-31 October 2019, Malang, Indonesia. https://doi.org/DOI: 10.4108/eai.23-10-2019.2293039

Sun, D., & Gao, Y. (2022). Real-time water usage monitoring in hospitals. *Environmental Monitoring and Assessment*, *194*(2), 1–12.

Sunyer, J., Jarvis, D., Gotschi, T., Garcia-Esteban, R., Jacquemin, B., Aguilera, I., Ackerman, U., de Marco, R., Forsberg, B., & Gislason, T. (2006). Chronic bronchitis and urban air pollution in an international study. *Occupational and Environmental Medicine*, *63*(12), 836–843.

Surendiran, J., & Meena, M. (2022). *Classification of glaucoma using K-mean clustering with optic disk and cup segmentation*. In *Proceedings of the International Conference on Recent Trends in Microelectronics, Automation, Computing and Communications Systems (ICMACC)* (pp. 97–102). IEEE. DOI: 10.1109/ICMACC54824.2022.10093284

Suresh Babu, C. V., & Auroshaa, A. (2024). Influence of Data Analysis Tools in Teaching and Learning Economics. In Scott, B., & Fox, M. E. (Eds.), *Cases on Economics Education and Tools for Educators* (pp. 229–248). IGI Global., DOI: 10.4018/978-1-6684-7583-6.ch010

Suresh Babu, C. V., Vinayagamoorthy, S., & Muthumanikavel, V. (2023). Impact of Business Analytics Tools in Statistical Arbitrage Models in Trading. In Gharoie Ahangar, R., & Napier, M. (Eds.), *Advancement in Business Analytics Tools for Higher Financial Performance* (pp. 260–270). IGI Global., DOI: 10.4018/978-1-6684-8386-2.ch013

Tabbakh, A., Al Amin, L., Islam, M., Mahmud, G. I., Chowdhury, I. K., & Mukta, M. S. H. (2024). Towards sustainable AI: A comprehensive framework for Green AI. *Discover Sustainability*, *5*(1), 408.

Tan, L., Singi, A., & Cross, A. (2025). AI-Driven Innovation For A Sustainable Future: Transforming Healthcare. *Metallurgical and Materials Engineering*, 1432–1439.

Tang, M. C. S., Teoh, S. S., & Ibrahim, H. (2022). *Retinal vessel segmentation from fundus images using DeepLabv3+*. In Proceedings of the 18th IEEE International Colloquium on Signal Processing & Applications (CSPA) (pp. 377–381). IEEE. DOI: 10.1109/CSPA55076.2022.9781891

Tan, L. A., Rodriguez, J., Lee, H., & Patel, V. (2024). Development and utility of an interactive online dashboard for monitoring adolescent health survey data. *Journal of Public Health Management and Practice*, *30*(4), 19–22. DOI: 10.1097/PHH.0000000000002045 PMID: 38870377

Tantum, L. K., Mahamane, E., Bauza, V., Mahamadou, K. O. B., Sanoussi, E. Y., Salzberg, A., & Anderson, D. M. (2024). Environmental Infrastructure Maintenance Bottlenecks in Healthcare Facilities and Coping Strategies Among Healthcare Workers in Niger. *Environmental Health Insights*, *18*. Advance online publication. DOI: 10.1177/11786302241271554 PMID: 39148586

Tanveer, S., Ahmad, M. I., & Khan, T. (2024). Technological progression associated with monitoring and management of indoor air pollution and associated health risks: A comprehensive review. *Environmental Quality Management*, *34*(1), e22236.

Tariq, M. U. (2025). Integrating Advanced Technologies for Multi-Stakeholder Collaboration: Driving Sustainability in Supply Chains Through Industry 4.0. In Frichi, Y., & Jawab, F. (Eds.), *Multi-Stakeholder Collaboration for Sustainable Supply Chain* (pp. 313–334). IGI Global Scientific Publishing., DOI: 10.4018/979-8-3693-8925-6.ch014

Tariq, M. U. (2025). Machine Learning Techniques for Personalized Rehabilitation: Enhancing Patient Outcomes Through Predictive Algorithms. In Korupalli, V., Ranasinghe, P., & Feldman, D. (Eds.), *Predictive Algorithms for Rehabilitation and Assistive Systems* (pp. 221–252). IGI Global Scientific Publishing., DOI: 10.4018/979-8-3373-0194-5.ch009

Tariq, M. U. (2025). Strategic Place Marketing in Cross-Border Regions: Enhancing Territorial Cooperation and Economic Growth. In Sousa, B. (Ed.), *Cross-Border Regions Cooperation and Implications for Organizations* (pp. 107–136). IGI Global Scientific Publishing., DOI: 10.4018/979-8-3373-1912-4.ch004

Tariq, M. U. (2025). The Challenge of Artificial Intelligence in Environmental Sustainability: Opportunities, Risks, and Policy Implications. In Ahmadi, A., & Mna, A. (Eds.), *Nexus of Environmental Quality and Technology Innovation* (pp. 267–292). IGI Global Scientific Publishing., DOI: 10.4018/979-8-3373-1822-6.ch012

Tech CEOs: Grab the Competitive Advantage with Agentic AI | Gartner Webinars. (n.d.). Gartner. Retrieved July 28, 2025, from https://www.gartner.com/en/webinar/721397/1619143

Tenepalli, D., & T M, N. (2024). A Systematic Review on IoT and Machine Learning Algorithms in E-Healthcare. *International Journal of Computing and Digital Systems*, *15*(1), 279–294. DOI: 10.12785/ijcds/160122

Thazha, S. K., & Cruz, J. P.. (2022). Infection prevention and control awareness, attitudes, and practices among healthcare professionals in South India. *BMC Health Services Research*, *22*(1), 272. DOI: 10.1186/s12913-022-07673-4

Topol, E. (2018). *Deep Medicine*. https://www.hachettebookgroup.com/titles/eric-topol/deep-medicine/9781541644649/?lens=basic-books

Tsang, T. W., Wong, L. T., & Mui, K. W. (2024). Experimental studies on airborne transmission in hospitals: A systematic review. *Indoor and Built Environment*, *33*(4), 608–640.

Tseng, C.-J., & Lin, S.-Y. (2024). Role of artificial intelligence in carbon cost reduction of firms. *Journal of Cleaner Production*, *447*, 141413.

Tundjungsari, V., Ernawati, K., & Mutia, N. (2020). *Public Health Surveillance to Promote Clean and Healthy Life Behaviours Using Big Data Approach (An Indonesian Case Study)*. Springer., DOI: 10.1007/978-3-030-23162-0_69

Turner, S. (2021). The Role of Iot In Smart Healthcare Facilities: Improving Operational Efficiency. *American Journal Of Internet Of Things*, *2*(5), 1–7.

U.S. EIA. (2022). *Commercial Buildings Energy Consumption Survey (CBECS)*. U.S. Energy Information Administration.

Udendhran, R., Sasikala, R., Nishanthi, R., & Vasanthi, J. (2023). Smart Energy Consumption Control in Commercial Buildings Using Machine Learning and IOT. *E3S Web of Conferences, 387*, 02003. https://doi.org/DOI: 10.1051/e3sconf/202338702003

Ueda, D., Walston, S. L., Fujita, S., Fushimi, Y., Tsuboyama, T., Kamagata, K., & Naganawa, S. (2024). Climate change and artificial intelligence in healthcare: Review and recommendations towards a sustainable future. *Diagnostic and Interventional Imaging*. PMID: 38918123

Ulrich, R., Zimring, C., & Quan, X. (2022). The impact of healthcare design on staff well-being: A review of evidence. *Health Environments Research & Design Journal, 15*(4), 75–92. DOI: 10.1177/19375867221103256

van Dijk, J., Meijer, A., & Schmidt, K. (2022). Embedding IoT-based monitoring systems for staff safety in European hospitals. *Safety Science, 153*, 105792. DOI: 10.1016/j.ssci.2022.105792

van Wynsberghe, A. (2021). Sustainable AI: AI for sustainability and the sustainability of AI. *AI and Ethics, 1*(3), 213–218. DOI: 10.1007/s43681-021-00043-6

Velicka, J., Pies, M., Hajovsky, R., Barnova, K., & Martinek, R. (2025). Smart oxygen monitoring in hospitals: A pilot study during COVID-19. *Scientific Reports*. Advance online publication. DOI: 10.1038/s41598-025-87665-6

Verdejo Espinosa, Á., Lopez Ruiz, J. L., Mata Mata, F., & Estevez, M. E. (2021). Application of IoT in Healthcare: Keys to Implementation of the Sustainable Development Goals. *Sensors (Basel), 21*(7), 2330. DOI: 10.3390/s21072330 PMID: 33810606

Verma, A., Saleem, A. M., Ranadive, J. P., Chouhan, A. P. S., & Singh, V. (2024). Artificial Intelligence in Smart Healthcare. In *IoT, Machine Learning and Data Analytics for Smart Healthcare* (pp. 42-56). CRC Press.

Verma, J. K. (2021). Healthcare dashboards for sustainable monitoring: A case study. *IEEE Access : Practical Innovations, Open Solutions, 9*, 54321–54329.

Verma, S., & Singh, A. (2021). Low-cost workplace safety interventions in rural Indian hospitals: A pilot study. *Indian Journal of Public Health, 65*(2), 123–128. DOI: 10.4103/ijph.IJPH_1058_20

Vincent, J.-L. (2003). Nosocomial infections in adult intensive-care units. *Lancet*, *361*(9374), 2068–2077.

Visser, E. H., Brakema, E. A., Slootweg, I. A., Vos, H. M. M., & Adriaanse, M. A. (2024). *Patients' perspectives on ecologically sustainable healthcare in general practice*. https://doi.org/DOI: 10.1101/2024.10.18.24310602

Vonderlin, R., Biermann, M., Bohus, M., & Lyssenko, L. (2020). Mindfulness-based programs in the workplace: A meta-analysis of randomized controlled trials. *Mindfulness*, *11*(3), 2020. DOI: 10.1007/s12671-019-01391-5

Wafula, S. T., Musiime, J., & Oporia, F. (2019). Health care waste management among health workers and associated factors in primary health care facilities in Kampala City, Uganda: A cross-sectional study. *BMC Public Health*, *19*(1), 203. DOI: 10.1186/s12889-019-6528-4 PMID: 30777034

Wang, J. (2023). AI and smart materials in healthcare. *Nature Reviews. Materials*, *8*(1), 37–53. DOI: 10.1038/s41578-022-00535-5

Wani, A. K., Rahayu, F., Ben Amor, I., Quadir, M., Murianingrum, M., Parnidi, P., Ayub, A., Supriyadi, S., Sakiroh, S., & Saefudin, S. (2024). Environmental resilience through artificial intelligence: Innovations in monitoring and management. *Environmental Science and Pollution Research International*, *31*(12), 18379–18395.

Wassie, B., Gintamo, B., Mekuria, Z. N., & Gizaw, Z. (2022). Healthcare Waste Management Practices and Associated Factors in Private Clinics in Addis Ababa, Ethiopia. *Environmental Health Insights*, *16*. Advance online publication. DOI: 10.1177/11786302211073383 PMID: 35095276

Watts, N., Amann, M., Arnell, N., Ayeb-Karlsson, S., Belesova, K., Berry, H., Bouley, T., Boykoff, M., Byass, P., & Cai, W. (2018). The 2018 report of the Lancet Countdown on health and climate change: Shaping the health of nations for centuries to come. *Lancet*, *392*(10163), 2479–2514.

Wei, Y., Cui, M., Ye, Z., & Guo, Q. (2021). Environmental challenges from the increasing medical waste since SARS outbreak. *Journal of Cleaner Production*, *291*, 125246. DOI: 10.1016/j.jclepro.2020.125246 PMID: 33250588

WHO. (2018). *Health-care waste. Fact Sheet*. World Health Organization.

Windfeld, E. S., & Brooks, M. S. (2015). Medical waste management - A review. *Journal of Environmental Management*, *163*, 98–108. PMID: 26301686

Wooldridge, M. (2002). *An Introduction to Multi-Agent System*. John Wiley & Sons. LTD.

World Health Organization. (2021). Urban health. https://www.who.int/health-topics/urban-health)

World Health Organization. (2022). *Ethical considerations for digital health monitoring in workplaces*. WHO Press., DOI: 10.26719/9789240053456

Wu, N. (2023). Research on the emissions of diesel engine and the selection of suitable diesel engine additives to reduce particulate emissions. *Journal of Physics: Conference Series*, *2608*(1), 012053. DOI: 10.1088/1742-6596/2608/1/012053

Xu, W., Mei, K., Gao, H., Tan, J., Liang, Z., & Zhang, Y. (2025). A-mem: Agentic memory for llm agents. *arXiv Preprint arXiv:2502.12110.*

Yang, J., He, M., Zhang, X., Ning, Q., Chen, Y., & Mazinan, M. A.-S. Z. (2025). *Climate-Adaptive Energy Efficiency Modeling: A Generalized Additive Approach for Optimizing Building Performance Across Chinese Climate Zones*. https://doi.org/DOI: 10.21203/rs.3.rs-6152814/v1

Yao, Z., & Yu, H. (2025). *A survey on LLM-based multi-agent ai hospital*. OSF.

Yassaie, R., & Brooks, L. (2025). Reassessing 'good' medical practice and the climate crisis. *Journal of Medical Ethics*, *51*(6), 365–370. DOI: 10.1136/jme-2023-109713 PMID: 38871401

Zbyrad, B., Zaborniak, M., Kochmański, Ł., Jasik, K., Kluczyński, J., Budzik, G., & Turek, P. (2025). Evaluation of High-Temperature Sterilization Processes: Their Influence on the Mechanical Integrity of Additively Manufactured Polymeric Biomaterials. *Materials (Basel)*, *18*(6), 1356. DOI: 10.3390/ma18061356 PMID: 40141640

Zengyu, C., Luqi, W., Yuan, F., & Jianwei, Z. (2021). Research and Progress on Data Security Based on Medical Information System. *Proceedings of 2021 The 11th International Workshop on Computer Science and Engineering*, 1–5. https://doi.org/DOI: 10.18178/wcse.2021.06.001

Zhang, R., Tang, S., Liu, Y., Niyato, D., Xiong, Z., Sun, S., Mao, S., & Han, Z. (2025). Toward agentic ai: Generative information retrieval inspired intelligent communications and networking. *arXiv Preprint arXiv:2502.16866.*

Zhang, Y., Liu, Q., & Chen, H. (2021). A survey of physics-informed AI for complex urban systems. arXiv. (https://arxiv.org/html/2506.13777v1)

Zhang, H., & Wang, M. (2022). Predictive maintenance using environmental data analytics in medical infrastructure. *International Journal of Medical Informatics*, *160*, 104–111.

Zhang, M., Shao, F., Zheng, R., Liu, M., & Ji, Z. (2023). An Efficient Encryption Scheme with Fully Hidden Access Policy for Medical Data. *Electronics (Basel), 12*(13), 2930. DOI: 10.3390/electronics12132930

Zhang, T., Wang, L., & Hu, X. (2022). Psychological stress and burnout in healthcare workers under digital monitoring systems. *BMC Health Services Research, 22*(1), 945. DOI: 10.1186/s12913-022-08456-3

Zhang, Y., Chen, X., Lao, Y., Qiu, X., Liu, K., Zhuang, Y., Gong, X., & Wang, P. (2023). Effects of the implementation of intelligent technology for hand hygiene in hospitals: Systematic review and meta-analysis. *Journal of Medical Internet Research, 25*, e37249. DOI: 10.2196/37249

Zhang, Z., Chen, L., Xu, P., Wang, Q., Zhang, J., Chen, K., Clements, C. M., Celi, L. A., Herasevich, V., & Hong, Y. (2022). Effectiveness of automated alerting system compared to usual care for the management of sepsis. *NPJ Digital Medicine, 5*, 134. Advance online publication. DOI: 10.1038/s41746-022-00650-5

Zhao, L., Wang, H., & Xu, J. (2023). Research on the impact of urban innovation on public health. *Frontiers in Public Health, 11*, 1535932. DOI: 10.3389/fpubh.2024.1535932 PMID: 39835317

Zhou, H., Wang, T., Zhou, F., Liu, Y., Zhao, W., Wang, X., Chen, H., & Cui, Y. (2019). Ambient Air Pollution and Daily Hospital Admissions for Respiratory Disease in Children in Guiyang, China. *Frontiers in Pediatrics, 7*. Advance online publication. DOI: 10.3389/fped.2019.00400 PMID: 31681705

Zlateva, P., Ivanov, M., & Terziev, A. (2024). Analyses of the energy efficiency enhancement in Bulgarian health care premises. *E3S Web of Conferences, 551*, 01002. https://doi.org/DOI: 10.1051/e3sconf/202455101002

About the Contributors

Ciufudean Calin Horatiu is Professor, Ph.D. Eng. with "Stefan cel Mare" University of Suceava, Faculty of Electrical Engineering and Computer Science, Department of Computers, Control Systems, and Electronics. - Courses and laboratories: Industrial Control Systems Diagnosis, Discrete Event Systems; – Researcher in discrete event systems, environment and sustainable development; – Researcher in the teams and director of over 34 research projects (national and international); – Author of over 160 scientific papers published in scientific journals and conferences proceedings abroad and in Romania; – Author of 11 books published in Romania and abroad; – Author or co-author of 32 inventions. - Technical Expert of the Romanian Ministry of Justice. - President of the Romanian Society of Electrical & Control Engineering, Suceava Branch. - He is a member of the editorial boards of several international scientific journals and conferences of control systems and electric engineering science. He was designated chairmen and/or key note speaker at 29 international conferences.

***

Guddo is an Assistant Professor of Social Work at Lovely Professional University, Punjab, with a PhD in Social Work from IGNTU. A Gold Medalist and UGC-NET/JRF qualifier, he specialises in psychiatric social work, disaster management, and tribal welfare. With numerous publications in Scopus-indexed journals, he has extensive experience in teaching, research, and fieldwork coordination. Her expertise spans mental health, climate change, and social interventions, making his a dedicated contributor to academia and social work practice.

Kholis Ernawati (51 years old) is a permanent lecturer at the Bachelor of Medicine Study Programme, Faculty of Medicine, YARSI University. The author completed his S1 and S2 studies at Airlangga University and then S3 at the

University of Indonesia. The author's area of expertise is Public Health, focusing on Environmental Health. Teaching at the Faculty of Medicine, YARSI University since 2006 - now. The author actively writes scientific articles and is published in national and international proceedings and journals, compiling modules and books. Activities other than teaching are as a LAM PTKes Public Health Study Program Assessor, BKD Assessor, Study Program Evaluator at the Kemdikbud Institution, and Reviewer of articles in several national and international journals.

Renu Mishra is presently working as an Associate Professor at Sharda University, Greater Noida, U.P. She obtained Ph.D. from the School of IT, Rajiv Gandhi Proudyogiki Vishwavidyalaya (RGPV), Bhopal, India. She holds an M-Tech (Honors) from RGPV, Bhopal (M.P.), and a B-Tech from Uttar Pradesh Technical University (UPTU), Lucknow, U.P. With 18 years of teaching experience, Dr. Renu's research interests include Blockchain Technology, Mobile Ad-hoc Networks, Computer Networks, Wireless Sensor Networks, Cryptography, and Network Security. She has also made significant contributions to the academic community by publishing various books and book chapters.

N. Rajavel, is a principal of Selvamm Arts and Science College (Autonomous), Namakkal. He completed his Ph.D. at Bharathiyar University (Coimbatore) and his M.S. (Education) at Alagappa University. He has started his teaching career since 1999. He has been an elected senate member of Periyar University, Salem, since 2007. The specialized subject areas of Dr. N. Rajavel are marketing, Human Resource Management and Finance. He is recognized to guide for MBA, M.Phil., and Ph.D scholars. He has guided more than 100 MBA candidates and 12 M.Phil. candidates. He has presented various research articles on various topics at 32 National and International Conferences to his credit. He is one of the Authors for five books, namely Marketing, Production & Materials Management, Service Marketing, Human Resource Management, and Principles of Management Practices. He has published 12 research articles in National and International Journals and received the Best Programme Officer Award, Best Citizens of India Award, and Pride of India Award from various national agencies.

Mamta Narwaria is an assistant professor in the School of Computing Science & Engineering, Sharda University, Greater Noida. She has more than 20 years of academic experience. She is Post graduate in Computer Science & Engineering from Rajiv Gandhi Prodyougiki University, Bhopal, India. She has broad research interests in AI/ML,Federated learning, Image processing. She has published 05 papers in reputed conferences and refereed journals.

SC Vetrivel is a faculty member in the Department of Management Studies, Kongu Engineering College (Autonomous), Perundurai, Erode Dt. Having experience in Industry 20 years and Teaching 16 years. Awarded with Doctoral Degree in Management Sciences in Anna University, Chennai. He has organized various workshops and Faculty Development Programmes. He is actively involved in research and consultancy works. He acted as a resource person to FDPs & MDPs to various industries like, SPB ltd, Tamilnadu Police, DIET, Rotary school and many. His areas of interest include Entrepreneurship, Business Law, Marketing and Case writing. Articles published more than 100 International and National Journals. Presented papers in more than 30 National and International conferences including IIM Bangalore, IIM Kozhikode, IIM Kashipur and IIM Indore. He was a Chief Co-ordinator of Entrepreneurship and Management Development Centre (EMDC) of Kongu Engineering College, he was instrumental in organizing various Awareness Camps, FDP, and TEDPs to aspiring entrepreneurs which was funded by NSTEDB – DST/GoI

Sneha Sinha is a Computer Science researcher at Sharda University with a passion for innovation. My major projects include Blockchain-Enabled Security for healthcare Image Processing. Her work primarily focuses on AI, computer vision, and cybersecurity to address practical, real-world challenges.

C.V. Suresh Babu is a pioneer in content development. A true entrepreneur, he founded Anniyappa Publications, a company that is highly active in publishing books related to Computer Science and Management. Dr. C.V. Suresh Babu has also ventured into SB Institute, a center for knowledge transfer. He holds a Ph.D. in Engineering Education from the National Institute of Technical Teachers Training & Research in Chennai, along with seven master's degrees in various disciplines such as Engineering, Computer Applications, Management, Commerce, Economics, Psychology, Law, and Education. Additionally, he has UGC-NET/SET qualifications in the fields of Computer Science, Management, Commerce, and Education. Currently, Dr. C.V. Suresh Babu is a Professor in the Department of Information Technology at the School of Computing Science, Hindustan Institute of Technology and Science (Hindustan University) in Padur, Chennai, Tamil Nadu, India.

Muhammad Usman Tariq has more than 17+ year's experience in industry and academia. He is a prolific author of research articles, case studies, book chapters, and academic books, with work spanning a wide range of disciplines. His contributions also include several patents. He is founder and CEO of The Case HQ, a unique repository for courses, narrative and video case studies. Additionally, he is President of Gulf Higher Education (Gulf HE) focused on advancing academic practice. He has been working as a consultant and trainer for industries representing six sigma, quality, health and safety, environmental systems, project management, and information security standards. His work has encompassed sectors in aviation, manufacturing, food, hospitality, education, finance, research, software and transportation. He has diverse and significant experience working with accreditation agencies of ABET, ACBSP, AACSB, WASC, CAA, EFQM and NCEAC. He is a Principal Fellow of Advance HE UK, Senior Fellow of SEDA UK, and Chartered Fellow of CIPD UK other than Senior Member IEEE.

Corneliu Octavian Turcu received his B.Sc. (1991) and Ph.D. (1999) degrees in Automatic Systems from the University of Ia i, Romania, and an M.Sc. in Informatics from tefan cel Mare University of Suceava. Since 1991, he has been with the Faculty of Electrical Engineering and Computer Science at tefan cel Mare University of Suceava, where he is a Full Professor of System Theory and Intelligent Systems. He also serves as Head of the Programmes Management Department and supervises both Ph.D. and M.Sc. theses. Dr. Turcu has authored more than 100 research papers and four books. His research interests include intelligent systems, web technologies, the Internet of Things, and automatic control.

Cristina Elena Turcu is a Professor and currently the Vice-Dean of the Faculty of Electrical Engineering and Computer Science, and also the President of the Scientific Council of the tefan cel Mare University of Suceava, Romania. During the period 2004–2011, she was the Head of the Computer Science Department. Her research interests include software engineering, intelligent systems, and the Internet/ Web of Things. She was an Editor for six books. She has served on various Program Committees of conferences in computing and the Internet of Things. She has also served as a reviewer for numerous refereed journals and conferences. She is an Associate Editor of the International Journal of Engineering Business Management. She has published over 100 publications in books or book chapters, refereed journals, technical reports, and refereed conference/workshop/seminar proceedings.

V.P. Arun is a driven and accomplished professional with a diverse educational background and extensive hands-on experience across various industries. Graduating with honors, Arun earned his Master of Business Administration (M.B.A) with a specialization in Human Resources and Marketing from the renowned Sona School of Management in Salem in 2018, where he excelled academically with an impressive 8.3 Cumulative Grade Point Average (CGPA).Throughout his academic journey, Arun displayed an unwavering commitment to learning and personal growth, actively seeking opportunities to expand his knowledge and skills beyond the confines of traditional education. He sought practical experiences to complement his theoretical understanding, such as a 45-day summer internship focused on conducting a feasibility study for R-Doc Sustainability in the market. Additionally, Arun broadened his horizons through a 7-day industrial visit to Malaysia and Singapore, immersing himself in diverse cultural and professional environments. Arun's academic pursuits were further enriched by his involvement in hands-on projects, including a comprehensive study on Employee Job Satisfaction at Roots Cast Private Limited. His professional trajectory includes serving as a Growth Officer at Parle Agro Private Limited, where he played a crucial role in driving sales growth and market expansion. Arun is a dedicated professional, currently employed at JKKN Engineering College in the Management Studies Department. He holds expertise in his field and has contributed significantly to academia through the publication of two journal articles. Arun's work focuses on advancing knowledge and understanding in management studies, making valuable contributions to the academic community.

Index

A

Agentic AI 49, 51, 53, 54, 56, 57, 61, 62, 68, 74, 75, 76, 77, 78, 79, 80, 81, 82, 83, 84, 85, 86, 87, 88
AI 34, 35, 39, 40, 45, 49, 51, 52, 53, 54, 55, 56, 57, 58, 59, 60, 61, 62, 65, 67, 68, 74, 75, 76, 77, 78, 79, 80, 81, 82, 83, 84, 85, 86, 87, 88, 89, 90, 91, 96, 97, 98, 99, 100, 106, 108, 109, 110, 111, 112, 113, 114, 115, 116, 118, 121, 124, 125, 127, 128, 129, 131, 132, 133, 134, 137, 139, 140, 143, 144, 145, 146, 147, 148, 149, 150, 156, 157, 158, 164, 166, 167, 169, 170, 171, 173, 174, 176, 178, 180, 181, 182, 184, 207, 219, 225, 226, 227, 228, 229, 230, 234, 235, 236, 238, 256

C

Compliance 8, 17, 25, 28, 30, 31, 33, 36, 44, 50, 51, 56, 58, 61, 65, 67, 68, 69, 70, 71, 72, 73, 74, 76, 94, 96, 99, 100, 101, 102, 105, 112, 119, 120, 122, 123, 124, 125, 128, 130, 131, 133, 135, 157, 165, 168, 169, 170, 171, 172, 173, 174, 176, 177, 178, 179, 180, 181, 182, 183, 184, 215, 216, 222, 223, 224, 225, 226, 227, 230, 233, 236, 238
CPS 17, 19, 20
Cybersecurity 17, 34, 35, 36, 100, 101, 102, 111, 112, 133, 165, 184

D

Data Protection 64, 72, 76, 100, 101, 108, 131, 133, 157, 166, 168, 182, 223, 224, 225, 232, 235, 239
Disaster Mental Health 241, 243, 245, 252, 254, 255, 256, 257, 258, 259, 262, 267

E

Energy Efficiency 5, 12, 13, 23, 24, 29, 31, 46, 47, 53, 74, 79, 96, 105, 109, 112
Environmental Monitoring 17, 19, 20, 21, 27, 28, 29, 31, 32, 33, 37, 42, 44, 49, 50, 51, 52, 58, 59, 60, 61, 62, 65, 66, 68, 74, 75, 77, 78, 79, 81, 85, 89, 91, 106, 121, 137, 139, 148, 227, 230, 238
Environment Monitoring 117, 118, 211, 213, 230
Eye Disease 190, 196

G

GDPR 64, 67, 72, 76, 94, 96, 100, 101, 102, 108, 133, 146, 148, 157, 158, 166, 168, 169, 170, 172, 174, 176, 177, 178, 179, 180, 182, 183, 223, 225, 236
Glaucoma Detection 189, 192, 193, 194, 195, 196, 197, 198, 199, 200, 201, 202, 204, 208
Green AI 53, 87
Greenhouse Gas Protocol 2, 9

H

Healthcare 1, 2, 3, 4, 5, 6, 7, 8, 9, 10, 11, 12, 14, 15, 16, 17, 18, 19, 20, 21, 22, 23, 24, 25, 26, 27, 29, 30, 31, 32, 33, 34, 35, 36, 37, 39, 40, 41, 42, 43, 44, 45, 46, 49, 50, 51, 52, 53, 54, 55, 56, 57, 58, 59, 60, 61, 62, 65, 68, 74, 75, 76, 77, 78, 79, 81, 82, 83, 84, 85, 86, 87, 88, 89, 90, 92, 93, 94, 95, 96, 97, 98, 99, 100, 101, 102, 103, 104, 105, 106, 107, 108, 109, 110, 111, 112, 113, 114, 115, 116, 117, 118, 119, 120, 121, 122, 123, 124, 125, 126, 127, 128, 129, 130, 131, 132, 133, 134, 135, 136, 137, 139, 140, 142, 144, 145, 146, 148, 149, 151, 154, 155, 156, 157, 158, 159, 160, 162, 163, 164, 165, 166, 167, 168, 169, 170, 171, 172, 173, 174, 175, 176, 177, 178, 179, 180, 181, 182, 183, 184, 186, 187, 192, 194, 211, 212,

213, 214, 215, 216, 217, 218, 219, 220, 221, 222, 223, 224, 225, 226, 227, 228, 229, 230, 231, 232, 233, 234, 235, 236, 237, 238, 239, 240, 245, 254, 255
Healthcare Sustainability 1, 12, 40, 125, 129, 137
HIPAA 64, 67, 72, 76, 94, 96, 100, 102, 112, 133, 146, 148, 157, 158, 166, 168, 169, 172, 174, 177, 178, 179, 183, 223

I

Image Segmentation 189, 190, 193, 207
intelligent decision support 117, 120, 123, 128, 134
Interactive Visualization 140, 160
Internet of Medical Things 52, 83, 84, 85, 86, 89, 100, 166, 167, 175
Intervention Frameworks 241, 251, 252
IoMT 52, 55, 56, 67, 68, 69, 71, 73, 79, 83, 84, 85, 89, 90, 100, 101, 102, 111, 112, 166, 167, 168, 169, 170, 177, 178, 180, 181, 182, 183, 184
IoT 17, 19, 20, 21, 27, 28, 29, 30, 31, 32, 33, 34, 35, 36, 37, 38, 39, 41, 42, 43, 44, 45, 46, 52, 56, 58, 59, 62, 63, 66, 67, 69, 71, 73, 78, 79, 81, 82, 83, 86, 87, 88, 99, 113, 114, 115, 116, 118, 121, 122, 125, 127, 129, 130, 131, 133, 140, 141, 142, 144, 147, 148, 149, 150, 151, 155, 157, 165, 166, 167, 168, 169, 170, 171, 172, 173, 174, 175, 177, 178, 179, 180, 181, 182, 183, 184, 186, 187, 211, 216, 217, 219, 220, 221, 222, 226, 227, 229, 230, 231, 235, 237, 239, 240
IoT Governance 165, 166, 169, 170, 171, 178, 179, 183, 184

M

Medical Care Systems 229
Medical Waste 5, 7, 14, 16, 17, 18, 19, 20, 22, 23, 24, 26, 27, 31, 33, 42, 44, 46, 119, 134
Multi-Agent System 49, 61, 88
Multi-Criteria Decision Analysis 1, 2

O

Occupational Health 214, 219, 220, 229, 230, 233, 237, 239
One Health 17, 19, 20, 40

P

Post-Traumatic Stress Disorder 243, 247, 248, 253, 261, 262, 265, 267
predictive maintenance 61, 118, 122, 132, 134, 137
Privacy 34, 35, 36, 52, 60, 66, 67, 69, 70, 71, 72, 74, 76, 79, 91, 100, 101, 102, 109, 111, 131, 132, 133, 145, 146, 148, 155, 157, 165, 166, 168, 169, 170, 171, 172, 173, 174, 175, 176, 177, 178, 180, 181, 182, 183, 184, 186, 187, 217, 219, 223, 225, 232
Psychological Resilience 241, 242, 243, 244, 246, 257, 258
Public Health 2, 17, 20, 21, 22, 23, 25, 26, 27, 28, 29, 31, 32, 39, 42, 45, 46, 58, 61, 76, 78, 81, 82, 83, 84, 87, 95, 105, 119, 135, 140, 143, 144, 146, 148, 150, 151, 154, 155, 156, 157, 159, 160, 161, 162, 163, 164, 168, 232, 234, 235, 236, 237, 238, 239, 240, 241, 260, 262, 264, 267, 268

R

real-time dashboards 99, 159
Real-Time Monitoring 30, 31, 36, 37, 49, 52, 55, 59, 62, 69, 87, 100, 107, 110, 122, 126, 140, 141, 142, 143, 154, 166, 168, 221, 223, 226, 233
Real-Time Patient Tracking 183
Retinal Imaging 191, 195

S

Security 21, 34, 35, 36, 37, 39, 43, 47, 49, 52, 57, 64, 67, 69, 70, 71, 72, 73, 74, 76, 79, 84, 85, 91, 93, 95, 96, 97, 100,

101, 102, 107, 108, 111, 145, 146, 148, 158, 165, 166, 167, 168, 169, 170, 171, 173, 174, 175, 177, 178, 179, 180, 181, 182, 184, 186, 187, 236, 249
Smart hospitals 84, 89, 96, 114, 118, 124, 128, 130, 137
Smart Sensors 17, 19
Staff Safety 211, 212, 216, 217, 220, 221, 222, 223, 224, 225, 226, 227, 229, 230, 238, 240
Sustainability 1, 12, 13, 14, 15, 18, 21, 23, 25, 26, 27, 28, 30, 31, 40, 41, 43, 49, 50, 53, 54, 56, 57, 58, 59, 62, 65, 66, 67, 69, 70, 73, 74, 76, 77, 78, 79, 81, 82, 83, 84, 85, 86, 87, 88, 95, 97, 103, 105, 106, 111, 112, 113, 114, 115, 116, 118, 119, 120, 121, 122, 123, 124, 125, 126, 127, 128, 129, 130, 131, 132, 134, 135, 136, 137, 140, 143, 144, 159, 160, 178, 213, 219, 222, 227, 228, 230, 231, 234, 236, 256
Sustainable Environmental Monitoring 49, 51, 58, 61, 66, 77, 79
Sustainable healthcare 15, 17, 30, 46, 49, 59, 76, 78, 113, 115, 120, 121, 122, 123, 126, 127, 128, 130, 133, 136, 137, 139, 158, 219, 226, 230, 232
Sustainable healthcare systems 133, 232

T

TOE Framework 19

V

Vulnerable Populations 24, 184, 241, 245, 255, 256

W

Waste Management 6, 7, 12, 16, 18, 19, 21, 22, 23, 24, 27, 28, 30, 32, 33, 40, 42, 44, 46, 58, 107, 121, 137, 222
Well-being 90, 92, 99, 102, 103, 104, 105, 211, 212, 213, 215, 217, 218, 219, 221, 222, 223, 224, 225, 226, 227, 228, 229, 230, 231, 232, 233, 235, 236, 238, 239, 240, 242, 251, 252

www.ingramcontent.com/pod-product-compliance
Lightning Source LLC
LaVergne TN
LVHW060003031026
849161LV00025B/1344